AF443706

ESSENTIALS OF CHILD NEUROLOGY

Suresh Kotagal, M.D.
Associate Professor of Neurology and Pediatrics
Director, Section of Child Neurology
St. Louis University Medical Center
St. Louis, Missouri

Ishiyaku EuroAmerica, Inc.
St. Louis • Tokyo

Book Editor: Gregory Hacke, D.C.

Ishiyaku EuroAmerica, Inc.
716 Hanley Industrial Court, St. Louis, Missouri 63144

Library of Congress Catalogue Number 90-080094

Suresh Kotagal
Essentials of Child Neurology

ISBN 0-912791-37-3

Ishiyaku EuroAmerica, Inc.
St. Louis • Tokyo

Composition by HiTec Typeset, Columbia, Missouri
Printed by Rose Printing, Tallahassee, Florida

Acknowledgements

I am grateful for the perseverance and diligence of Dr. Greg Hacke and Mr. Manuel Ponte of Ishiyaku EuroAmerica, Publishers, in guiding this work to its completion. I thank my wife Nirmala for her patience and understanding. Ms. Barbara Tournour and Ms. Penny Bird were of invaluable assistance in compilation of the illustrations and typing of the manuscript, respectively.

Suresh Kotagal, M.D.

Notice

Medicine is an ever-changing science. As new research and clincal experience broaden our knowledge, changes in treatment are required. The editors and the publisher of this work have made every effort to ensure that the procedures herein are accurate and in accord with the standards accepted at the time of publication, but the final authority in all cases is the professional judgement of the attending physician.

Preface

There are a number of excellent textbooks in the field of Child Neurology—some concise and others very comprehensive. However, books of intermediate length of utility to practitioners, residents, allied health personnel and medical students are lacking. It is this void that *Essentials of Child Neurology* tries to fill. Wherever possible, an attempt has been made to present a practical, symptom–oriented approach to childhood neurological disorders. Algorithms have been incorporated in some chapters to guide management. Cross references appearing throughout the text have also been utilized to avoid repetitions.

Suresh Kotagal, M.D.
Saint Louis, Missouri
19th March, 1990

Contents

CHAPTER I

CLINICAL ASSESSMENT

History Taking

Neonatal Neurological Examination

Neurological Examination: Infants, Toddlers and Young Children

Glossary of Commonly Observed Neurological Manifestations

HISTORY TAKING

I. Chief complaint and history of present illness. Attempt to determine whether symptoms are episodic (stroke, seizure, or syncope) or constant; whether static, progressive or resolving; also, localize the symptoms using historical information, e.g., cerebral cortical, white matter, brain stem, spinal cord or neuromuscular system involvement. Intellectual dysfunction and seizures are seen with cerebral cortical involvement. A combination of hemisensory and motor disturbances suggest dysfunction in the hemispheric white matter. Brainstem disorders are frequently accompanied by diplopia, dysphagia, dizziness, impaired equilibrium, and altered consciousness. Cerebellar disorders are associated with impaired equilibrium in the trunk or extremities. Diseases of the spinal cord frequently result in dissociation of motor and sensory function below a certain altitudinal level as well as bowel and bladder dysfunction.

II. Neurological review of systems. History of breath holding leading to syncope, difficulties in memory, orientation, language, affect, and mood; disturbances of coordination and gait; bulbar disturbances (dysarthria, dysphagia, drooling, etc.); disturbances of sensorimotor function such as paresthesia, excessive falling, unsteady gait, fatigue on exertion, muscle cramps.

III. Review of other systems.

IV. History of previous illnesses.

V. Pregnancy and birth history. Maternal age, gravida, parity, complications during pregnancy, e.g., hypertension, diabetes, toxemia, exposure to drugs or radiation; gestational age, duration of labor, intrapartum alterations in heart rate, instrumentation during labor, presentation, route of delivery, APGAR scores, birth weight, need for resuscitation, neonatal seizures, hyperbilirubinemia, feeding difficulties, alterations in sleep-wake cycles, need for blood transfusions.

VI. Developmental history. Outline age at acquisition of various motor, intellectual and social milestones; indicate developmental arrest or regression. The Denver Developmental Screening Test-Revised is recommended for this purpose.

NEONATAL NEUROLOGICAL EXAMINATION

Introduction

Owing to continuous maturation of the central nervous system, normal examination findings vary with the neonatal gestational age, which in turn conforms to the length of pregnancy. Gestational age is best estimated from the mother's date of the last menstrual period as well as by assessing certain external characteristics, e.g., number of plantar creases, degree of maturation of the external genitalia, and the ear cartilage. Radiological studies to determine appearance of time-specific ossification centers in the long bones are also helpful. Post-conceptional age refers to the gestational plus postnatal age.

Maturation of the EEG is linked closely with the postconceptional age. Neonatal neurological examination findings vary with the state of the infant: wakefulness, active, or quiet sleep. As a consequence, one may find muscle tone diminished in active sleep relative to that during wakefulness or quiet sleep. The ideal time for an examination is when the neonate is awake but not crying, generally 15-30 minutes after a feed. Serial neurological examinations are often necessary to confirm suspected neurologic deficits.

Outline

1. In all neonates, length, weight, and head circumference should be plotted against the gestational age to determine the rate of intrauterine growth. Small for gestational age babies have frequently been exposed to placental insufficiency, intrauterine infections, toxins or may have chromosomal anomalies.

2. Dysmorphic facial features such as hypotelorism, hypertelorism, small palpebral width, epicanthal fold, and low set ears are generally a clue towards associated central nervous system malformations.

3. The skin should be examined for petechiae (seen in systemic cytomegalovirus infections), vesicles (herpes simplex infections), whorled hyperpigmented lesions (incontinentia pigmenti) and facial nevus (Sturge-Weber syndrome).

4. Estimate the level of alertness. Using behavioral and EEG criteria, wakefulness can be differentiated from sleep by 28 weeks postconceptional age. By 32 weeks, infants demonstrate periods of spontaneous eye opening and eye closure. Differentiation of sleep into active and quiet states becomes apparent between 30-32 weeks post-conceptional age. Periods of wakefulness, spontaneous activity, and the level of reactivity to environmental stimuli gradually increase with age. Normal awake and quiet full-term neonates habituate to auditory, visual, and tactile stimuli by the fourth or fifth repetition of the stimulus and cease to respond in a stereotypic manner as stimulus trials are continued beyond this number.

5. Resting posture. Muscle tone develops initially in the flexor muscles, and in a gradual, caudal-cephalad sequence. At 28 weeks postconceptional age, infants have flaccid, fully extended extremities; flexion at the hips and knees appears by 32 weeks post-conceptional age; by 36 weeks, all four extremities are kept at rest in weak flexion. Strong flexion of all four limbs becomes apparent by full term or 40 weeks post-conceptional age.

Truncal muscle tone is assessed in the prone position and also by pulling the infant from the supine to the sitting position. A term infant is able to briefly keep the head almost in line with the trunk during the latter maneuver and may even by able to support the head upright in the sitting position for 2-3 seconds. Hypotonia may be secondary to either diffuse cerebral cortical, cerebellar, or neuromuscular disorders. Persistent fisting of the hands in an awake but quiet term infant suggests corticospinal tract dysfunction. Arching of the neck and trunk (opisthotonos) indicates uninhibited activity of the reticulospinal and vestibulospinal systems owing to failure of cortical inhibitory mechanisms. All infants should be examined in the supine, prone, and erect positions in order to check for abnormalities in muscle tone. The head should be kept in the midline when appendicular muscle tone is assessed in order to avoid activation of the asymmetric tonic neck reflex, which may spuriously increase tone on the side towards which the face is turned.

6. Ocular findings. Pupillary and blink reflexes in response to light appear by 27-28 weeks conceptional age, transient visual fixation and optokinetic nystagmus by 34 weeks. Doll's eye movements (brisk movement of the head in one direction eliciting conjugate eye movements in the opposite direction) are present in most neonates during wakefulness and sleep. Pupils are generally 2-3 mms in size and reactive to light. Mydriasis is generally seen with sympathetic overactivity (in mild hypoxic encephalopathy). An asymmetric, constricted pupil may be secondary to Horner's syndrome from brachial plexus injury. A unilaterally dilated, poorly reactive pupil in a comatose patient suggests uncal herniation. Cataracts may be visualized in patients with Lowe (oculocerebrorenal) syndrome, congenital rubella syndrome, and galactosemia; chorioretinitis (irregular areas of dark pigmentation) may suggest congenital intrauterine infections. Optic nerve hypoplasia (the optic disc

head is one third to one half the normal size) may be seen in septo-optic dysplasia.

7. In examination of other cranial nerves, absent corneal reflexes may suggest either V or VII cranial nerve dysfunction. Infants with upper motor neuron VII involvement (facial paresis) have weakness only of the contralateral lower half of the face, whereas lower motor neuron VII nerve lesions will affect both upper and lower halves of the face. Infants with deafness may fail to demonstrate an alerting response to auditory stimuli administered in a quiet room. The gag reflex may be absent in neonates with IX or X cranial nerve involvement. Soft palatal movements are diminished (or absent) in those with X nerve lesions. Swallowing difficulties, especially nasopharyngeal reflux, are also frequently associated. Examination of the accessory (XI) cranial nerve is difficult. The tongue may protrude towards the side of the XII nerve lesion; in Werdnig-Hoffmann disease, the tongue may be atrophic, and actively degenerating portions demonstrate fasiculations (slow, undulating, ripple-like movements), which are best visualized in good light with the tongue resting on the floor of the mouth.

8. Developmental reflexes are generally mediated at lower levels of the neuraxis (brainstem and spinal cord), with each having a precise age for appearance. They disappear, or are incorporated into involuntary motor activity at definite ages owing to progressive maturation of descending cortical inhibitory projections. Abnormal central nervous system function should be suspected when a developmental reflex is absent at an age when it should be normally present, when it persists unduly beyond the time by which it should have normally disappeared, or if it is asymmetric. The most commonly tested developmental reflexes include:

Moro. With the infant lying supine, lifting the head off the bed by 1-2 inches and letting it gently fall backwards elicits opening of the palms, a cry, extension and abduction of the upper extremities followed by adduction at the shoulders.

Asymmetric Tonic Neck. Rotation of the head to one side elicits reflex extension of the extremities towards which the face is turned and flexion in the opposite upper extremity ("fencing posture").

Placing. Contact of the dorsum of the foot with the edge of a table elicits placement of foot on table.

Rooting. Stroking the perioral region elicits head turning towards the side of stimulation; most prominent in a hungry child, least apparent in a well-fed infant.

9. Tendon reflexes elicitable in the neonatal period include the jaw, biceps, and knee reflexes. Altitudinal changes in the amplitude of tendon reflexes are commonly seen with bilateral parasaggital hemispheric lesions or spinal cord dysfunction, whereas asymmetry in the amplitude suggests lateralized cerebral pathology.

10. The spine should be examined for midline fusion defects such as meningomyelocele and sacral dermal sinus.

11. The occipitofrontal head circumference should be measured and plotted on the growth chart. The normal rate of growth in head circumference is discussed in Chapter X. Microcephaly at birth may be secondary to congenital intrauterine infections, malformations of the central nervous system, or exposure to intrauterine toxins. Macrocephaly at birth frequently accompanies congenital hydrocephalus (secondary to aqueductal stenosis). The anterior fontanelle may be bulging in the presence of increased intracranial pressure, enlarged in size (beyond 1″x1″) in hypothyroidism and Zellweger syndrome, and small in patients with microcephaly.

DIAGNOSTIC YIELD OF THE NEONATAL NEUROLOGICAL EXAMINATION

Results of the neonatal neurological examination may be classified as normal, "suspect", or abnormal. Those with a normal neurological examination usually have a normal developmental outcome. Infants with "suspect" neurological examinations may either revert to normal upon reexamination or develop frank abnormalities.

Table 1-1. Commonly tested developmental reflexes

REFLEX	DESCRIPTION
Moro	
Appearance:	Partially by 28-32 weeks conceptional age. Well developed by 36-37 weeks.
Disappearance:	By age 6 months.
Abnormality:	Absence in the neonatal period; Asymmetry beyond 6 months; Persistence beyond age 6 months.
Asymmetric Tonic Neck	
Appearance:	Partially by 35-36 weeks conceptional age. Fully developed by 40 weeks.
Disappearance:	By 3-4 months later.
Abnormality:	Absence in a term neonate or 40-48 weeks postconceptional age; Obligatory ATNR (present at rest) Persistence beyond 5-6 months.
Placing	
Appearance:	Partially by 37 weeks.
Disappearance:	By 48-50 weeks conceptional age.
Abnormality:	Absence in a term neonate or asymmetry.
Rooting	
Appearance:	30-32 weeks, conceptional.
Disappearance:	Resolves by 6-8 months.
Abnormality:	Absence at time when it should be present.

While isolated, abnormal signs in the neonatal period have little diagnostic significance; neurologic impairment is likely when they occur in a combination, with approximately 16% in the latter category going on to develop cerebral palsy. Persistence of neurological abnormalities beyond the first week in a term infant is usually predictive of future developmental delay. Prechtl and Beintema, who were the first to identify combinations of abnormal neurological findings in the neonate, have identified the following syndromes:

1. **Apathy and coma syndromes.** A generalized suppression of alertness and reflexes.

2. **Hyperexcitability syndrome.** Presence of tremulousness and an unduly easily elicitable Moro response.

3. **Hemisyndrome.** Asymmetry in posture, movements, and reflexes.

Apathy and coma syndromes carry the worst prognosis. In one particular study, 73% of 150 neonates with one or more syndromes in the neonatal period had persistent neurological abnormalities between 2-4 years of age.

NEUROLOGICAL EXAMINATION: INFANTS, TODDLERS, AND YOUNG CHILDREN

General Principles

With toddlers, the initial steps of the examination are best conducted while the child is seated in the parent's lap. This minimizes apprehension which in turn may alter testing of higher functions, muscle tone, and reflexes. It is advisable to defer uncomfortable parts of the examination such as fundoscopy, checking of the gag reflex and inspection of the tympanic membranes till the very end.

Observation of infants and toddlers during play (e.g., while stacking blocks or playing with age-appropriate toys) will frequently provide valuable information about the child's attentiveness, gross and fine motor coordination, and problem solving ability.

Certain findings in the general physical examination may provide clues to the nature of the underlying neurological disorder, e.g., adenoma sebaceum and hypopigmented patches in tuberous sclerosis, cafe-au-lait patches in neurofibromatosis, facial hemangioma in Sturge-Weber syndrome, coarse facial features and coarse texture of the hair in the mucopolysaccharidoses, hepatosplenomegaly in certain lysosomal storage disorders, cardiac murmurs or bradycardia in patients with syncope, dysmorphic facial features in malformations of the central nervous system.

A thorough history of development of the various motor, intellectual, and social milestones is helpful in determining abnormal function of the nervous system. An attempt should be made to determine whether the clinical course is progressive, static, or improving. Some common developmental milestones include:

Fixes gaze briefly	Birth
Smiles responsively	1 month
Visual tracking to 180 degrees	2 1/2 - 3 months
Rolls over; holds head upright	3 months
Reaches for objects	3 - 4 months
Sits unsupported	6 months
Thumb-finger grasp	8 months
Crawls	9 months
Walks with support	10 months
Pincer grasp	12 months
Walks unsupported	12 - 14 months
Says 3 words other than "mama" & "dada"	13 months
Climbs steps	17 months
Pedals tricycle	36 months
Forms 2-3 word declarative sentences	30 - 36 months
Asks questions	36 months

THE EXAMINATION

HIGHER FUNCTIONS

6-12 Months. Awareness of surroundings, interaction with the examiner, e.g., social smile; habituation, consolability, inquisitiveness in playing with toys (after 4-5 months' age), ability to make complex defensive maneuvers when the face is covered with a cloth (after 4-5 months), non-specific or specific Mama or Dada sounds after 8 months.

12-36 Months. Development of an 8-12 word vocabulary, ability to comprehend simple one-step commands and pointing to body parts by age 18 months; naming of 2-3 body parts by age 24 months; use of phrases and simple declarative sentences between 18-24 months; asking questions by age 36 months; concept of self (referral to "I", knowledge of own name, age) between 24-30 months.

36-72 Months. Counting three objects, understanding prepositional concepts (over, under), naming three colors and use of interrogative sentences between 36-42 months; copying of a cross and a square by 48-60 months respectively; counting three objects correctly by age 48 months; repeating four digits (1 of 3 trials) by 54 months; copying of a triangle and counting correctly to 10 by 60 months; copying a diamond, spelling monosyllabic words, adding serial fives correctly and knowing left from right by 72 months.

Beyond 72 months. Concepts of reading, spelling, abstract calculation ability, general knowledge, geography, and reasoning in abstract terms evolve progressively.

CRANIAL NERVES

I. Response to alcohol or peppermint.

II. Visual acuity, visual fields on confrontation, fundoscopy, optokinetic nystagmus, pupillary response to light (direct and consensual), accommodation.

III, IV, VI. Extraocular movements in appropriate directions.

V. Tactile facial sensation, corneal response, masseter strength.

VII. Symmetry of the nasolabial folds, taste sensation over anterior two thirds of the tongue, strength in orbicularis oculi and orbicularis oris muscles.

VIII. Response to the sound of a bell or rattle in an infant; discrimination of whispered numerals with masking of sound simultaneously in the contralateral ear in an older child.

IX, X. Swallowing function, soft palatal movements, gag reflex, hoarseness of voice (X nerve).

XI. Strength in trapezius and sternomastoid muscles.

XII. Tongue position upon protrusion, voluntary movements, fasiculations, apraxia.

MOTOR SYSTEM

Abnormalities of the resting posture (fisting of the hands, opisthotonos, athetosis, obligatory asymmetric tonic neck reflex, abducted hips when supine), axial and appendicular muscle tone, power, abnormal movements (tremor, myoclonus, chorea, seizures), atrophy, pseudohypertrophy, myotonia, fasiculations.

SENSORY SYSTEM

Temperature, touch, joint and vibratory sense, two point discrimination, Romberg's sign.

REFLEXES

a. Tendon (jaw, biceps, triceps, supinator, Hoffman's, knee, ankle).

b. Superficial (corneal, abdominal cremasteric, plantar).

c. Developmental (Moro, asymmetric tonic neck, positive supporting, stepping, parachute).

SKULL

OFC-cms, percentile, head shape, anterior fontanelle (whether bulging), flat or sunken, riding of sutures, bruit, tenderness.

SPINE

External defects: tuft of hair, sinus, midline mass, scoliosis.

CEREBELLAR SYSTEM

Dysmetria, hypotonia and broad based gait, pendulous tendon reflexes.

MENINGEAL IRRITATION

Neck stiffness.

Kernig's sign: flexion of the lower extremity at the hips, knees, followed by gradual extension elicits low backache.

Brudzinski's sign: flexion of the neck elicits flexion at the hips or flexion at one hip elicits flexion at the other.

COMMONLY OBSERVED NEUROLOGICAL MANIFESTATIONS

Aniscoria. Asymmetry in pupillary size. A constricted pupil associated with ptosis, enophthalmos, and anhidrosis is seen in Horner's syndrome secondary to ipsilateral sympathetic denervation of the pupil. A unilaterally dilated, poorly reactive pupil in a comatose patient suggests uncal herniation, with extrinsic compression of the third cranial nerve by a temporal lobe mass.

Ataxia. Unsteadiness from difficulty in regulating the rate and range of muscle contraction. Ataxia most often develops following cerebellar dysfunction or altered sensory function, e.g., with peripheral nerve disease or dorsal column involvement (sensory ataxia). Midline cerebellar dysfunction leads to truncal and gait ataxia which is not significantly altered by eye closure. Sensory ataxia, on the other hand, is associated with a positive Romberg's sign (normal balance when feet are placed together while standing with eyes open, but loss of balance when the same maneuver is repeated with eyes closed).

Apraxia. Inability to perform a motor task upon command which can, however, be carried out reflexively without difficulty; generally secondary to parietal cortical dysfunction; most often affects speech, dressing, and gait.

Aphasia. An acquired disorder in which comprehension, formulation, or expression of language are impaired.

Astereognosis. Inability to identify objects placed in the hand using tactile manipulation, despite presence of normal touch sensation; usually seen with parietal cortical lesions.

Attentional Deficit Disorder. Easy distractibility, sometimes accompanied by impulsivity, motor restlessness (hyperactivity); may occur independently or along with learning disabilities and may lead to poor school performance.

Akinetic Mutism. A chronic vegetative state secondary to diffuse bihemispheric cortical, white matter, or thalamic lesions in which the patient demonstrates clear sleep-wake cycles, but has no content whatsoever to consciousness.

Anxiety State. A feeling of fear or apprehension and excessive concern over danger that is either minor in degree or largely unrecognized; may be sometimes accompanied by autonomic disturbances, e.g., sweating, tachycardia.

Athetosis. Abnormal posture, with pronation and flexion of the distal extremity; generally seen with contralateral putaminal lesions.

Ballism. Flinging movements of the upper extremity, usually from a lesion in the contralateral subthalamic nucleus; may herald kernicterus, or basal ganglionic dysfunction due to hemorrhage or hypoxia.

Coma. State of decreased consciousness in which vigorous stimuli either evoke minimal or only non-purposive responses.

Chorea. Involuntary movements, characterized by rapid, semipurposive movements of the proximal segments of the body.

Cataplexy. Sudden loss of extensor muscle tone which may result in fall to the floor; consciousness is preserved throughout; precipitated by fright, anxiety, anger, or laughter; represents intrusion of REM sleep phenomena into wakefulness and is seen in patients with narcolepsy.

Catatonia. A form of schizophrenia in which the patient remains mute and motionless.

Confusion. State of decreased consciousness in which the patient has difficulty comprehending the environment, has poor memory, and tends to misinterpret external stimuli.

Delirium. Confusion combined with agitation, hallucinations, and anxiety; generally seen along with toxic, febrile, or drug withdrawal states.

Dysphagia. Difficulty in swallowing which may be a consequence of pseudobulbar or bulbar dysfunction, neuromuscular or structural diseases affecting the pharynx, or psychological disturbances.

Dysarthria. Defective enunciation of speech owing to dysfunction in the peripheral mechanisms involved in speech articulation, e.g., cleft lip, cleft palate, or facial muscle weakness.

Dysdiadochokinesis. Impaired rapid, to and fro movements of a segment of the body (pronation-supination, flexion-extension of the wrists) owing to cerebellar disease.

Dystonia. Abnormal contorted postures affecting either segments or the entire body, arising as a consequence of simultaneous cocontraction of agonist and antagonist muscles.

Dysmetria. Difficulty in regulating the rate and range of muscle contraction due to cerebellar disease, leading to nystagmus, intention tremor, rebound phenomenon, and gait ataxia.

Echolalia. Involuntary repetition by an individual of the terminal syllables or words addressed to the individual; usually present in patients with poor language comprehension.

Equinovarus and Equinovalgus Deformities. Flexion deformity at the ankle along with internal or external rotation respectively; most often develops in children with cerebral palsy as a consequence of defective motor control.

Fasiculations. Spontaneous contraction of motor units due to active denervation, visible in the form of ripple-like movements of muscles. Most commonly seen in children with infantile spine muscular atrophy (Werdnig-Hoffman disease). They are best visualized in these patients over the edges of the tongue while it is at rest.

Flapping Tremor (Asterixis). Myoclonus of the forearm muscles resulting in an abrupt, flexion-extension movement of the wrist; generally accompanies metabolic encephalopathies, e.g., hepatic or uremic coma.

Finger Agnosia. Inability to indicate which finger was touched or to name it in the absence of any primary sensory deficit; a sign of left parietal brain damage.

Finger-Nose Test. When seated with elbows fully extended and arms in a horizontal plane, the patient is asked to touch the index finger to the nose with the eyes closed and then return to the starting position. Cerebellar deficits will impair performance on the test.

Gait Disturbances. Best visualized while having the patient walk down a long corridor. A hemiparetic gait is associated with circumduction and impaired flexion at the knee; those with peripheral neuropathy may drag the foot while walking; a slow, waddling gait is seen in those with myopathies; a broad-based gait is indicative of ataxia.

Gower's Sign. Propping of the hands against the floor or lower extremities for assistance while coming erect from the sitting position; indicative of bilateral proximal muscle weakness in the lower extremities.

Heel-Knee Test. While lying in the supine position, the patient is asked to run the posterior aspect of one heel over the opposite shin to and fro between the knee and ankle in one smooth motion. Patients with cerebellar disorders and peripheral neuropathy will demonstrate clumsiness during the maneuver.

Hemianopsia. Loss of vision in one half of the field in each eye; when the same, corresponding halves of vision are lost in each eye, i.e., right or left, the disorder is termed homonymous hemianopsia, and may accompany lesions in the optic tract or radiation. Bitemporal hemianopsia is generally present with lesions in the midline of the optic chiasm.

Hemiparesis/Plegia. Weakness of one half of the body; may be secondary to cerebral hemispheric or brainstem lesions.

Hypotonia. Decreased resistance during movement, frequently associated with hyperextension at the joints; may be secondary to cerebral cortical, cerebellar, spinal, or neuromuscular disorders.

Hypertonia. Increased resistance to movement of the limbs. It may be secondary to either pyramidal (spasticity) or extrapyramidal lesions (rigidity).

Hemiatrophy. Smallness of one half of the body as a consequence of contralateral cerebral infarction in infancy or early childhood.

Hemihypertrophy. Enlargement of one half of the body, generally seen along with Wilm's tumor or the Beckwith-Wiedemann syndrome (macroglossia, omphalocele, visceromegaly, and neonatal hypoglycemia).

Hoarse Cry. Seen along with congenital hypothyroidism, ectodermal dysplasia, Farber's lipogranulomatosis, de Lange syndrome, vocal cord polyps, and unilateral vocal cord paralysis.

Jaw Jerk. With the jaw held partially open, the examiner places a finger over the chin and taps it lightly with a hammer; this should elicit partial closure of the jaw; both afferent and efferent impulses are through the trigeminal nerve; this is the only tendon reflex to be mediated above the plane of the foramen magnum; most commonly exaggerated in pseudobulbar states.

Jitteriness. Exaggerated stretch responses in neonates and young infants which can be abolished by relaxing the involved limb; not associated with any impairment of consciousness or head segment automatisms; may be mistaken for seizures; commonly observed along with hypocalcemia, hypomagnesemia, hypoxia, and drug withdrawal states.

Joint Sense. With the patient's eyes closed, his/her great toes and thumbs are moved upwards or downwards and the patient asked to indicate the direction of movement; patients with disease of the large myelinated peripheral nerve fibers or dorsal columns will have difficulty with the task.

Learning Disability. Scholastic underachievement in the absence of generalized cognitive incompetence, lack of motivation, or lack of educational opportunity.

Macrocephaly. Occipito-frontal head circumference greater than the 90th percentile for age.

Microcephaly. Occipito-frontal head circumference of less than the 10th percentile for age; invariably associated with micrencephaly or small brain size.

Minimal Cerebral Dysfunction. See Attentional Deficit Disorder.

Mental Retardation. Generalized cognitive incompetence combined with maladaptive social behavior; while psychometric tests are not always an accurate gauge of intellectual function, mentally retarded subjects generally have Intellectual Quotients of less than 70.

Muscle Strength Assessment. Generally carried out by having the patient resist pressure initiated by the examiner. In the system devised by the General Medical Council of Great Britain, Grade 0/5 indicates complete lack of voluntary movement, Grade 1/5 a flicker of movement, Grade 2/5 movement with gravity eliminated, Grade 3/5 movement against gravity, Grade 4/5 movement against gravity and some external resistance, Grade 5/5 movement against gravity and good resistance (normal).

Nystagmus. Rhythmic eye movements which may be horizontal, vertical, rotatory, or mixed; three to four beats of nystagmus upon extreme lateral gaze are physiological. Pendular nystagmus is generally seen with ocular or cerebellar disease; sustained nystagmus upon lateral gaze associated with vertigo suggests impairment of the vestibular system. Vertical nystagmus suggests either brainstem dysfunction or drug intoxication.

Ocular Bobbing. Intermittent, usually conjugate, brisk downward eye movement followed by a slow drift back to the primary position; may occur in comatose patients with destructive caudal pontine lesions, but also occasionally with metabolic encephalopathies or extrinsic compression of the brainstem, e.g., in hydrocephalus.

Oculogyric Crisis. Spasmodic deviation of the eyes, usually upwards lasting minutes to hours; most frequently seen in post-encephalitic Parkinsonism or phenothiazine intoxication.

Optokinetic Nystagmus. Physiological phenomenon; movement of a tape marked with solid parallel bars in front of the patient from the patient's left to the right elicits quick jerky movements of the eyes to the left, and vice versa. It is at least partially dependant upon preservation of visual fixation. Loss of optokinetic nystagmus is generally indicative of a hemispheric lesion behind the central sulcus. An abnormal optokinetic response is often associated with, but not dependant upon, a homonymous field defect.

Optic Atrophy. Alteration in the color of the optic disc to light pink, gray, or white, along with decreased visual acuity.

Optic Nerve Hypoplasia. Congenital smallness of the optic disc which may be unilateral or bilateral; associated with normal or impaired vision and occasional central nervous system malformations, e.g., septo-optic dysplasia.

Ptosis. Drooping of the upper eyelid, resulting in encroachment upon the pupillary margin; may be seen along with myopathies, Horner's syndrome, or local eyelid pathology, e.g., neurofibroma.

Pseudobulbar State. Bilateral interruption of corticobulbar fibers in the region of the centrum semiovale, internal capsule, diencephalon or mesencephalon with resultant dysphagia and defective articulation; bilateral pyramidal signs and emotional lability are frequently present also; most often observed in quadriparetic forms of cerebral palsy.

Papilledema. Choking of optic nerve axoplasmic flow and retinal venous return from increased intracranial pressure; the initial manifestation is enlargement of the blind spot. This is followed by loss of venous pulsations, blurring of the disc margins, obliteration of the physiological cup and subsequently, retinal hemorrhages and exudates.

Rebound Phenomenon. Observed in cerebellar disorders, due in part to loss of synergistic control by opposing groups of muscles. Under normal circumstances an outstretched arm returns promptly without oscillation to the original position when it is depressed slightly by the examiner. The presence of the rebound phenomenon, on the other hand, is associated with overshooting before the limb can be finally brought to rest at the original position.

Rigidity. A form of hypertonicity seen in extrapyramidal disorders in which alternating contraction of agonist and antagonist muscles frequently confers a "cog-wheel" feeling to the muscles. Tendon and plantar reflexes remain unaltered with pure rigidity.

Root Pain. Sharp shooting pain over a certain dermatome from pressure or irritation of a nerve root that is frequently made worse by maneuvers that increase intraspinal pressure, e.g., coughing, bending.

Spasticity. A form of hypertonicity secondary to pyramidal dysfunction and the resultant abnormal lengthening-shortening reaction. The resistance to movement is greatest in the very initial and terminal phases of a movement ("clasp-knife" phenomenon).

Tics. Habit spasms; stereotyped, repetitive body movements which are usually associated with a compulsive urge to carry them out.

Tremor. Involuntary movement characterized by rhythmic oscillation of the distal extremity due to alternating contraction of agonist and antagonist muscles. Resting tremor of a coarse amplitude is seen in patients with Parkinson's disease and intention tremor (upon movement) with cerebellar disease. Fine tremor apparent at rest while the limb is kept extended is frequently of the essential (familial) type.

SUGGESTED READING

1. Touwen BC. Examination of the child with minor neurological dysfunction. In: Clinics in Developmental Medicine. No. 71, Heinemann Publishers, London, 1979.

2. Nelson KB and Ellenberg JH. Neonatal signs as predictors of cerebral palsy. Pediatrics 64:225-232, 1979.

3. Volpe JJ. The neurological examination: normal and abnormal features. In: Neurology of the Newborn. WB Saunders, Philadelphia, 1987; 70-96.

4. Golden GS. Practical Guidelines for the Routine Neurological Examination of Children. Health Sciences Consortium Inc. Chapel Hill, North Carolina, 1982.

5. Clinical Examinations in Neurology. 5th ed. Mayo Clinic and Mayo Clinic Foundation. WB Saunders, Philadelphia, 1981.

6. Knobloch H and Pasamanick B, eds. Gesell and Amartruda's Developmental Diagnosis. 3rd ed. Harper and Row, Hagerstown, Maryland, 1974.

7. Sarnat HB. Anatomic and physiologic correlates of neurologic development in prematurity. In: Surnat HB, ed. Topics in Neonatal Neurology. Grune and Stratton, Orlando, 1984.

CHAPTER II

DEVELOPMENT OF THE NERVOUS SYSTEM AND ITS ABERRATIONS

Phases of Development

Disorders of Dorsal Organ Induction

Disorders of Ventral Induction

Disorders of Neuronal and Glial Proliferation and Migration

Disorders of Myelination

PHASES OF DEVELOPMENT

An orderly sequence of events, some of them overlapping, is involved in the formation and organization of the nervous system. While certain elements of the nervous system are quite mature at full term, others continue their development throughout infancy and childhood. Knowledge of developmental anatomy and physiology is fundamental to understanding some pediatric neurological disorders.

Organ Induction

Around the 16th day of life, the embryo is composed of three layers: the ectoderm, mesoderm, and endoderm. By the 18th day, the notochordal mesoderm induces thickening in the central portion of the ectoderm to form the neural plate (Fig. 2-1). Under the continuous inductive influence of the mesoderm, the lateral margins of the neural plate approximate dorsally to complete formation of the neural tube by the 28th day. A process of segmentation and cavitation follows at the rostral end soon thereafter, resulting in separation into the forebrain, mid, and hind brain segments, each then going on to develop a central vesicle. The vesicles are the anlage of the ventricular system.

Table 2-1. Important events in the formation of the central nervous system

EVENT	TIME OF OCCURRENCE
Organ induction	2 1/2-6 weeks gestation
Neuronal proliferation and migration	2-5 months gestation
Glial cell proliferation and migration	6 months prenatally to 6 months postnatally
Myelination	2nd month prenatally through 3rd decade
Synaptogenesis	20-24 weeks prenatally through most of the the learning portion of one's life

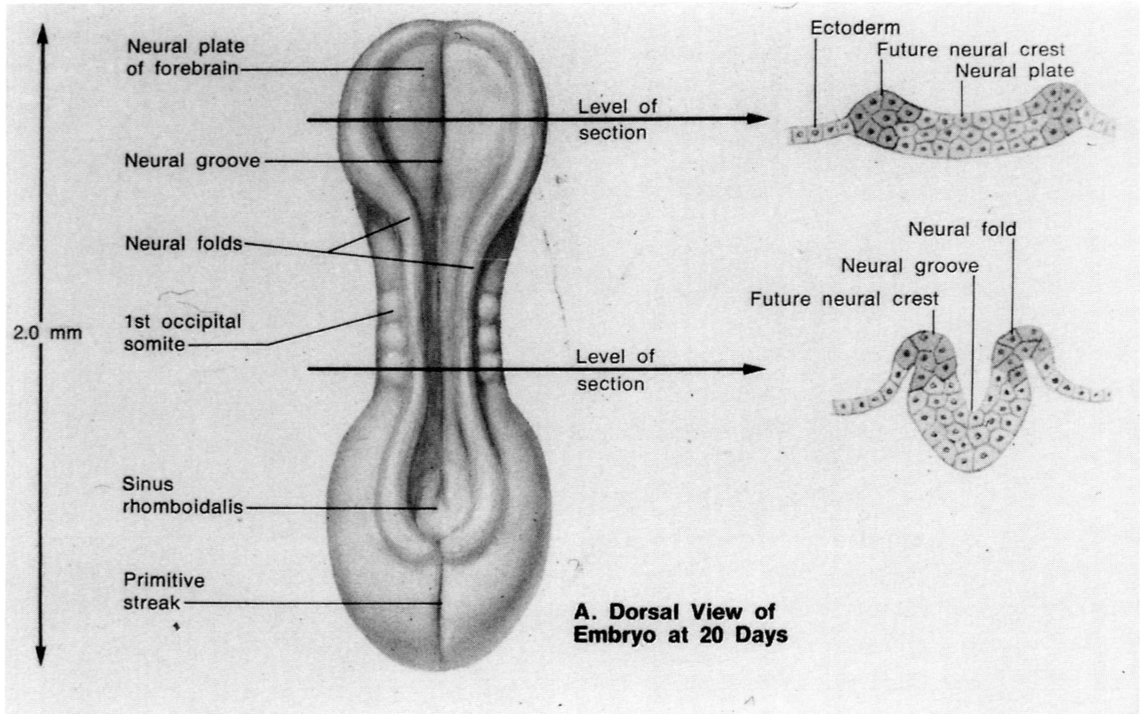

Fig. 2-1. Dorsal view of the embryo at 20 days age, demonstrating differentiation of the ectoderm into the neural plate and neural crest. Copyright 1974. CIBA-GEIGY. (Reproduced with permission from Clinical Symposia, by Frank H. Netter, M.D. All rights reserved.)

Neuronal Proliferation and Migration

Between the 2nd and 5th months of gestation, primitive cells in the periventricular region (germinal matrix) proliferate to form neurons. The neurons migrate outwards in a centrifugal, and subsequently tangential manner to ultimately form the hemispheric deep gray matter, cerebral and cerebellar cortices. Development of cerebral and cerebellar convolutions reflects progressive neuronal migration. Sulci and gyri form in a specific sequence related to gestational age.

Glial Cell Proliferation and Migration

Glial cells (astrocytes and oligodendrocytes) also evolve from the multipotent cells of the periventricular germinal matrix, maximally between the 6th month of intrauterine life to about the 6th month postnatally, and migrate centrifugally. Amongst other functions, glial cells regulate myelination and the blood-brain barrier.

Synaptogenesis

Appropriate cell-to-cell connections are prerequisite to the development of normal motor and intellectual function. Dendritic, synaptic and neurotransmitter proliferation is most active between 20-30 weeeks gestation, being reflected in progressive maturation of the EEG in the preterm infant (e.g., evolution from a discontinous pattern at 28 weeks gestation into a continuous pattern by 34 weeks, along with sleep-wake and sleep state differentiation). Axodendritic synapses are generally excitatory, whereas axosomatic and axoaxonal synapses are inhibitory in function. In the neocortex and hippocampus, inhibitory pathways undergo a preferentially earlier development than excitatory circuits. It is believed that the capacity to form or alter synapses continues in some way throughout the learning portion of our lives and that synaptic fixity or loss result in an inability to learn.

Myelination

This process begins in the early second trimester and extends into adult life. Myelination within the central nervous system is accomplished by oligodendroglial cells, and in the peripheral nervous system by Schwann cells. The ventral and dorsal spinal nerve roots and the medial longitudinal fasiculus are some of the earliest structures to myelinate, whereas certain commisural (connecting the two hemispheres) and association (connecting structures within the same hemisphere) pathways are about the last to myelinate. Myelination of neural pathways is important because it provides insulation of individual axons and enhances the speed of impulse conduction. Conduction velocity is a factor in enabling a neuron to deliver a critical number of impulses per unit time, thus allowing the appropriate release of neurotransmitters and maintaining stable motor and sensory functions. Evolution in posture of a preterm infant from passive extension at 30 weeks conceptional age to strong flexion at 40 weeks conceptional age is a visible example of progressive maturation on account of myelination of the descending motor pathways. These pathways can be grouped physiologically into the corticospinal, medial subcorticospinal, and lateral subcorticospinal systems. The terms "medial" and "lateral" refer to the location of the pathways in the brainstem relative to the midline. Each pathway incorporates several anatomically distinct tracts such as the rubrospinal and vestibulospinal tracts. The infant of 30 weeks conceptional age lies with passive extension of all four limbs, as myelination at this age is restricted only to the medial subcorticospinal system, the action of which induces extension of the proximal extremities. The lateral subcorticospinal system subserves flexion in the proximal extremities. Myelination of this system results in gradual evolution to a flexed posture by 36-40 weeks conceptional age.

DISORDERS OF
DORSAL ORGAN INDUCTION

Anencephaly. Failure of closure of the rostral aspect of the neural tube; the timing of the insult is usually no later than the 26th day of gestation. Polyhydramnios are frequently noted in the mothers. Approximately 75% of affected children are stillborn, while the remainder die in the neonatal period. Both environmental and genetic factors are responsible.

Spina bifida occulta. Asymptomatic condition characterized by failure of fusion of the vertebral arches without any neurologic deficit; occurs in approximately 5% of the population.

Encephalocele. Protrusion of cerebral tissue through a cranial defect which is usually located in the frontal or occipital regions. The herniated tissue is generally non-viable. The disorder occurs at the time of closure of the anterior neuropore, i.e., usually prior to the 26th day of gestation. Most of the time the encephalocele is the only major congenital malformation in the child. CT scanning with coronal, saggital, and transaxial reconstruction, magnetic resonance imaging, and cranial neurosonography help assess the extent of the encephalocele. Unless ethical considerations dictate otherwise, surgical closure of the defect in the neonatal period is recommended.

Meningocele. Herniation of the meninges into a cyst located generally over the dorsum of the spine; neurologic deficit in the extremities may be minimal; the external covering of the cyst may be intact or ulcerated. In the latter instance, there may be leakage of cerebrospinal fluid and a significant risk of the child contracting bacterial meningitis.

Meningomyelocele. Herniation of meninges, nerve roots, and spinal cord through a dorsal vertebral defect. Malformations of the spinal cord and Arnold-Chiari malformation (downward displacement of the cerebellar tonsils, with or without the medulla and 4th ventricle, into the cervical spinal canal) frequently accompany the meningomyelocele. Hydrocephalus from the associated Arnold-Chiari malformation or aqueductal stenosis occurs in 63 to 90% of the cases. Approximately 80% of meningomyeloceles occur in the thoracolumbar, lumbar, or lumbosacral region. Varying degrees of paraparesis, bowel, and bladder dysfunction are the rule.

Management of Neural Tube Defects

Operative repair of encephalocele, meningocele, and meningomyelocele is required to reduce viable portions of the dorsally displaced nervous tissue into the cranial cavity or spinal canal, to repair any breach in continuity of the meninges, and to cover the areas of the defect with available skin, fascia, or muscle. Rapid exacerbation of associated hydrocephalus following meningomyelocele repair is common and cranial CT should be repeated 1-2 weeks after the surgical procedure. Surgery in the neonatal period for neural tube defects is only the beginning of management—coordinated care through multidisciplinary myelodyplasia clinics with participation of neurosurgeons, pediatric neurologists, urologists, orthopedists, psychologists, physical and occupational therapists, and social workers is necessary for most children with neurologic deficits.

The atonic neurogenic bladder is evacuated in the neonatal period by the Crede maneuver (gentle pressure on the suprapubic region). Periodic monitoring for urinary tract infections and calculi is essential. If significant adynamic urinary tract obstruction is noted over time, surgical procedures for urinary diversion may be necessary. The patient should also be monitored for intellectual deficits and seizures, usually from associated migrational defects in the cerebral cortex. As the patient becomes older, psychometric evaluation, placement in academically appropriate school programs, and supportive psychotherapy may become necessary.

Antenatal Diagnosis of Neural Tube Defects

In most affected children with neural tube defects, no malformations are noted outside of the central nervous system and the inheritance is multifactorial, i.e., dependent upon a polygenic genetic predisposition combined with environmental influences. With one affected offspring in the family, the risk for having additional children with neural tube defects is 5%. Recurrence risk with two affected offspring is approximately double that figure. Prenatal diagnosis of neural tube defects can be established by documentation of elevated amniotic fluid alpha fetoprotein levels using aminocentesis between the 16th and 17th weeks of gestation. If elevated, the test should be repeated within a week to confirm. If the alpha fetoprotein level remains elevated at the second determination, abdominal ultrasound studies are obtained to exclude false positives from multiple pregnancy or wrong gestational dates. Anencephaly may also be detected upon maternal abdominal ultrasound studies.

DISORDERS OF VENTRAL INDUCTION

Between the 5th and 6th weeks of embryonic life, the prechordal mesoderm induces changes in the ventral aspect of the rostral neural tube to give rise to the paired cerebral hemispheres, lateral ventricles, and diencephalon. This interaction influences formation of the forebrain as well as the face, hence the association of facial anomalies with disorders of development occuring at this stage.

Arhinencephaly is the simplest disorder of ventral induction, characterized by bilateral absence of the olfactory bulbs and tracts, manifesting with anosmia in the neonatal period.

Holoprosencephaly (Fig. 2-2) is characterized by arhinencephaly, presence of a single lateral ventricle, single forebrain and thalamus. It occurs in approximately 1 in 13,000 live births, but the incidence is fifty-fold greater in spontaneously aborted embryos. Facial anomalies, such as hypotelorism are frequently present. Using conventional chromosomal studies, approximately half the patients have a normal karyotype, whereas the remaining half demonstrate trisomy 13-15, mosaic trisomy 13-15, trisomy 18, deletion 18, or ring 18 abnormalities. Familial cases, probably recessive, have also been reported. When holoprosencephaly is associated with presence of a single median eye, the disorder is termed **cyclopia**. **Septo optic dysplasia** is another common ventral induction defect that is characterized by hypoplastic optic discs, absence of the septum pellucidum, hypothalamic dysfunction, seizures, and occasional intellectual dysfunction.

DISORDERS OF NEURONAL AND GLIAL PROLIFERATION AND MIGRATION

Neuronal and glial proliferation and migration are most active in the second trimester. During this period therefore, they are especially vulnerable to metabolic, toxic, and infectious insults which may result in microcephaly, intellectual dysfunction, or seizures. Histologically, the cerebral cortex in most microcephalic patients has fewer neurons, with disruption of the normal laminar cellular arrangement (Fig. 2-3) and alteration in cell-to-cell connections.

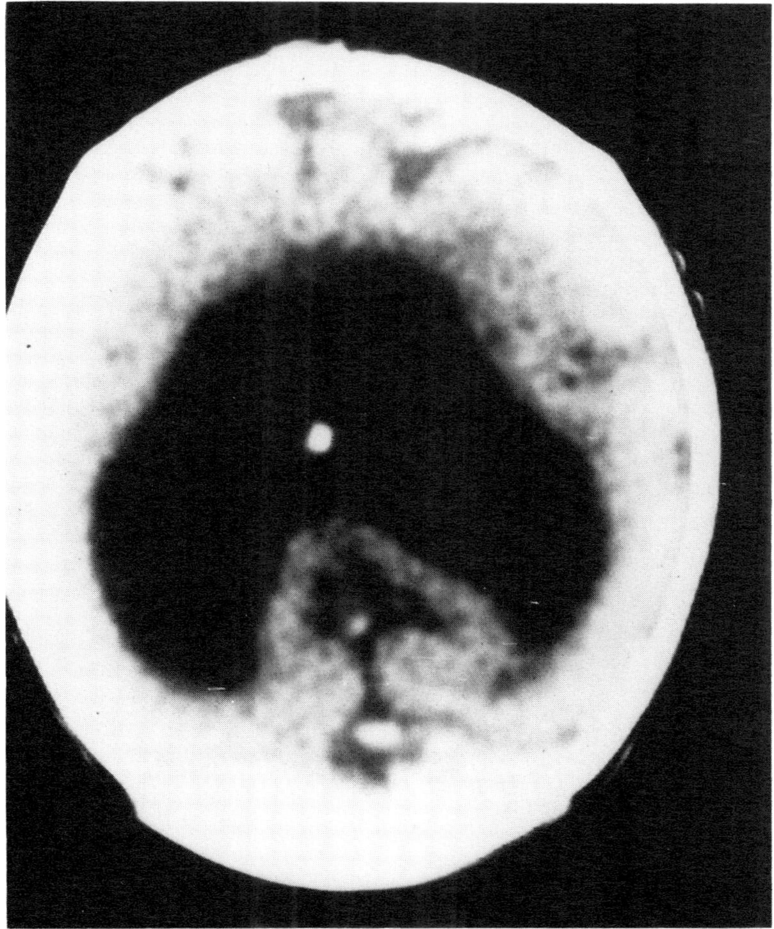

Fig. 2-2. Semilobar holoprosencephaly in a three-month-old; there is a single lateral ventricle and absence of the septum pellucidum.

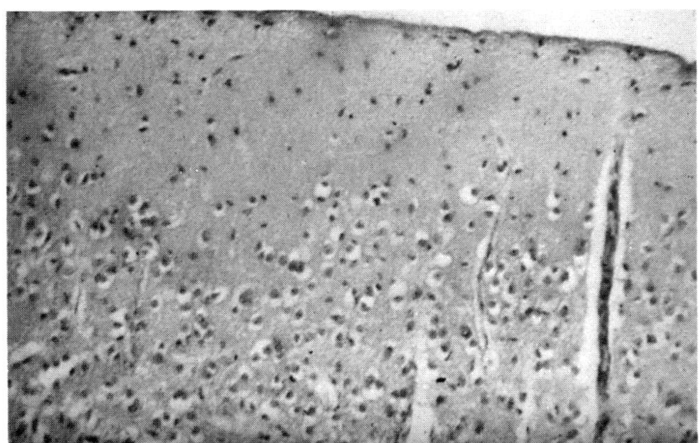

Fig. 2-3. Cerebral cortex in a patient with microcephaly; there is a paucity of neurons and failure of development of the normal laminar arrangement of cellular elements.

Heterotopic neurons arrested in the deep white matter during the course of their centrifugal migration are also seen. Some of the common clinical disorders in this category include:

Congenital intrauterine infections. Toxoplasmosis, rubella, cytomegalovirus, herpes simplex, and syphilis.

Chromosomal disorders. Down's syndrome, trisomy 18, deletion of the short arm of chromosomes 4 or 18, deletion of the long arm of 13 or 18.

Fetal alcohol syndrome. Characterized frequently by pre and postnatal growth deficiency, intellectual dysfunction, microcephaly, short palpebral fissures, maxillary hypoplasia, and strabismus.

Microcephaly vera. The micrencephaly is not related to any intrauterine infection, metabolic or toxic insult. There are no chromosomal abnormalities and no gross derangements of other events in the development of the nervous system. In contrast to other microcephalic infants, seizures and major neurologic deficits are noted only infrequently in the neonatal period, but become

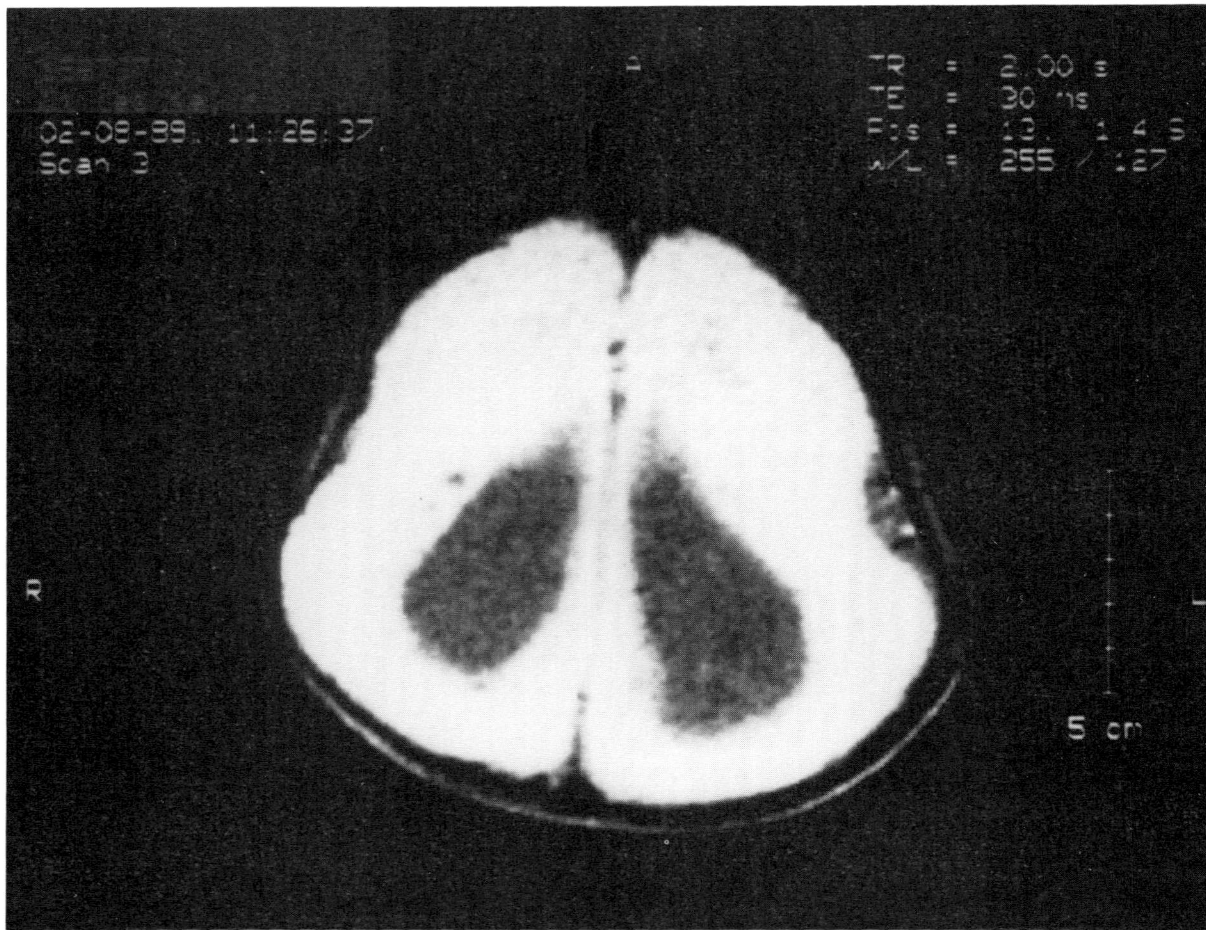

Fig. 2-4. Magnetic resonance image demonstrating agyria in a patient with Miller-Dieker syndrome. The cortical surface is smooth, without presence of any gyri or sulci. Routine and high resolution banding chromosome studies were normal in this patient, but molecular genetic investigations disclosed a characteristic small deletion on the distal part of the short arm of chromosome 17.

apparent as the child grows older. Sporadic X-linked and autosomal recessive transmission have all been described.

Lissencephaly. In this first trimester disorder, the brain has very few or no gyri, and its surface presents a smooth appearance with minimal convolutions. Severe neurologic dysfunction is manifest at birth or early infancy in the form of extreme opisthotonic posturing, difficult to control seizures, microcephaly, and developmental delay. The CT scan helps to establish the diagnosis, demonstrating paucity of gyri and sucli and a failure in closure of the operculum. The EEG is markedly abnormal, with presence of a discontinuous pattern and generalized or multifocal epileptiform discharges. Sporadic and autosomal recessive forms have both been reported. Association of lissencephaly with facial anomalies

(anteverted nares, micrognathia, depressed nasal bridge, low-set malformed pinnae) is termed the Miller Dieker syndrome, and some patients with this syndrome have a ring chromosome 17 or an unbalanced 17p13 translocation (Fig. 2-4).

Schizencephaly. This severe malformation usually develops in the second month of gestation, and is characterized by the presence of bihemispheric, fluid-filled clefts; the overlying cortex has abnormal gyral development. Seizures and severe mental retardation are common.

Micropolygyria. Increased numbers of small gyri, particularly in temporoparietal regions. The onset is most likely in the second trimester. While most cases are free standing, micropolygyria may also accompany the Zellweger syndrome (cerebro-hepato-renal syndrome), a disorder of peroxisomal function.

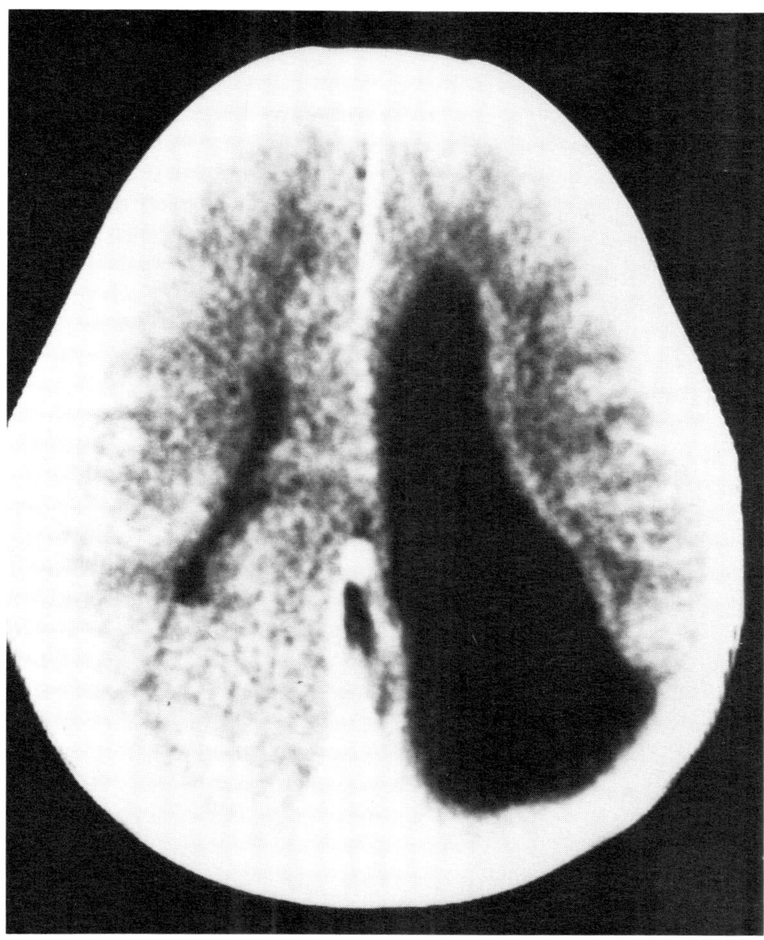

Fig. 2-5. Three-year-old with porencephaly who had intractable focal seizures, hemiparesis and hemianopsia.

Porencephaly. A focal area of liquefaction necrosis and cyst formation of vascular (infarction or hemorrhage), infectious, or traumatic etiology (Fig.2-5). The cyst may or may not communicate with the ventricular system. The lesion develops in the second or third trimesters or early infancy. Some focal neurologic deficits become apparent in infancy and early childhood, e.g., hemiparesis, hemisensory deficits, and visual field deficits, whereas others like hemiatrophy and scoliosis are detectable only in later childhood. Seizures may occur at any age. The EEG frequently discloses spike and slow wave complexes overlying in the region of porencephaly. The diagnosis can be readily established using CT or cranial ultrasound studies.

Hydranencephaly. Replacement of major portions of the cerebral hemispheres by paired, cystic lesions, usually due to bilateral infarction in the distribution of the internal carotid vessels in the second trimester (Fig. 2-6). These infants frequently display normal brainstem function (e.g., sucking, swallowing) but fail to develop any higher level functions. The head size is frequently normal at birth, but the markedly increased transillumination and CT scan help establish the diagnosis in the neonatal period or early infancy.

Agenesis of the Corpus Callosum. The corpus callosum normally develops between the 10th and 12th weeks of embryonic life and carries commisural pathways between the hemispheres from the 3rd and 4th cortical layers. The occurrence may be sporadic, or X-linked, isolated, or in conjunction with other cerebral malformations. Seizures may be noted in some during infancy, while others subsequently manifest intellectual dysfunction from impairment of the interhemispheric transfer of information. The diagnosis can be readily established on cranial CT, which discloses a characteristic high-riding 3rd ventricle, wedged in between two widely separated lateral ventricles.

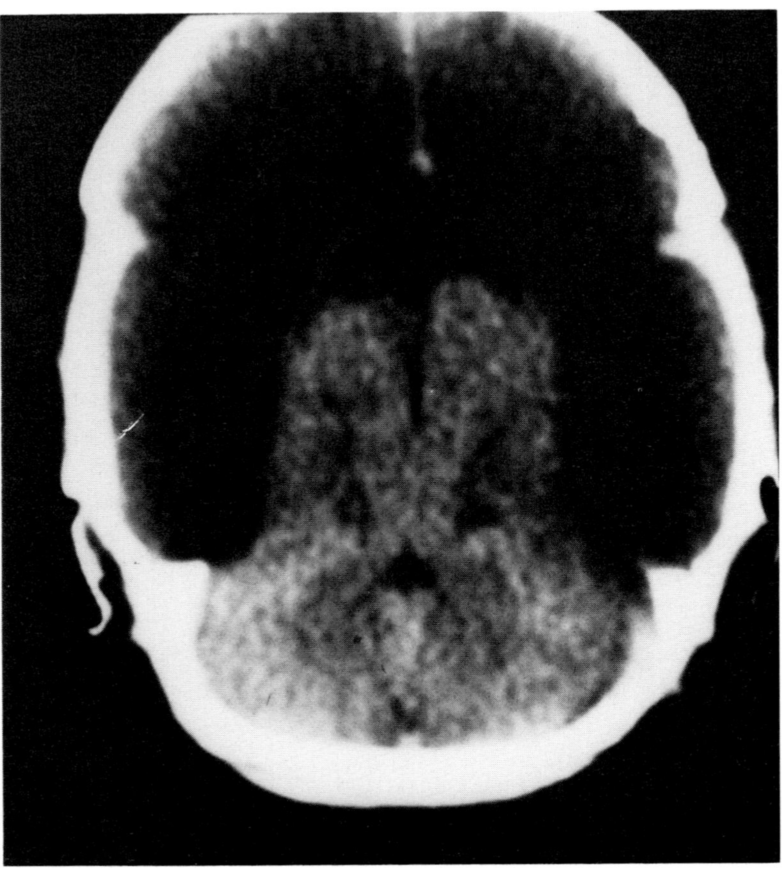

Fig. 2-6. Neonate with hydranencephaly; a hypodense, cystic structure occupies the region of distribution of the anterior and middle cerebral arteries.

DISORDERS OF MYELINATION

Primary cerebral white matter hypoplasia, perinatal undernutrition, severe maternal malnutrition during pregnancy, certain leukodystrophies (e.g., Canavan's and Alexander's diseases), congenital intrauterine infections, and amino acidurias can all lead to disruption of myelination within the central nervous system, resulting in abnormalities of muscle tone, stretch reflexes, visual function, and motor development.

SUGGESTED READING

1. Dobbing J and Sands J. Quantitative growth and development of human brain. Arch Dis Child 48:757-767, 1973.

2. Garcia CS, Dunn D and Trevor R. The lissencephaly (agyria) syndrome in siblings. Arch Neurol 35:608-611, 1978.

3. Gilles FH. Myelination in the human brain. Hum Pathol 7:244-248, 1976.

4. Huttenlocher PR. Dendritic development in neocortex of children with mental defect and infantile spasms. Neurology 24:203-210, 1974.

5. Karfunkel P. The mechanisms of neural tube formation. Int Rev Cytol 38:245-271, 1974.

6. Sarnat HB. Topics in Neonatal Neurology. Grune and Stratton, Orlando 1984; 1-26.

7. Sidman RL and Rakic P. Neuronal migration, with special reference to the developing human brain: a review. Brain Res 62:1-35, 1973.

8. Volpe JJ. Neurology of the Newborn. 2nd ed. W.B. Saunders Company, Philadelphia, 1987; Chapters 1 and 2, 2-68.

CHAPTER III

COMMON NEURODIAGNOSTIC PROCEDURES

Lumbar Puncture

Subdural Taps

Electroencephalography(EEG)

Evoked Potentials

Magnetic Resonance Imaging (MRI)

Computerized Axial Tomography (CAT)

Comparison of CAT and MRI Scans

Cerebral Angiography

Skull X-Rays

Ultrasonography

Radionuclide Brain Scanning

LUMBAR PUNCTURE

Indications

Diagnostic; for suspected:

1. Bacterial meningitis
   Viral meningitis/meningoencephalitis
   Fungal meningitis
   Neoplastic meningeal infiltration
2. Demyelinating diseases
3. Subarachnoid hemorrhage (frankly bloody with xanthochromia of the centrifuged supernatant fluid)
4. Pseudotumor cerebri (CSF opening pressure increased above 200 mm)
5. Myelography

Therapeutic

1. Instillation of intrathecal chemotherapeutic agents (e.g., methotrexate in leukemia).
2. Withdrawal of CSF in pseudotumor cerebri.

Contraindications

A. Increased intracranial pressure from mass lesions. As a general rule, in febrile patients with papilledema or focal neurological signs, a brain imaging procedure (CT scan) rather than lumbar puncture should be obtained for establishing a diagnosis, since both manifestations are infrequent in meningitis, but common with focal intracranial mass lesions (e.g., abscess, neoplasm).

B. Presence of infection locally at the lumbar puncture site.

Technique

1. Sedation in an apprehensive patient immediately prior to lumbar puncture is helpful in allaying anxiety and minimizing movement during the procedure. Chloral hydrate in a single 50-75 mg/kg dose approximately 30 minutes prior to the test is recommended.

2. The patient is placed in the left lateral decubitus. An assistant is necessary in order to immobilize the patient. The spine, hips, and neck should be kept fully flexed in order to widen the interspinous spaces and facilitate needle entry. The table upon which the patient is placed should be firm; the patient's back should be perpendicular to the horizontal surface of the table throughout the procedure.

3. The back is cleaned with an antiseptic solution using a sterile technique. The lumbar region is then covered with a sterile drape that has a central perforation.

4. Local anesthesia is generally not necessary in neonates, but is essential in older children. It is administered under the skin and deep into the interspinous space selected for the procedure. The L4-5 or L3-4 spaces are preferred.

5. A 21 or 22 gauge needle with stylet (1 1/4″ length in young children, 2 to 2 1/2″ in adolescents) is inserted into the space, directed slightly cephalad with the bevel facing up. The stylet is withdrawn after every 2-4 mm of insertion in order to check entry into the subarachnoid space. The cerebrospinal fluid will flow freely once the needle tip is fully in the space. The stylet is then reinserted while preparations are being made to record the opening pressure.

6. The stylet is withdrawn and the manometer connected to the head of the lumbar puncture needle using a three way stopcock and preferably a silastic tubing. The stopcock is turned so that the CSF flows directly into the vertical limb of the manometer. The neck and hips of the patient are at this point gradually extended so that they come to lie in a semi-flexed position; there should be no pressure on the neck veins or the abdomen; the patient should be quiet and breathing normally.

   The opening pressure is read off the manometer once the upper meniscus has stopped fluctuating. The normal opening pressure is less than 180 mm of CSF; readings between 180-200 mm are suspicious of increased intracranial pressure, and those above 200 mm are diagnostic.

7. When increased intracranial pressure is encountered unexpectedly during the course of a diagnostic lumbar puncture, the stop-cock should be immediately closed to the patient so that no further CSF is allowed to drain. Spinal fluid already present in the manometer should be adequate for some essential diagnostic tests such as culture and cell count.

8. Only the minimum amount of CSF necessary for studies (generally 4-5 ml) should be withdrawn in a diagnostic lumbar puncture.

9. Following completion of specimen collection, the stylet is reinserted into the hollow needle and then both gradually withdrawn from the back. In order to prevent development of a post-lumbar puncture headache, the patient is advised to lie flat in bed for 6-8 hours following the procedure.

Normal Cerebrospinal Fluid

Normal CSF is crystal-clear, with less than 5 WBCs/cubic mm (all lymphocytes). The CSF protein is between 15-30 mg/dl. In newborns, however, the protein content may be as high as 120 mg/dl, dropping to 15-30 mg/dl by 5-6 weeks after birth. The CSF glucose value is generally two thirds of the blood glucose value.

Complications of Lumbar Puncture

Post-lumbar puncture headache. This most likely occurs as a consequence of CSF leakage from the puncture site with resultant lowering of intracranial pressure and traction on pain-sensitive structures like the dura. It is worsened by assuming an erect posture, relieved by lying down, and may last for 2-14 days. Bed rest and analgesics are the only effective therapy.

Backache. This occurs at the site of the procedure.

Spinal epidural hemorrhage. Patients with bleeding disorders may develop localized epidural hemorrhage, which can result in paraplegia. Lumbar puncture should be avoided in hemophiliac patients having Factor VIII/IX levels below 30% of normal or when the platelet count is less than 30,000/c.mm. A significantly prolonged prothrombin time should also be corrected.

Brain herniation. Cerebellar tonsillar herniation can develop when a lumbar puncture is carried out in the presence of increased intracranial pressure. It generally occurs 4-6 hours following the

procedure and is heralded by deterioration in the level of consciousness, opisthotonic posturing, and apnea. Mannitol should be administered immediately intravenously, along with intensive cardio-respiratory support. If patients are properly selected for lumbar punctures, this unfortunate complication can be generally avoided.

Alternative to Lumbar Puncture

When study of cerebrospinal fluid is absolutely essential for establishing a diagnosis (e.g., cryptococcal meningitis) and there is a significant risk of inducing brain herniation with lumbar puncture due to the presence of increased intracranial pressure, neurosurgical assistance should be sought in order to obtain the CSF specimen via a cisterna magna tap. As the cisternal tap decompresses the subarachnoid space above the plane of the foramen magnum,it is less liable to lead to tonsillar herniation.

SUBDURAL TAPS IN INFANCY

Aspiration of fluid from the subdural space in infants is a relatively simple procedure due to the presence of an open anterior fontanelle which serves as an easy route of access. Once the fontanelle has closed, however, neurosurgical assistance for insertion of a cannula through a twist drill hole becomes necessary.

Indications

Post-meningitic subdural effusions and empyema. This is usually characterized by delayed resolution of meningitis, with persistent lethargy, fever, excessive cranial enlargement, a tense anterior fontanelle, and generally (not always) increased cranial transillumination. Low density extracerebral fluid collections with concavity applied to the surface of the brain are visible on the CT scan.

Chronic subdural hematoma of infancy. This is secondary to indirect, whiplash-type shaking trauma, with resultant tearing of veins that normally bridge the dura and the superior saggital sinus. Infrequently, the venous hemorrhage may be secondary to birth trauma. Macrocephaly, palpably split cranial sutures, a tense anterior fontanelle, vomiting, and lethargy are the most common clinical manifestations. Associated linear retinal hemorrhages and fractures in various stages of healing on a skeletal radiological survey are strongly indicative of child abuse. The cranial transillumination may or may not be increased.

Technique

1. Bleeding disorders must be excluded prior to the subdural tap.

2. Scalp hair overlying the side of the fontanelle requiring the tap is shaved, the skin cleaned with an antiseptic solution and covered with a sterile drape.

3. A 21 or 20 gauge subdural tap needle is selected. Subdural needles generally have short bevels which minimize the likelihood of injury to the underlying cerebral cortex.

4. The needle is inserted through the skin surface in the anterior fontanelle, as far laterally and close to the coronal suture as possible, and directed towards the subdural collection. The needle is advanced only 2-3 mm at a time. The stylet of the needle is periodically withdrawn in order to check for entry into the subdural space, which is usually felt by a slight give in resistance 0.5-1.0 cm deep to the skin surface.

5. Fluid from the subdural space will automatically trickle out once the needle is in place. Subdural fluid is generally thick, straw colored, and with a high protein content (at least 30 mg/dl more than lumbar CSF). Between 15-20 ml of fluid may be withdrawn safely from each subdural tap. The needle should be periodically withdrawn a few mms and redirected in another plane in order to tap any loculated collections.

6. If the subdural collection is bilateral, an identical procedure is needed on the opposite side.

7. Daily taps for 8-12 days may be necessary in order to completely drain the chronic subdural fluid collection.

ELECTROENCEPHALOGRAPHY

The electroencephalogram is a sensitive test for determination of altered cortical function secondary to a variety of disorders.

Technique

An array of 18-20 electrodes is applied to the scalp surface using collodion or electrode paste. The site of electrode placement is standardized, and in most laboratories, conforms to the International "10-20" System[2]. The cortical action potential difference between each two adjacent electrodes is amplified and displayed on a strip of moving paper.

Sampling of cortical activity from homologous areas of the scalp is necessary during both wakefulness and sleep, as well as following activation procedures like photic stimulation and hyperventilation. Both the technician and electroencephalographer need to be familiar with biological and extraneous artifacts on the tracing which mimic EEG abnormalities, as well as the normal maturational changes. Sleep induction during the test enhances the yield of abnormalities and is best accomplished by sleep deprivation for 4-6 hours on the night prior to the test. Sedatives should be used to induce sleep only as a last resort, as they tend to induce high frequency activity (18-20 Hz beta), which can mask epileptiform abnormalities.

The Normal EEG

Familiarity with normal developmental changes in the electroencephalogram is a prerequisite for accurate interpretation of the record. The EEG of children is characterized by a mixture of activity in the delta (1-4 Hz), theta (4.5-7.5 Hz), alpha (8-13 Hz) and beta (14-22 Hz) ranges. Newborns have a predominance of slower frequency activity. With maturation, the resting activity during wakefulness shifts into the faster (theta, then alpha) frequencies (Fig. 3-1 and Fig. 3-2). Sleep spindles (12-16 Hz rhythmic fast activity in the central regions) appear by 6-8 weeks of age during non-

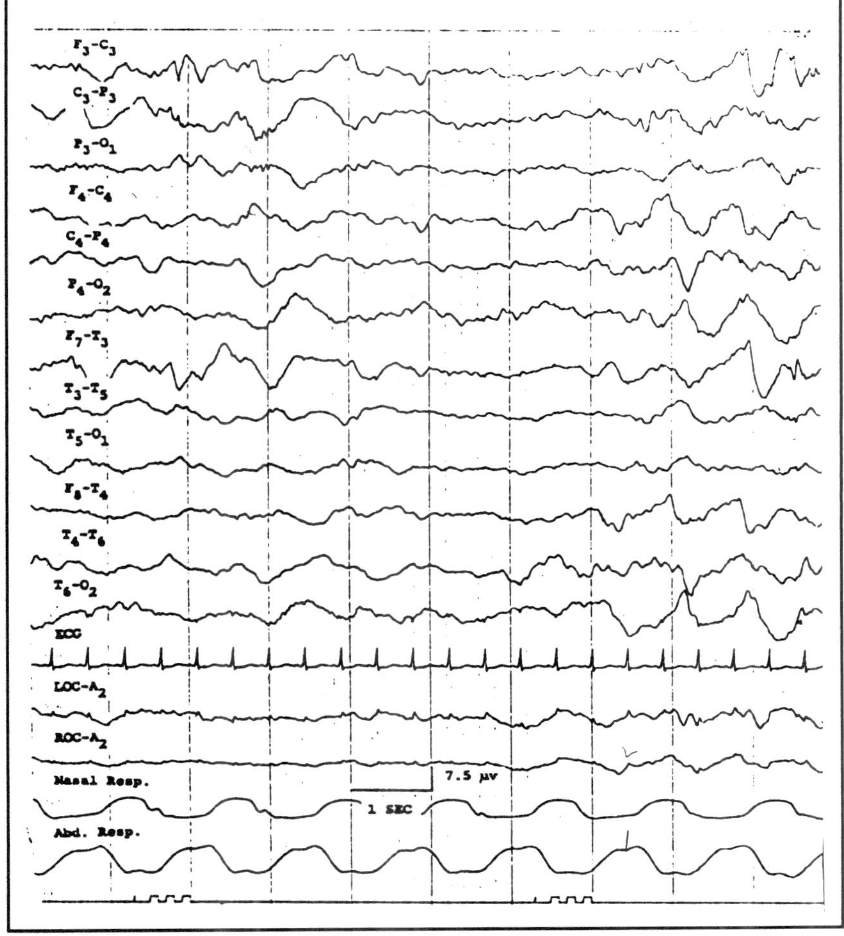

Fig. 3-1. Normal electroencephalogram in a full term (40 week conceptional age) infant demonstrating tracé alternans (alternating periods of high and low ampiltude activity characteristic of quiet sleep).

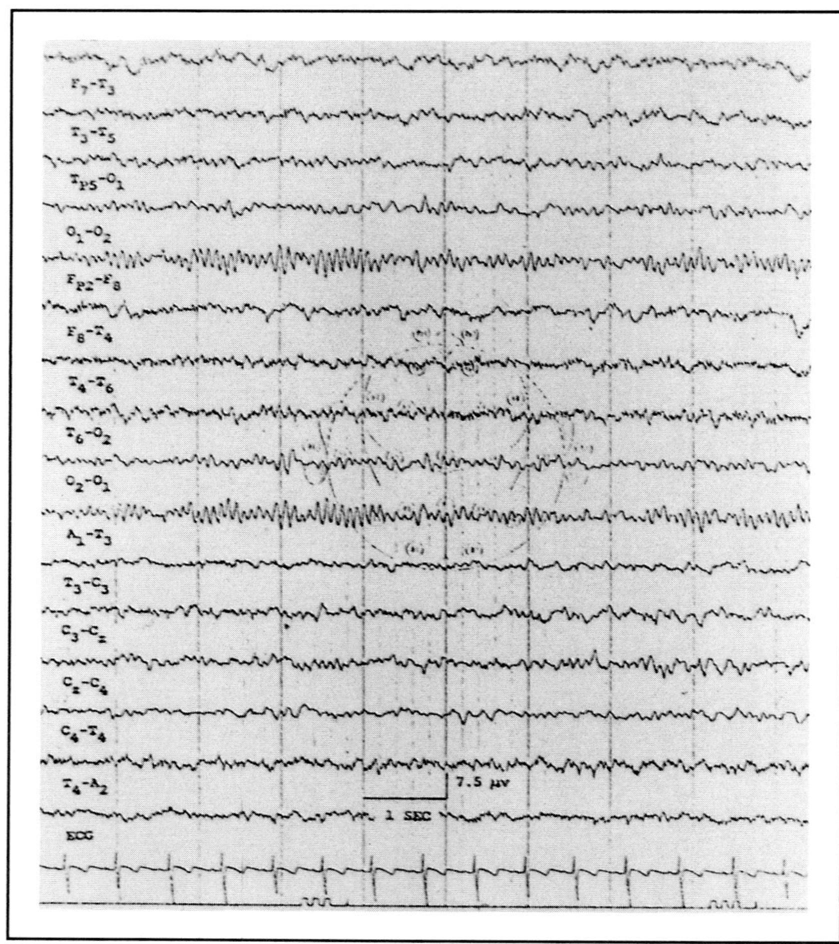

Fig. 3-2. Normal electroencephalogram in a six-year-old, demonstrating a normal 9-10 Hz frequency in the posterior quadrants (01-A1, 02-A2).

REM sleep. Owing to differences in the rates of normal cortical maturation, there may be considerable intersubject variation at a given age.

EEG Abnormalities

The distribution of the EEG abnormality may be focal (localized to a small area over one hemisphere), lateralized (extensively localized over one hemisphere), or generalized. The most common types of abnormalities are paroxysmal (spikes or sharp waves, Fig. 3-3), slowing in frequency (Fig. 3-4), attenuation in amplitude, lack of reactivity to stimuli, and immature patterns for age. Combined focal spike and slow complexes, and continuous focal polymorphous delta slow wave activity correlate significantly with underlying structural lesions.

Applications of the EEG

Investigation of patients with seizures. The test helps determine whether an epileptiform abnormality is present and if it is focal or generalized. Also, certain types of seizure disorders can be specifically diagnosed owing to their association with characteristic patterns such as the 3 Hz spike and wave discharges of absence seizures, the 2-2.5 Hz spike wave discharges seen with myoclonic-atonic or atypical absence seizures of early childhood (Fig. 3-5), and hypsarrythmia of infantile spasms (Fig. 3-6).

Detection of focal cerebral dysfunction that is secondary to inflammatory disorders such as herpes simplex encephalitis. This also includes traumatic or neoplastic disorders.

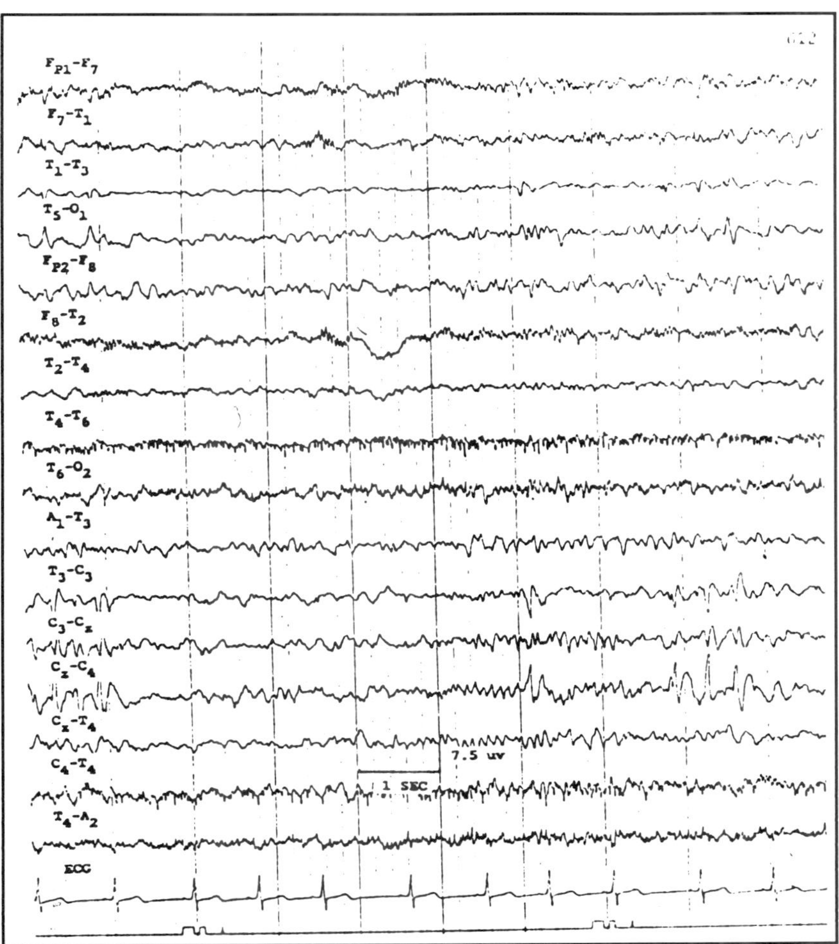

Fig. 3-3. Focal left central epileptiform discharges in a six-year-old with partial seizures.

Investigation of neurodegenerative disorders. Gray matter storage disorders (poliodystrophies) are associated with rather marked EEG abnormalities (multifocal spikes, spike and wave discharges) even early in the course of the illness. White matter storage diseases (leukodystrophies), on the other hand, induce mild to moderate generalized slowing. Periodic (suppression-burst) patterns are seen in patients with subacute sclerosing panencephalitis (SSPE), a slow virus central nervous system infection.

Evaluation of patients in coma. Preservation of reactivity to external stimuli and sleep spindle activity in the electroencephalogram of comatose patients generally indicates viability of thalamocortical projections and a favorable prognosis. In the absence of hypothermia or CNS depressant medications, periodic and isoelectric (flat) EEG patterns carry a poor prognosis for survival or the quality of survival.

Patients with metabolic, toxic, and inflammatory insults may have diffuse (occasionally focal) slow or paroxysmal abnormalities.

While in most instances coma is associated with slowing in the background EEG frequency, the alpha coma pattern (invariant activity in the 8-13 Hz range) suggests that recovery beyond a chronic vegetative state is unlikely. Periodic lateralized epileptiform discharges (PLEDs) may be seen in coma following herpes simplex encephalitis, and occasionally after head trauma or cerebral infarction.

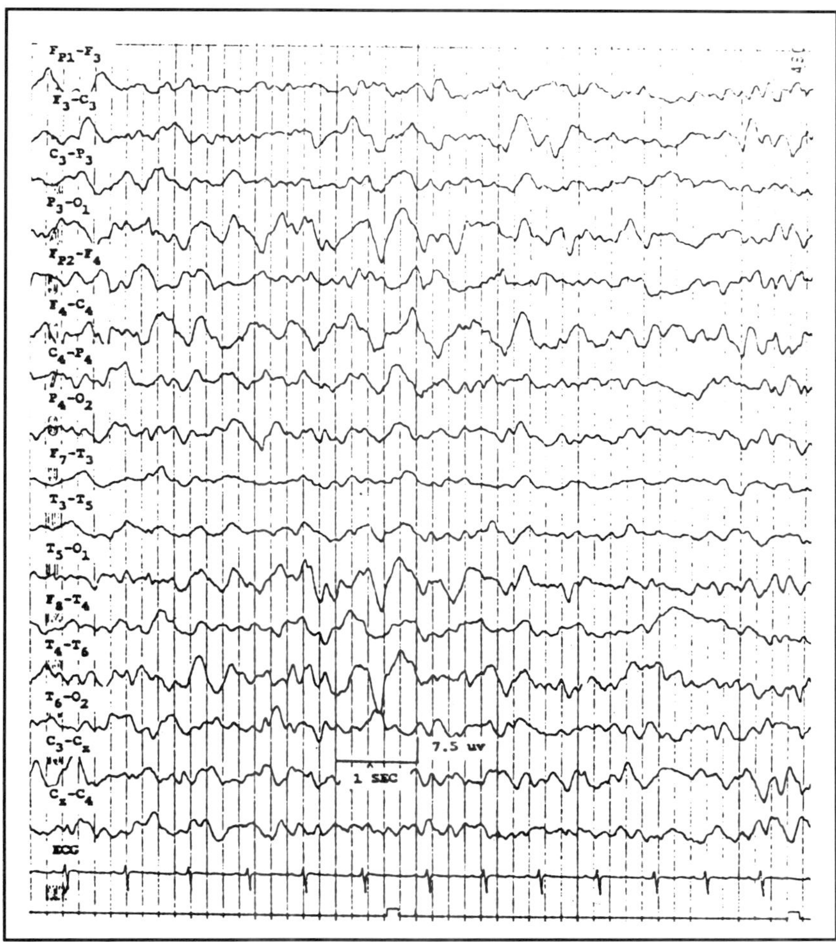

Fig. 3-4. Continuous generalized slow wave activity in the 2-5 Hz range in a six-year-old with metabolic encephalopathy. The slowing is slightly more prominent over the right hemisphere than over the left.

Determination of death. In the absence of hypothermia and sedative/hypnotic overdose, iso-electric EEG patterns on two successive studies 6 hours apart, combined with serial neurological examinations indicative of complete absence of brain function, are diagnostic of death. The protocol laid down by the American EEG Society for EEG technicians and electroencephalographers for this purpose must be rigidly adhered to.

Investigation of patients with headache. A brain imaging procedure (CT, radionuclide, or MRI scan) is far more informative than the EEG in evaluation of children with headaches. However, patients with migraine may display focal/generalized slowing, or paroxysmal changes due to alterations in cortical blood flow. The presence of paroxysmal abnormalities in migraine patients generally augurs a favorable prophylactic response to phenytoin.

EVOKED POTENTIALS

Evoked potential (response) studies are non-invasive neurophysiological procedures useful in assessing the function of the auditory, visual, and somatosensory pathways.

Technique

It has been observed that action potentials indicative of depolarization of the auditory nerve could be recorded from the human scalp. The

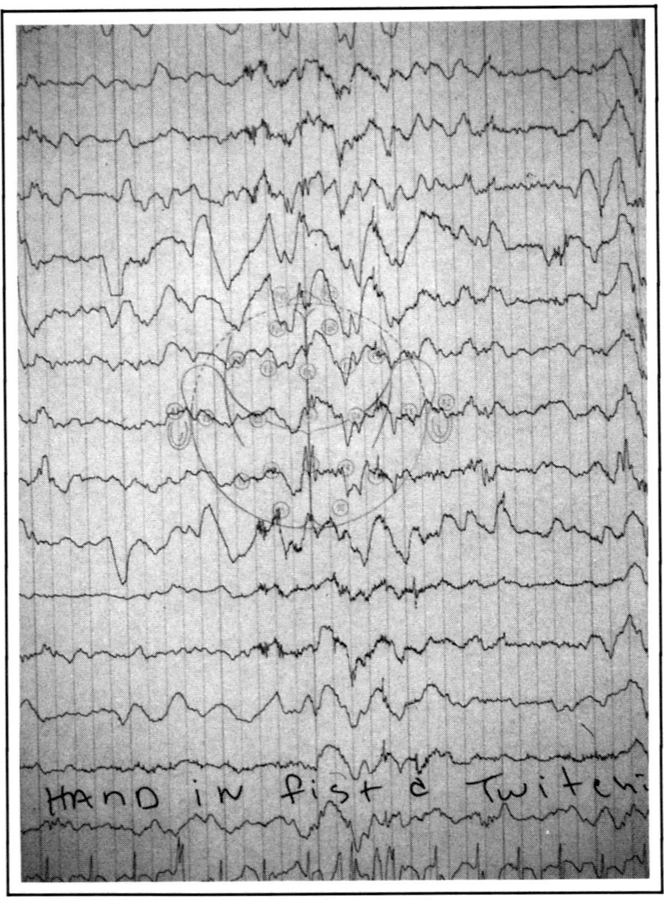

Fig. 3-5. Generalized 2-2.5 Hz spike and slow wave discharges in a 3 year old with atypical absence and generalized tonic-clonic seizures.

depolarization response, which is "time-locked" to an auditory stimulus, is termed the auditory evoked potential. It is normally masked by ongoing EEG activity. In evoked response studies, this "time-locked" signal is amplified up to 100,000 times, along with the background EEG activity. The computer then averages out (cancels) unwanted EEG activity, leaving only the amplified evoked response, which is composed of a series of positive-negative waves that indicate sequential depolarization of the auditory pathway in the auditory nerve and brainstem. Waveform latency and amplitude are altered in pathological states. The same basic principles that are used in studies of the auditory pathway are also valid in visual and somatosensory evoked potential studies.

BRAINSTEM AUDITORY EVOKED RESPONSE (BER)

The waveform complex is composed of a series of waves generated by sequential activation of the auditory nerve and brainstem auditory pathway. The stimulus (intensity of which can be varied) is usually a pure tone or click delivered into the ear using a headphone. Two trials of approximately 1500-2000 stimuli are averaged from each ear. The BER occurs within 8-10 seconds of stimulus delivery and is composed of five distinct wave forms. Initial studies had suggested that wave I, with a latency of approximately 1.5 m.sec., is generated in the auditory nerve, wave II in the cochlear nuclei (medulla), wave III in the superior olivary complex (pons), and waves IV

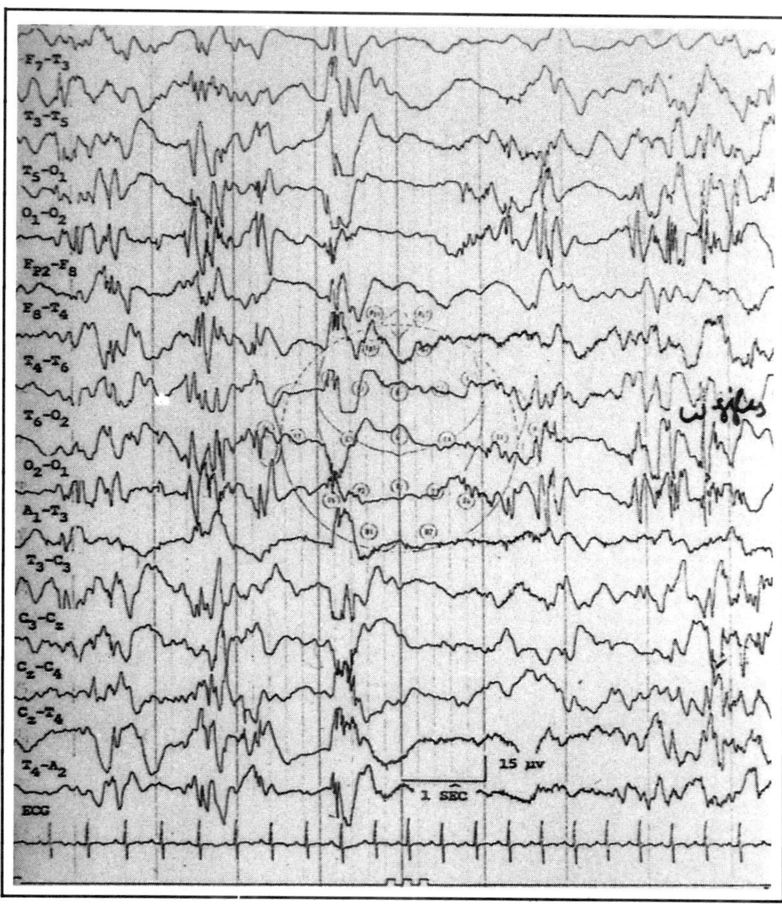

Fig. 3-6. Hypsarrythmia in a child with infantile spasms; the background activity is extremely disorganized, with superimposition of generalized spikes.

and V in the inferior colliculi (midbrain). It now appears that there may be more than one generator for some wave forms.

Application

Assessment of peripheral hearing in infants and young children. The advantage of the technique lies in the need for little or no patient cooperation. Absence of wave form I or the prolongation of its latency beyond normal is generally indicative of hearing impairment. The test is therefore quite valuable in follow-up of infants recovering from bacterial meningitis, or those who have received ototoxic medications (Fig. 3-7).

Detection and localization of brainstem lesions in neoplasms, or leukodystrophies. There may be prolongation in the interwave latencies (especially the V-I difference) or attenuation in the amplitude of individual wave forms.

VISUAL EVOKED POTENTIALS

Technique

The principles are similar to those for auditory evoked potential studies. The stimulus, however, is a flashing strobe light or an illuminated checkerboard pattern displayed on a television screen with rhythmic changes in contrast between adjacent squares. The recording electrodes are placed over the central and occipital head regions. Approximately 150-200 stimuli are averaged. The normal wave form complex consists of a negative deflection at approximately 75 msec and a positive wave at approximately 100 msec following the stimulus.

Application

The major value in children lies in the detection of disease of the anterior visual pathway,

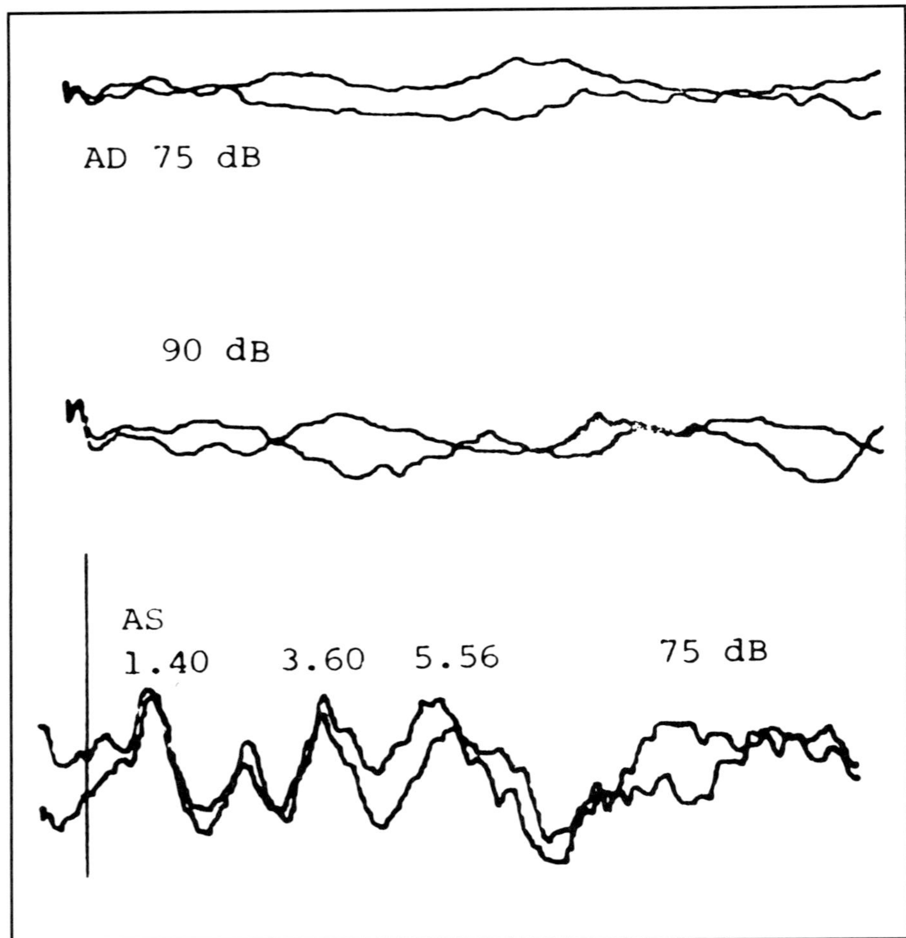

Fig. 3-7. Brainstem auditory evoked response in a child recovering from bacterial meningitis at 75 dB HL. No response is elicited with stimulation of the right ear; left ear stimulation evokes a response characterized by normal peripheral (wave I) latency but suppression in amplitude of waveform V, which is generated at the level of the inferior colliculi in the midbrain.

especially optic nerves and chiasm. Prolongation of latency and attenuation in amplitude may be seen in such instances.

SOMATOSENSORY EVOKED

RESPONSES (SER)

These are typically elicited by electrical stimulation of the peripheral nerve trunks and recording the evoked response over the limbs, spine, and scalp.

The measurement of peripheral sensory nerve conduction prior to obtaining the SER is a necessary prerequisite. Stimulation of the median nerve at the wrist elicits a positive-negative response at 15, 20, and 28 seconds following stimulation. The initial positive component is often difficult to obtain with stimulation of the lower extremities.

Neural pathways that need to be intact in order to be able to record somatosensory potentials over the scalp include the peripheral nerve trunk, dorsolateral columns, cuneate nucleus, thalamus, thalamocortical projections, and the cerebral cortex. Individuals with anteromedian cord lesions that produce weakness and loss of pain and temperature functions have normal somatosensory evoked potentials, whereas those with dorsolateral spinal cord diseases that produce loss of vibration and position sense may have altered somatosensory evoked potentials. Intraoperative monitoring of spinal evoked potentials during spine surgery may detect compression/ischemia of the dorsal cord during the procedure.

Application

1. In the diagnosis of traumatic and degenerative spinal cord diseases.

2. Monitoring of spinal cord function in the operating room in patients undergoing spinal surgery (e.g. for scoliosis)

3. In the diagnosis and monitoring of progression in degenerative diseases that affect the dorsolateral spinal cord, e.g., Friedreich's ataxia, ataxia-telangiectasia.

4. In coma; studies obtained upon admission in comatose patients indicate that bilaterally absent cortical SEP responses correlate with death or severe spastic quadriparesis. Unilaterally abnormal cortical SEPs are predictive of a residual hemiparesis. Patients with normal or mildly abnormal cortical SEPs have a favorable outcome.

5. In demyelinating diseases; SEPs may be more sensitive than BERs in the diagnosis leukodystrophies. Carriers of adrenoleukodystrophy may also demonstrate abnormalities.

6. Miscellaneous; SEP studies may also be useful in the evaluation of patients with perinatal brachial plexus lesions and suspected cervicomedullary junction compression.

MAGNETIC RESONANCE IMAGING

Nuclear magnetic resonance imaging (or Magnetic Resonance Imaging) has been used for obtaining images in humans since the mid 1970's. Improvements in technology have recently led to rapid advances in the field. The images in many ways provide greater detail than those obtained with a CT scanner. This, coupled with the inherent lack of exposure to ionizing radiation, has made Magnetic Resonance Imaging (MRI) the diagnostic procedure of choice for a variety of neurological disorders.

Technical Principles

A number of naturally occurring elements in the human body possess measurable magnetic properties. Hydrogen is at present the most commonly exploited magnetic element for MR imaging owing to its abundance in almost every organ of the body. In understanding the MR phenomenon, it is useful to consider groups of hydrogen protons as small magnets.

When the brain (and therefore these hydrogen molecules) are placed in an external magnetic field, the hydrogen molecules align themselves parallel to the magnetic field. They are at this point exposed to radiofrequency waves of characteristic frequencies and consequently begin to resonate at a specific frequency, hence the term "nuclear magnetic resonance." A variety of images from a sector of tissue can be obtained by varying the sequence of pulses emitted by the radiofrequency transmitter-receiver. The most commonly employed pulse sequences are called "spin-echo" and "inversion-recovery."[11]

After cessation of the radiowave pulse, the excited nuclei tend to return (relax) to their equlibrium state. While doing so, they emit radiowave pulses identical in frequency to the stimulation pulse. Because of differences in hydrogen concentration between various parts of the brain, the rate of decay of resonance will vary for different regions. The observed loss of signal strength is a product of two factors: 1) the loss of kinetic energy, as well as, 2) the influence of the decaying phase relationship. The time constant defining the former in MRI terminology is called T1 and the latter, T2. Computer-assisted frequency analysis and spatial localization techniques are then employed in order to construct a proton map or MR image of the brain. Absolute signal intensity increases with short T1 relaxation times, long T2 relaxation times, and increased proton (Hydrogen) density. Fatty tissues therefore display a high signal intensity on account of their high proton density and short relaxation time. Increasing the repetition time (TR) of the radiofrequency pulse and decreasing the echo delay will in most cases also enhance the signal intensity.

A routine MRI study generally includes multiple images of the same anatomical segment using T1 as well as T2 weighted images, with reconstruction in the saggital, coronal, and transverse planes. Advanced techniques now permit spatial resolution of up to 1-2 mm.

The appearance of a structure on the MRI scan is related to the intensity of the signal emitted by protons within the tissue. Areas providing a more intense signal appear white, whereas those

Table 3-1. Comparison of CT and MRI scanning techniques

	CT	MRI
Underlying principle	Exposure to ionizing radiation(X-ray)	No exposure to ionizing radiation; magnetic property of protons in tissues is exploited
Scanning time	30-45 minutes	30-120 minutes; similar to CT with newer systems
Gray-white matter differentiation	Fair	Excellent
Visualization of posterior fossa structures	Fair to good (bone artefact is a limitation)	Excellent
Visualization of mass lesions	Good	Excellent
Contrast agents	Iodinated compounds to enhance tissue density	Paramagnetic agents to enhance proton relaxation (gadopentetate dimeglumine)
Cost	Less expensive	More expensive

emitting a less intense signal appear gray or black. Signal intensity is a function of two sets of parameters: One is intrinsic to the tissue being examined (e.g., T1, T2, proton density, and blood flow). The other set is machine parameters, which can be regulated by the operator. Using the appropriate pulse sequence (inversion recovery or spin-echo), the white matter can be easily distinguished from the gray matter. As white matter has shorter T1 and T2 than gray matter, it appears brighter on the T1 weighted images and less bright on the T2 weighted images. Blood vessels with normal or high flow velocities normally appear dark, whereas areas with decreased flow velocity (e.g., distal to an occlusion) give a more intense signal. Fatty tissue, by virtue of its short T1, usually has high intensity.

Clinical Applications

MRI is extremely sensitive in the **detection of white matter lesions** such as leukodystrophies and multiple sclerosis plaques. In contrast to CT **scanning of the posterior fossa**, where bone artefact may obscure anatomical detail, MRI can outline such structures with great clarity. Consequently, Arnold Chiari malformations, cerebellar hypoplasia, and posterior fossa mass lesions are clearly visualized. Owing to the extreme sensitivity of MRI to increases in brain water concentration, **cerebral infarction** and **focal inflammatory disturbances** are detected in very early stages as areas of increased signal intensity on T2 weighted images. **Brain tumors** can also be well defined. Owing to differences in proton density between benign and malignant tumors, the ability to determine the nature of a tumor may also ultimately become possible.

The test also provides excellent information in the developing brain about the **degree of myelination**, which normally proceeds in a caudal to cranial sequence in the central nervous system. By one month of age, myelin should have appeared in the posterior limb of the internal capsule; by three months, in the optic radiations; by eight months, in the parietal and frontal white matter; and by one year, in the temporal white matter. By two years there should be additional branching in the subcortical white matter.

Limitations of MRI

The procedure is contraindicated in patients with cardiac pacemakers, those with ferromagnetic aneursymal clips, and mechanical life support devices owing to the potential for magnetization and displacement of such devices. The procedure is also relatively time consuming and therefore not ideal for use in neurological emergencies.

COMPUTERIZED AXIAL TOMOGRAPHY

Technical Principles

The CAT (or CT) technique scans the head in successive layers, using a narrow beam of x-rays, in such a manner that transmission of the x-ray photons across a particular layer of tissue is measured, and by means of a computer, used to construct a picture of the internal structure.

On the white-gray scale employed to depict organ density, the most dense structures (bone, fresh blood, and calcification) appear bright, whereas less dense tissues such as cerebrospinal fluid appear dark; gray and white matter densities are intermediate. Pathological lesions are associated with alteration in density. Tissue density may be artificially enhanced by the intravenous injection of iodinated contrast material. This is especially useful in delineating vascular structures such as normal blood vessels, arteriovenous malformations and the vascular rim of a neoplasm or abcess.

Major Clinical Applications

1. In the initial evaluation of a patient presenting with non-metabolic or non-toxic **coma**. In most instances, e.g., following head trauma, a non-contrast CAT scan may suffice. Brain edema (focal density attenuation, effacement of sulci), hydrocephalus, acute epidural, subdural, subarachnoid, or intracerebral hemorrhage can be readily recognized.

2. Evaluation of patients with suspected **neurological disorders of inflammatory** (e.g., brain abcess), **neoplastic or degenerative** (e.g., leukodystrophy) **etiology**. Chronic subdural hematomas and intracranial cystic lesions can also be clearly delineated.

3. Patients with chronic **headache** may require CAT scan examination to exclude an intracranial mass lesion. As a general rule, however, if a thorough neurological examination is normal, the CT scan is also normal in such instances. Acute onset of excruciating headache and neck stiffness may accompany subarachnoid or extradural hemorrhage. CT studies are diagnostic for these lesions.

4. Assessment of infants suspected of having **congenital malformations of the central nervous system**, such as agenesis of the corpus callosum, lissencephaly, and porencephaly.

5. Evaluation of patients with **seizures**. Approximately 65% of children with seizures who have focal slowing on the electroencephalogram and focal neurological findings on examination have underlying structural lesions. Disorders causing generalized seizures may also sometimes manifest CT abnormalities such as periventricular calcification in tuberous sclerosis. CT scanning of patients with seizures is indicated in all infants with seizures of a non-metabolic etiology when the seizure control is poor (to exclude a progressive neurological disorder), and in order to establish etiology of the seizures (e.g., for detection of periventricular calcific lesions in a child with suspected tuberous sclerosis).

CEREBRAL ANGIOGRAPHY

This procedure is of value in the detailed delineation of intracranial vascular lesions, e.g., arteriovenous malformations, aneurysms, vascular occlusion, and vasculitis. It requires the selective catheterization of carotid or vertebral arteries under fluoroscopy, using a transfemoral or transbrachial arterial approach. General anesthesia is usually required in children. Contrast material is injected and high speed X-ray films obtained in the anteroposterior, lateral, and oblique planes. A contrast CAT scan should be obtained prior to proceeding with cerebral angiography in order to be certain about the likelihood of a vascular lesion and to localize the area of interest.

With the transfemoral technique, the complication rate is approximately 3%, and consists of transient neurologic deficit in 1%, local hematomas in 1% and intramural or subintimal injection in 0.3%. The major complications (infarction, seizures) average about 0.5%. The incidence of complications in children under the age of 10 years is twice as high as compared to those above 10 years of age.

SKULL X-RAYS

With the increased availability of brain imaging procedures like CAT, MRI, and radionuclide scans, skull x-rays have become less important in investigation of intracranial pathology. However, they are still a valuable aid whenever the other imaging procedures are unavailable. They are also useful in the initial assessment of some patients with head trauma.

Techniques

The six standard projections routinely employed are the anteroposterior, straight posteroanterior, inclined posteroanterior, right and left lateral, and submentovertical. In addition, other special projections designed to demonstrate specific portions of the cranial anatomy can also be used.

Indications

Investigation of patients with head trauma. Especially when there is a clinical suspicion of a fracture involving the base of the skull or temporal regions and if it appears compound or depressed. Lateral views of the cervical spine should also be obtained simultaneously in order to exclude coexisting fracture/dislocation of the cervical spine.

Increased intracranial pressure and macrocephaly. In such instances there may be an increased craniofacial ratio (normally 3:1 to 4:1), splitting of sutures, thinning out of the calvarium, erosion of the anterior or posterior clinoid processes, and increased digital markings.

Detection of intracranial calcification. Congenital intrauterine infections and tuberous sclerosis. If the calcific lesion is not significantly dense, it may be inapparent on skull x-ray, but be visualized readily on a CAT scan.

Investigation of bone lesions. Osteomyelitis of the skull, dermoid cysts burrowing into the skull, osteomas, histiocytosis X, metastatic neoplasms, achondroplasia, basilar impression, and craniosynostosis.

ULTRASONOGRAPHY

Technique

Ultrasound studies of the head (neurosonograms) are primarily utilized in neonates and young infants with an open anterior fontanelle. Real-time B-mode scanning requires the application to the scalp surface of a 3.5 to 5.0 mHz transducer with a good internal focussing beam in order to obtain adequate sonic penetration and image quality. Images are obtained in the coronal and saggital planes. The ventricular system, corpus callosum, periventricular white matter, parenchymal hemorrhage or edema can be easily visualized (Fig. 3-8). The recent availability of the transcranial doppler equipment has now made it possible to non-invasively monitor cerebral blood flow in patients of all ages.

Advantages

1. The technique is non-invasive, and unlike CT scanning, there is no exposure to radiation.

2. The equipment is portable and serial studies can be obtained on sick newborns at the bedside.

3. Lower cost than CT scanning.

4. No artifacts from metallic clips and motion.

Indications

1. Prenatal diagnosis of some central nervous system lesions, e.g., hydrocephalus, anencephaly.

2. Monitoring of preterm infants for intraventricular hemorrhage at the bedside.

3. Serial studies are of value in following ventricular size in neonates with post-hemmorrhagic hydrocephalus.

4. Detection of parenchymal lesions, e.g., cerebral infarction, hemorrhage, agenesis of the corpus callosum.

5. In the determination of death; large cerebral vessels can be studied to determine absence of blood flow that is characteristic of cerebral death.

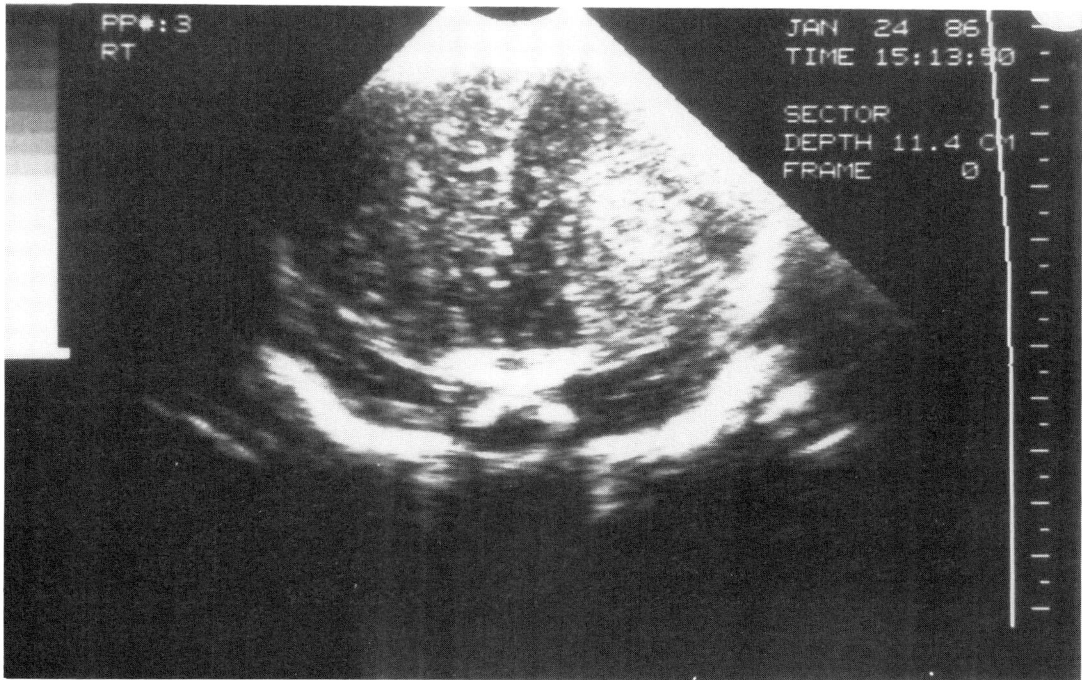

Fig. 3-8. Coronal image of a neurosonogram from a full term neonate, demonstrating an echodense lesion in the left hemisphere which was subsequently identified on CT scan as infarction.

RADIONUCLIDE BRAIN SCANNING

Technique

Prior to advent of the CT scan, the radionuclide scan was for many years the only available non-invansive brain imaging procedure. Also termed the "brain scan," the technique requires intravenous injection of the isotope 99M Technecium-pertechnetate. This tracer does not penetrate into the normal brain, but does cross areas with breakdown of the blood-brain barrier (e.g., abcess, infarction, inflammation, tumor) that are apparent as areas of increased uptake when pictures are taken in the antero-posterior and lateral planes using a gamma scintillation camera. A high rate of flow of the isotope may also be seen in areas with increased vascularity (e.g., arteriovenous malformation). Images are obtained immediately after isotope injection (flow study) and subsequently at periodic intervals, up to 4 hours after injection (static scan).

Indications

1. In the evaluation of supratentorial mass lesions (abcess or neoplasm). The diagnostic yield is comparable to that of the CT scan (85-90%).

2. Investigation of cerebrovascular disease; cerebral infarcts and arteriovenous malformations can be easily visualized.

3. In the determination of death; cerebral death is consistently associated with loss of cerebral blood flow ("no-flow phenomenon"). Portable equipment is used in the Intensive Care Unit for this purpose.

Limitations

1. The ventricular system, suprasellar region, and posterior fossa are poorly visualized.

2. The procedure is time consuming and may take up to 4 hours.

3. Cerebral lesions cannot be visualized in the absence of blood-brain barrier breakdown or alterations in regional blood flow.

New Developments

Radiolabelled amines which readily cross the blood-brain barrier and are taken up by the brain parenchyma for a period of time sufficient to allow tomographic imaging have now become available. Iodoamphetamine 123 is one such isotope. The

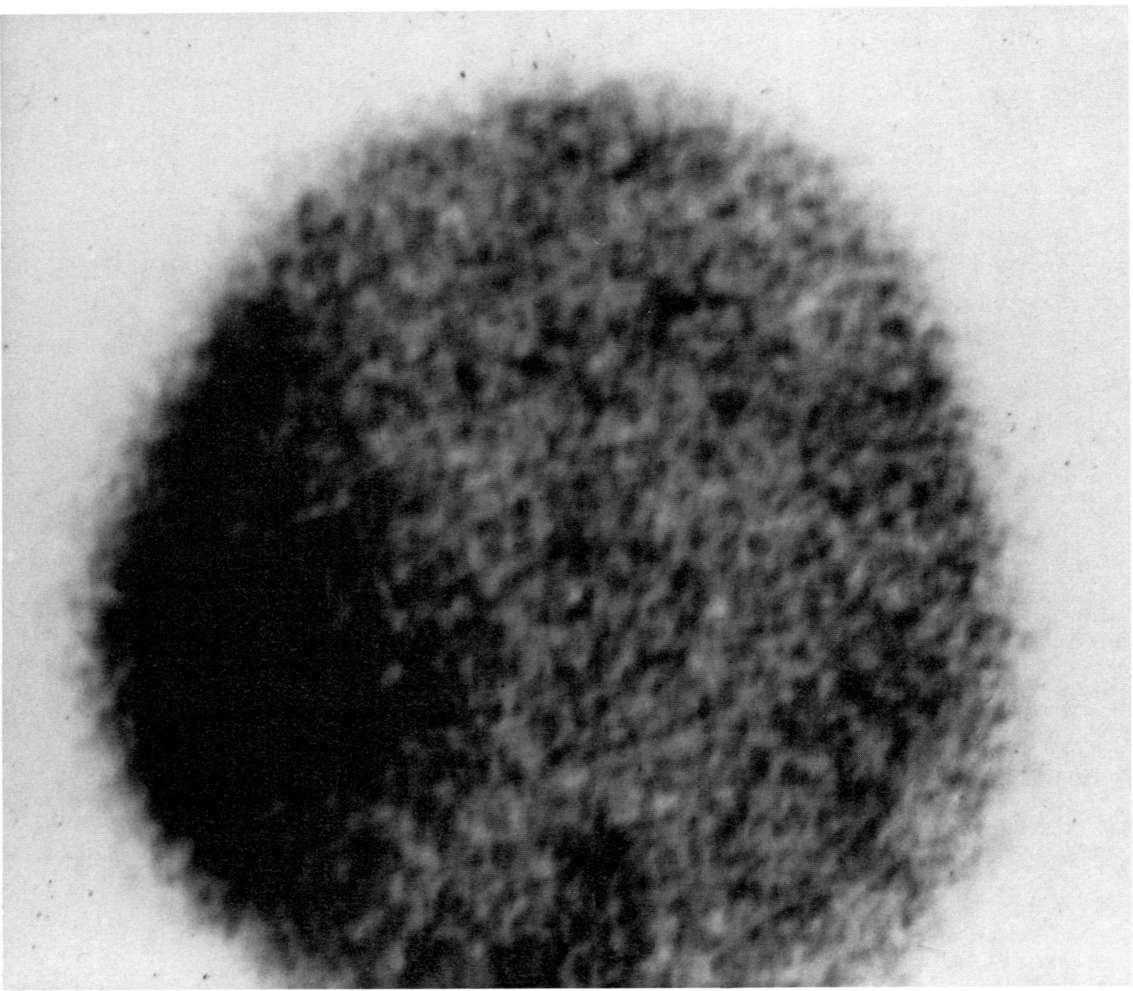

Fig. 3-9. Transverse view of Technitium-99 radionuclide brain scan in a patient with cerebral infarction, demonstrating increased uptake of the tracer in the temporo-parietal region due to local breakdown of the blood-brain barrier.

rate of blood flow and metabolism in a given area dictate the intensity of the signal emitted from that particular region (Single Photon Emission Tomography or SPECT scanning).

SUGGESTED READING

1. Mihorat TH. Subdural hematoma in infants and young children. In: Pediatric Neurosurgery. FA Davis Company, Philadelphia, 1978; 64-72.

2. Silverman D. The rationale and history of the 10-20 system of the International Federation. Amer J EEG Technol 3:17-22, 1963.

3. Remond A and Lairy GC, eds. The evolution of the EEG from birth to adulthood. In: Handbook of Electroencephalography and Clinical Neurophysiology, Vol 6B. Elsevier, Amsterdam, 1975.

4. Rowe JC, Holmes GL, Hafford J, Baboval D, Robinson S, Philips A, Rosenkrantz T and Raye J. Prognostic value of the electroencephalogram in term and preterm infants following neonatal seizures. EEG and Clin Neurophysiol 60:183-196, 1985.

5. Starr A. Sensory evoked potentials in clinical disorders of the nervous system. Ann Rev Neurosci 1:103-127, 1978.

6. Stockard JE, Stockard JJ, Westmoreland BF and Corfits JL. Brainstem auditory evoked responses. Normal variation as a function of stimulus and subject characteristics. Arch. Neurol. 36:823-831, 1979.

7. Celesia GG. Visual evoked potentials in neurologic disorders. Am J EEG Technol 18:47-59, 1978.

8. Chiappa KH. Evoked Potentials in Clinical Medicine. Raven Press, New York, 1983.

9. Brasch RC. Magnetic resonance imaging in pediatric practice. Pediatric Annals 15(5):386-393, 1986.

10. Gooding CA, Brasch RC and Lattemand DP. et al. Nuclear magnetic resonance imaging of the brain in children. J Pediatr 104:509-515, 1984.

11. Budinger TF and Lauterbur PC. Nuclear magnetic resonance technology for medical studies. Science 226:288-298, 1984.

12. Ambrose J. Computerized transverse axial scanning (tomography): Part 2. Clinical application. Brit J Radiol 46(552):1023-1047, 1973.

13. Abrams HL and McNeil BJ. Medical implications of computed tomography (CAT scanning). Parts I and II. N Engl J Med 298(5):255-260, 298(6):310-317, 1978.

14. Harwood-Nash DC and Fitz CR, eds. Neuroradiology in infants and children, Vols I and II. CV Mosby, St. Louis, 1976.

15. Babcock DS and Han BK. The accuracy of high resolution, real-time ultrasonography of the head in infancy. Radiology 139:665-676, 1981.

16. Elliot D. Ultrasonography of the neonatal brain. In: Sarnat HB, ed. Topics in Neonatal Neurology. Grune and Stratton, Orlando, 1984; 223-256.

17. Holman BL, Hill TC, Lee RGL, Zimmerman RE, Moore SC and Royal HD. Brain imaging with radio-labelled amines. In: Freman LM and Weissmann HS, eds. Nuclear Medicine Annual 1983. Raven Press, New York, 1983.

CHAPTER IV

CENTRAL NERVOUS SYSTEM INFECTIONS

Viral Infections

Bacterial Meningitis

Brain Abscess

Tuberculous Meningitis

Cryptococcal Meningitis

CSF Profile in Central Nervous System Infections

VIRAL INFECTIONS

Introduction

The spectrum of neurological disorders caused by viruses is broad, ranging from those disorders evolving over days to others that evolve over months or years. While certain viruses have a predilection for affecting only specific neural elements (e.g., polio virus affecting the anterior horn cells in the spinal cord and brain stem), other viruses cause wide-spread involvement of the nervous system (measles). Viruses are obligate intracellular agents. They are composed of a central core of nucleic acid (DNA and RNA) and are surrounded by a protein coat. They utilize host cell nucleic acids for their own propagation and lack energy-generating or biosynthetic mechanisms.

The route of invasion of the nervous system may be hematogenous (enteroviruses) or via direct extension from adjacent infected structures (rabies along peripheral nerves). Once the agent has gained access to the central nervous system, additional viral replication soon follows, with spread to previously uninfected cells. The clinical picture produced by some viral agents is benign and self-limiting, and in others, it is relentlessly progressive.

CLASSIFICATION

Congenital intrauterine infections

Rubella
Cytomegalovirus
Herpes simplex

Infections in immunologically competent hosts

ECHO, Coxsackie, and polio (aseptic meningitis/ meningoencephalitis/anterior horn cell disease) — Picornaviruses

St. Louis, California, Eastern, and Western equine encephalitis, yellow fever, Japanese B (acute encephalitis) — Togaviruses

Herpes simplex
Measles
Varicella
Rabies
Acute encephalitis

Mumps (aseptic meningitis/meningoencephalitis)
Lymphocytic choriomeningitis (aseptic meningitis)

Infections in immunologically compromised hosts

SV-40 virus (progressive multifocal leukoencephalopathy)
Subacute measles encephalitis
Herpes zoster
Reactivation of latent poliomyelitis
Subacute enterovirus and cytomegalovirus encephalitis

Slow virus infections

    Conventional (visually indentifiable) agents
      Progressive multifocal leukoencephalitis
      Progressive rubella panencephalitis
      Subacute sclerosing panencephalitis

    Unconventional (visually non-identifiable) agents
      Scrapie
      Transmissible mink encephalopathy
      Kuru
      Jacob-Creutzfeldt disease

    Unconventional (retrovirus)
      Acquired Immune Deficiency Syndrome (AIDS)

ACUTE VIRAL MENINGITIS

Also termed aseptic meningitis, this disorder is most frequently caused by enterovirus, adenovirus, mumps, or the lymphocytic choriomeningitis virus. The inflammatory process is usually restricted to the leptomeninges and is benign, resolving spontaneously within 3-5 days.

The principal clinical features are abrupt onset of fever, intense occipital and nuchal pain, vomiting, and photophobia. Neck stiffness and a Kernig's sign may be present. The mental status is usually normal and no other abnormalities are noted upon neurological examination.

The diagnosis can be readily confirmed by examination of the CSF, which discloses pleocytosis (WBC count of over 5/cu mm), mild to moderate increase in protein (generally between 40 and 100 mg/dl), normal glucose content, and negative bacterial cultures.

ACUTE VIRAL MENINGOENCEPHALITIS

Involvement of the brain along with the meninges in the viral inflammatory process is termed meningoencephalitis. Enteroviruses, adenoviruses, measles, varicella, herpes simplex, and arboviruses are some common causative agents.

Presence of altered sensorium (confusion/obtundation/coma), seizures, abnormalities in muscle tone, posture, movement, or tendon reflexes, together with an abnormal electroencephalogram distinguish viral meningoencephalitis from viral meningitis. The illness begins to resolve spontaneously after 7 to 14 days. Recovery may be gradual, continuing for a period of up to 2 years after onset. The outcome in infants of less than 12 months of age with meningoencephalitis is not as favorable as that in older children.

Herpes simplex encephalitis deserves special attention because:

a. It is the most common sporadic viral meningoencephalitis, occurring with a frequency of 1 in 200,000 individuals.

b. There is a focal inflammatory disturbance with edema, generally localized to one or both temporal lobes.

c. Untreated, the mortality is high, approaching 70%. With early institution of antiviral therapy, however, the mortality can be brought down to 30-40%. Approximately 50% of the survivors are left with major neurologic sequale.

d. At this point in time it appears to be the only acute viral encephalitis for which a specific treatment is available.

Management Approach in Acute Meningoencephalitis

1. Obtain a lumbar puncture to determine the presence of pleocytosis (cell count of more than 5/cubic mm). While a combination of neutrophils and lymphocytes is seen initially, by the end of the first week the cellular response becomes mainly lymphocytic. The CSF protein is usually elevated to the 50 to 200 mg/dl range, while glucose remains normal. In patients with suspected herpes simplex virus (HSV) encephalitis, a herpes antibody index of more than 1.9 is indicative of the diagnosis. The antibody index =

$$\frac{\text{CSF herpes antibodies titre/serum herpes antibody titre}}{\text{CSF albumin/serum albumin}}$$

If increased intracranial pressure is suspected prior to carrying out the lumbar puncture, a bolus of intravenous mannitol (0.25-1.0 gm/kg) may decrease the risk of brain herniation. The fluid should also be saved for viral titres (when necessary).

2. Obtain an electroencephalogram at the earliest; the presence of periodic lateralized epileptiform discharges (PLEDs) on the EEG, especially when localized to the temporal regions, is highly suggestive of herpes simplex encephalitis. In other forms of viral encephalitis, generalized or focal slow wave abnormality or multifocal spikes are more likely to be seen.

3. When focal abnormalities are present on neurological examination and the EEG demonstrates PLEDs, there is a strong likelihood of herpes simplex encephalitis. A radionuclide brain scan should be obtained in this situation in order to detect increased uptake in the temporal regions owing to local breakdown of the blood-brain barrier. CT evidence of a mass effect in the temporal lobe is further evidence in support of herpes simplex encephalitis. The magnetic resonance (MR) scan is superior to both CT and radionuclide scan in detecting early inflammatory changes.

4. If focal cerebral dysfunction is observed clinically in a patient with encephalitis and confirmed by EEG/CT scan/radionuclide scan, a brain biopsy may be obtained to confirm the diagnosis of herpes simplex encephalitis. Brain biopsy should be considered when the patient with suspected herpes encephalitis is not responding favorably to antiviral therapy (see below). The biopsy should be taken from the region suspected to be abnormal on the basis of EEG and CT scan/radionuclide scan. The tissue is sent for viral cultures, histopathology, electron microscopy, and immunofloresence studies.

5. Regardless of whether or not a cortical biopsy is obtained, if a clinical suspicion of herpes encephalitis is entertained, antiviral therapy should be commenced immediately after the EEG and CT/MR/radionuclide scan have been obtained. Acyclovir in a dose of 10 mg/kg/dose at 8 hourly intervals for 10 days is the drug of choice and is superior to adenine arabinoside (ARA-A). The patient should be monitored closely for hepatic and renal dysfunction with Acyclovir use. If cortical biopsy confirms the diagnosis of herpes encephalitis, treatment should be continued for the full 10 day course. If cortical biopsy results are negative for herpes encephalitis, the Acyclovir treatment may be discontinued. When a biopsy is not obtained, treatment should be continued until serological studies have failed to disclose a rising titre for herpes encephalitis or an alternative diagnosis has been established (usually in 5-6 days).

6. Supportive care in all patients with acute encephalitis includes treatment of seizures, monitoring fluid and electrolyte balance for inappropriate secretion of antidiuretic hormone, blood gases, and cardiopulmonary function. Monitoring intracranial pressure with epidural, subarachnoid, or intraventricular devices may be required in comatose patients who are deteriorating clinically; judicious use of intravenous mannitol (0.5-1.0 gm/kg bolus) is needed in patients with increased intracranial pressure .

Differential Diagnosis of Acute Viral Encephalitis

Partially treated bacterial meningitis. The CSF picture in this illness demonstrates pleocytosis, protein elevation, and normal or decreased glucose content. Bacterial antigen can be detected in urine or CSF using countercurrent immunoelectrophoresis, latex particle fixation, or enzyme-linked immunoabsorbent studies.

Fungal meningitis. Antigen from specific fungal agents (e.g., cryptococcus) can be readily detected in the CSF. Serial cerebrospinal fluid assays for fungal antigen and cultures enhance the diagnostic yield. Such infections generally occur in immunologically compromised individuals.

Brain abcess. A ring-shaped area of contrast enhancement is usually seen in the involved area on the CT scan. The EEG discloses a slow wave focus, and in contrast to herpes simplex encephalitis, PLEDs are rarely seen.

ACUTE ANTERIOR POLIOMYELITIS

Polio is an enterovirus with three distinct serotypes which may result in a syndrome of acute, flaccid weakness. Poliomyelitis is endemic in tropical countries and occurs in summer epidemics in the temperate regions. The virus is usually acquired via the oropharyngeal route, and proliferates in the gastrointestinal tract. Involvement of the central nervous system occurs following a period of viremia. The neurological disorder specifically involves the meninges and motor neurons in the spinal cord and brainstem; on occasions the reticular formation, hypothalamus, and cortical neurons of the precentral gyrus may also be affected. ECHO and Coxsackie viruses have been reported to also cause a clinically identical illness.

The clinical picture can be classified into the non-paralytic and paralytic forms. In the former, manifestations of aseptic meningitis predominate, with presence of fever, headache, neck stiffness, and a Kernig's sign. In the paralytic illness, the above clinical manifestations are followed within 3-5 days by intense muscular pain, patchy and asymmetric muscle paralysis. The weakness may be restricted to the limbs and trunk or extend to involve the bulbar musculature, resulting in respiratory insufficiency. Consciousness and sensory functions are preserved. Tendon reflexes are impaired in the late stages. Recovery from the paralytic illness commences after 2-3 weeks, and in the non-paralytic within a week. However, motor function returns to normal only rarely after the paralytic illness, with the prognosis in infants less than 12 months of age being particularly poor.

Diagnosis

The cerebrospinal fluid discloses a lymphocytic pleocytosis, with presence of 50-250 WBC/cu mm, mild to moderate protein elevation, normal glucose and bacterial cultures. Polio virus may be isolated from the CSF or rectal swab cultures. Convalescent titres may demonstrate a four-fold increase relative to the acute titres.

Poliomyelitis should be distinguished from acute infectious polyneuritis (Guillian-Barré syndrome), in which the CSF cell count is usually lower (always less than 50 WBC/cu mm and generally less than 12/c.m). Nerve conduction studies performed during the acute illness in the latter may show a slowing of conduction velocity (especially proximally), whereas nerve conduction velocity is normal in poliomyelitis.

Management

In the nonparalytic form, only analgesics and bedrest are indicated. In the acute phase of the paralytic illness, care of the skin, monitoring and support of respiratory function, and provision of parenteral alimentation for dysphagia are called for. In the convalescent phase of the paralytic illness, physical therapy and orthopedic consultation for management of joint abnormalities secondary to the weakness and hypotonia are required.

Prevention

The polyvalent oral (Sabin) and parenteral (Salk) vaccines, when administered according to standard immunization protocols through infancy and early childhood, are able to effectively prevent poliomyelitis and the consequent disabling long-term sequale.

CYTOMEGALOVIRUS ENCEPHALITIS

This DNA virus is generally found ubiquitously in the saliva and urine. It induces a characteristic change in infected cells—cellular enlargement and intranuclear inclusion bodies. The virus is of no major pathologic significance in healthy adults. In immunologically compromised individuals and the fetus, however, the infection is associated with serious neurological disturbances.

The clinical picture in immunologically impaired children and adults is one of gradual deterioration of intellectual function, lethargy, and seizures.

Congenital CMV infection usually develops after transplacental passage of the virus into the fetus. The consequences of this multisystem illness depend to some extent on the gestational age of the fetus at the time of acquisition of the infection; onset in early gestation is associated with the more serious sequale. As a general rule, the developmental process most active at time of infection will be the most impaired. The affected neonate is usually small for gestational age. Microcephaly, seizures, spasticity, nerve deafness, chorioretinitis, porencephaly or hydranencephaly may also result. Periventricular calcification is seen upon CT or skull x-ray examination. Hepatosplenomegaly, jaundice, thrombocytopenia, and petechial hemorrhages also frequently accompany the neurologic syndrome in the neonate. Older immunologically compromised patients with cytomegalovirus may demonstrate a gradually evolving dementia.

Diagnosis

The diagnosis can be established by obtaining IgM specific serological titres on the infant and the mother. In infected infants, the titre is usually higher than in the mother and may even rise over time. Cerebrospinal fluid and urine cultures for the virus may be positive, and in some instances, virus shedding may continue for months. Auditory evoked potentials and behavioral audiometry help diagnose hearing deficits.

Treatment

No treatment is available for cytomegalovirus infections, and the management is essentially symptomatic.

CONGENITAL RUBELLA

Infection by the rubella virus is innocuous to the pregnant mother, but transplacental passage of the virus causes a major illness in the fetus, with involvement of multiple organs. The risk of adverse fetal outcome when fetal infection has occurred prior to the 13th week of pregnancy exceeds 50%. The consequences are less serious if the infection is acquired later in the course of pregnancy.

The most common clinical manifestations are microcephaly, seizures, mental retardation, cataracts, chorioretinitis, nerve deafness, and spastic tetraparesis. Congenital heart defects which frequently accompany the neurological syndrome include pulmonary stenosis and septal defects.

The diagnosis can be confirmed by presence of an elevated and rising antibody titre against rubella on serial serum specimens. As in the case of cytomegalovirus, no specific treatment is available, and only symptomatic management is possible. Women of child-bearing age who are not pregnant should ensure that they have an adequate protective antibody titre against rubella, and if not, obtain active immunization at a time when they are definitely not pregnant.

RABIES

This is primarily a viral infection of animals. Humans are affected following an animal bite. The disease is prevalent worldwide.

Following a bite by a rabid animal, the virus gains entry into the central nervous system along the perineural spaces. The incubation period varies from 6 days to 6 months. The closer the bite is located to the head, the shorter the incubation period. A fulminant, generalized inflammation develops, with maximum change in the forebrain, limbic system, medulla oblongata, cerebellum, cranial nerve nuclei, and spinal ganglia. Eosinophilic intracytoplasmic inclusions (Negri bodies) may be seen upon histological examination.

The initial clinical manifestation is paresthesia at the site of the bite. It is followed by restlessnes, fever, headache, exaggerated sensitivity to sound and light, auditory and visual hallucinations. The most remarkable symptom, hydrophobia, is characterized by pharyngeal and laryngeal muscle spasm at the very sight of water. Respiratory muscle dysfunction and seizures may also occur. Although most cases are fatal, some possibility of survival exists with intensive nursing care.

Prevention of Rabies

1. If the animal can be observed for a period of 10 days following the human bite and does not die, it is highly unlikely that it is rabid. In this case, no prophylaxis is necessary for the human.

2. If the animal dies within 10 days or was wild and therefore unobservable, passive immunization with hyperimmune antirabies serum (40 I.U./kg) is recommended. Half the dose should be administered around the site of the bite and the remainder by the intramuscular route. This is followed by active immunization, preferably with the human diploid-cell vaccine, which is administered on days 0, 3, 7, 14 and 28, with booster doses 10 and 20 days later. It is recommended that all these injections be administered in the deltoid muscle. Immunization schedules may vary when the human diploid-cell vaccine is unavailable.

3. In all bites, thorough local cleaning with soap and water followed by application of a quarternary amine compound solution and a tetanus toxoid booster are also recommended.

SUBACUTE SCLEROSING PANENCEPHALITIS

Slow virus infections are characterized by a latent period of months to years between invasion of the nervous system by the agent and the actual onset of clinical manifestations. Once the disease becomes clinically apparent, however, it may progress rapidly and relentlessly.

Subacute sclerosing panencephalitis (SSPE) is the most common slow viral infection in children. It is caused by an atypical strain of measles virus. The incubation period varies from 1-6 years. The initial manifestations are relatively subtle, with alteration in behavior, decline in academic performance at school, poor concentration and memory loss. With time, myoclonic and generalized tonic-clonic seizures, ataxia, optic atrophy, and spasticity also develop. Death usually results from respiratory complications. The diagnosis can be established on the basis of elevated serum and cerebrospinal fluid measles titres and an elevated CSF gamma globulin concentration. The EEG demonstrates a generalized periodic (suppression burst) pattern.

No specific treatment is available.

ACQUIRED IMMUNE DEFICIENCY SYNDROME (AIDS)

Epidemiology

First described in 1981, this disorder is reaching near epidemic proportions worldwide. It is estimated that between 1 to 2 million people in the United States are presently infected with the viral agent. The three year mortality is close to 90%. Risk factors for developing AIDS in adults and adolescents include homosexuality, intravenous drug abuse, and hemophilia. In younger children, almost all cases are either congenital (secondary to birth to a mother with AIDS) or following receipt of infected blood or blood products.

Pathogenesis

AIDS is caused by the Human Immunodeficiency Virus (HIV), which is a unique RNA retrovirus with a specific predilection for attacking the T4+ helper/inducer lymphocytes in the body. After specific binding to these target cells, HIV enters the cell and becomes uncoated. The viral genomic RNA is then transcribed into DNA by a reverse transcriptase. This genomic DNA is subsequently incorporated into the host cell DNA, which is used for additional viral protein and genomic RNA synthesis. With additional HIV replication, the host T4+ cell eventually dies. The T4+ cell is a central figure in the immune response and its loss leads to a multitude of immunological deficits and consequent life threatening opportunistic infections.

Clinical Features

Approximately 60% of patients with AIDS have neurological symptoms. In about 10%, neurologic manifestations are the sole feature upon initial presentation. Between 80-90% of patients demonstrate neuropathological abnormalities. Clinical manifestations may result from actual invasion of the central nervous system by the HIV agent or consequent to opportunistic infections. The AIDS-Dementia complex is the most characteristic disorder and follows direct viral CNS involvement. It is characterized by progressive memory loss, inability to concentrate, and behavioral change that progress to a full-blown dementia within a year. CT, MRI, and spinal fluid findings are non-specific. Examination of the brain reveals central and cortical atrophy, gliosis and neuronal loss in the gray and white matter, demyelination, and presence of multinucleated giant cells.

The various neurological complications of AIDS are:

  I. Primary viral
     aseptic meningitis
     AIDS-Dementia complex
     vacuolar myelopathy
     congenital AIDS syndrome

  II. Opportunistic, viral
     herpes simplex encephalitis
     herpes varicella zoster meningoencephalitis
     cytomegalovirus encephalitis
     progressive multifocal leukoencephalopathy

  III. Opportunistic, non viral
     toxoplasmosis
     cryptococcal meningitis
     candidiasis
     syphilis
     atypical mycobacterial infections

  IV. Neoplastic
     primary CNS lymphoma
     systemic lymphoma metastatic to CNS
     Kaposi's sarcoma metastatic to CNS

  V. Cerebrovascular
     infarction
     hemorrhage

  VI. Peripheral Neuropathy
     distal symmetric polyneuropathy
     chronic inflammatory demyelinating neuropathy

Investigations

CT and MRI studies are used for detecting central nervous system involvement, localizing lesions for possible brain biopsy, and in follow-up to determine response to treatment of certain opportunistic infections. MRI studies appear to be more sensitive in detecting central nervous system involvement in AIDS. The AIDS dementia complex is generally associated with widespread cortical and white matter atrophy. Children with this complication may also manifest calcification in the region of the basal ganglia. Toxoplasmosis is the most common focal central nervous system lesion, demonstrating ring-shaped or nodular areas of contrast enhancement on CT scan.

The cerebrospinal fluid shows pleocytosis with normal to mildly elevated protein concentrations in patients developing aseptic meningitis. Moderate lowering of the CSF glucose, along with the pleocytosis and presence of cryptococcal antigen, suggests cryptococcal meningitis. A VDRL test may also be necessary in the adult.

Nerve conduction studies, sural nerve biopsy, and serum assay for circulating IgG antibodies to peripheral nerve tissue are recommended in those with distal muscle weakness, sensory deficit, or hyporeflexia.

Management

This consists mainly of treatment of certain opportunistic CNS infections as and when they develop (e.g., cryptococcosis, toxoplasmosis, syphilis), as well as providing emotional support to the child and family.

BACTERIAL MENINGITIS

Bacterial meningitis requires prompt diagnosis and initiation of appropriate therapy if associated mortality and morbidity are to be limited. The most common causative organisms are shown in Table 4-1.

Pathophysiology

The bacteria gain access to the central nervous system via the hematogenous route or by direct spread from adjacent infected structures (e.g.,

nasopharynx). The inflammatory process involves the leptomeninges extensively, with formation of purulent exudate and a polymorphnuclear cellular response. There is also inflammation of the underlying cerebral cortex. Involvement of the superficial cortical veins by the inflammatory process can lead to vascular thrombosis and cerebral infarction. Thrombosis of the vasa nervora and organization of the perineural fibrinous-purulent exudate can lead to cranial nerve paralysis. The 8th, 7th, 6th, and 3rd nerves are most frequently involved. Organization of the exudate in the superficial subarachnoid spaces may interfere with the normal transit and absorption of CSF, thereby leading to communicating hydrocephalus.

Table 4-1. Most common causative organisms in bacterial meningitis

Age	Causative Organism
Birth to age 2 weeks	Group B streptcoccus Escherichia coli Listeria monocytogenes Group D streptococcus Staphylococcus aureus
2 weeks to 2 months	Group B streptococcus Escherichia coli Hemophilus influenza Streptococcus pneumonia
Older infants and young children	Hemophilus influenza Niesseria meningitidis Streptococcus pneumonia
In the presence of an intracranial device (e.g., Ventriculo-peritoneal shunt)	Streptococcus viridans Coagulase negative staphylococcus

Clinical Features

In the neonate, fulminant septicemia and pneumonitis generally accompany meningitis. The infection may be acquired during the process of birth from aspiration of infected amniotic fluid, or nosocomially during the first two weeks after birth. Lethargy, poor feeding, respiratory distress, shock, and disseminated intravascular coagulation may be present. Signs of meningeal irritation (neck stiffness and a positive Kernig's sign) are rarely seen. Ventriculitis is a special feature of gram negative neonatal meningitis, and is frequently responsible for delay in resolution. It can be recognised by the presence of contrast enhancement of the ependymal lining of the ventricles on CT scan.

Signs and meningeal irritation may likewise be absent in young infants. Cerebral edema is a frequent accompaniment. Resistance of Haemophilus influenza to ampicillin has been noted in 20-30% of isolates in the United States.

Fulminant meningococcemia may be associated with generalized petechial, subcutaneous hemorrhage. A gram stain of scrapings of the skin lesions may disclose the organisms.

Inappropriate secretion of antidiuretic hormone occurs in about 80% of children with meningitis within the first 48-72 hours.

While seizures occuring at onset of the illness may be benign, those developing towards the end of the first week of illness generally signify infarction from venous thrombosis.

Excessive cranial enlargement and increased cranial transillumination are indicative of communicating hydrocephalus or subdural effusion, with the latter most frequently accompanying H. influenza meningitis.

The overall incidence of major sequlae following childhood meningitis is between 25-30%. They include hemiparesis, seizures, mental retardation, hydrocephalus, cranial neuropathies (most commonly VIII cranial nerve), and cortical blindness. The mortality has remained relatively constant over the past two decades and is about 5% for infections caused by *N. meningitides*, 10% for *H. influenzae* and 25% for *Streptococcus pneumoniae*.

Diagnosis

A high clinical index of suspicion of bacterial meningitis must be maintained in all instances of unexplained and abrupt onset of fever, lethargy, vomiting, and seizures in infancy and childhood.

The only definitive method of establishing the diagnosis is via examination of the cerebrospinal fluid (Table 4-2). This is accomplished in most instances by lumbar puncture. If the child has signs of increased intracranial pressure (e.g., coma with decerebrate posturing or loss of pupillary reaction), and services of a skilled neurosurgeon are available, CSF can be withdrawn via a cisterna magna tap. This circumvents the risk of sudden

decompression below the foramen magnum and consequent cerebellar tonsillar herniation. Whenever a lumbar puncture is carried out in a child with suspected meningitis, an effort should be made to obtain the CSF opening pressure, and only the minimal amount of fluid necessary for diagnostic studies should be withdrawn. If the opening pressure is elevated above 200 mm of CSF, a bolus of mannitol (0.25-0.5 mg/kg) should be administered immediately following the lumbar puncture to lessen the risk of brain herniation.

Table 4-2. The CSF profile as seen in bacterial meningitis

Test	Range
WBC count	Between 200-2000 cu mm, with predominance of neutrophils
Glucose	Markedly decreased; generally between 0-20mg/dl
Protein	Increased to between 200-1000mg/dl
Gram stain	Positive or negative
Latex agglutination (LA) Enzyme-linked immunoassay Countercurrent immuno-electrophoresis	Positive even in pretreated meningitis; LA is most rapid and simple

Management

1. Antibiotic therapy (Table 4-3); this should be age and agent-specific and initially designed as a combination in order to cover for all common causative organisms at a given age. Once culture and sensitivity results become available, monotherapy with the most specific and effective antibiotic can be initiated and others discontinued. The antibiotic should be administered via the intravenous route (except gentamicin, which also has excellent IM absorption), the frequency of administration being regulated by the antibiotic half-life. Periodic monitoring of serum antibiotic levels and for antibiotic-related toxic manifestations is necessary at all ages, but especially so in the neonate.

2. The fluid intake in the initial 24-72 hours should be limited to 1000 ml/meter^2 in order to compensate for inappropriate secretion of antidiuretic hormone which develops in

approximately 80% of patients. The serum sodium should be checked at least once a day during this period. If significant hyponatremia (below 130 meq/l) develops despite fluid restriction, more stringent limitation may be necessary.

Table 4-3. Suggested antibiotics at various ages

Age	Dosage

NEONATE

Initial

Ampicillin 150-200 mg/kg/day; 3 divided doses

PLUS

Gentamycin 5-7 mg/kg/day IM, IV; 2 divided doses

After culture results become available:

GRAM POSITIVE ORGANISMS

Ampicillin 150-200 mg/kg/day; 3 divided doses or Penicillin G 150,000-200,000 units/kg/day; 6 divided doses

OR

GRAM NEGATIVE ORGANISMS

Gentamycin 5-7 mg/kg/day IM, IV; 2 divided doses or Cefotaxine 100-150 mg/kg/day; 3 divided doses

2 WEEKS to 2 MONTHS

Suspected gram negative infection:

Ampicillin 300-400 mg/kg/day IV; 6 divided doses

PLUS

Chloramphenicol 50 mg/kg/day IV; 4 divided doses

OR

Cefotaxime 150-200 mg/kg/day IV; 6 divided doses

Suspected gram positive infection:

Ampicillin 300-400 mg/kg/day IV; 6 divided doses

OR

Penicillin 100, 000 units/kg/day; 6 divided doses

---

3. Daily monitoring of head circumference and the zone of cranial transillumination is indicated in order to assess for subdural effusion and hydrocephalus. If the child remains febrile beyond the first week of treatment and a subdural fluid collection is confirmed on CT scan, serial subdural taps through the open anterior fontanelle may be required for draining the fluid.

4. In all infants, hearing should be checked using Auditory Evoked Potentials studies prior to discharge from the hospital. If the results are abnormal, the test should be repeated in 2-3 months. If the abnormality persists, behavioral audiometry should be used for confirmation of hearing loss.

5. In the 8-10 months following meningitis, a close watch should be kept for excessive enlargement secondary to hydrocephalus, and if this is suspected, a CT scan should be obtained. Motor and intellectual development should be monitored and psychometric studies obtained whenever the child is suspected to be at risk for developing learning difficulties.

Prevention of H. Influenza Infections

Active immunization against this organism is recommended for children between the ages of 2 and 5 years. In children at high risk for developing such an infection (e.g., those attending a day-care center), the immunization may be initiated at age 18 months.

RECURRENT BACTERIAL MENINGITIS

Very often, the causative organism provides a clue towards the underlying cause for the recurrence. Repeated meningitis with coliform organisms is generally associated with a communicating tract between the bowel and the meninges. Recurrent meningococcal and gonococcal meningitis may be associated with deficiencies of C6, C7, or C8 complement; recurrent pneumococcal infections may accompany anatomic defects in the cranium (e.g., absence of the cribriform plate or petrous temporal bone defects), hypogammaglobulinemia, or absence of C2, C3, or C5 complement.

The patient should be investigated for the appropriate immunological disorder. Plain x-ray films of the skull, paranasal sinuses and spine; radionuclide or metrizamide cisternography; and thin-slice CT scanning of the head/spine help identify the cause of recurrence. If an anatomic defect is detected, it should be repaired surgically once the meningitis has resolved.

SHUNT INFECTIONS

In the presence of ventriculoperitoneal shunts, organisms causing bacterial meningitis may differ from those commonly encountered. Coagulase negative staphylococcus and streptococcus viridans are frequently isolated. The meningitis is unlikely to resolve unless the infected shunt is removed. Intracranial pressure may be controlled during the acute illness using serial ventricular or lumbar punctures.

BRAIN ABSCESS

Abscess formation in the brain usually occurs following spread of infection from an adjacent infected structure (e.g., sinus), a penetrating foreign body, or septicemia. Congenital cyanotic heart disease, with or without bacterial endocarditis, is most commonly associated with hematogenous spread. Following a period of cerebritis, a focal area of tissue destruction surrounded by intense vascular congestion and edema develops.

Headache, intermittent fever, and focal neurological deficits are seen initially. By the 2nd or 3rd week, papilledema and alteration in the level of consciousness appear. If untreated, the disorder progresses to brain herniation and death by the 3rd or 4th week.

The diagnosis should be suspected in any individual with subacute, progressive focal neurological deficit and manifestations of increased intracranial pressure. Contrast CT scanning readily confirms the diagnosis. Lumbar puncture is contraindicated owing to the presence of increased intracranial pressure and risk of producing herniation.

The treatment consists of surgical drainage combined with broad spectrum antibiotics (penicillin plus chloramphenicol) for 5-6 weeks. Intravenous mannitol may temporarily decrease intracranial pressure in the acute stage.

TUBERCULOUS (TB) MENINGITIS

Seen most frequently in developing countries, this subacute infection usually has a peak incidence in children between the ages of 6 months and 3 years. It generally commences 6-8 weeks following primary pulmonary infection or during the course of miliary tuberculosis. Arteritis with resultant infarction, a fibrosing adhesive arachnoiditis around the base of the brain that leads to

communicating hydrocephalus, and cranial neuropathies are the principal pathologic features.

In the first week of illness lethargy, fever, headache, and vomiting are the predominant manifestations. Signs of meningeal irritation, seizures, papilledema, and stupor develop during the second week. If untreated, there is relentless progression until coma and death by the end of the third week.

The illness should be suspected in any individual with prior personal or family history of tuberculosis who undergoes an unexplained, progressive alteration in mental status. The tuberculin skin test may sometimes be negative owing to anergy from associated suppression of cell-mediated immunity.

The CSF is straw colored, with 50-200 WBC/cu mm, protein elevation to 100-300 mg/dl, and a moderate reduction in glucose to 15-30 mg/dl. Tubercular antigen may be rapidly detected in CSF using enzyme-linked immunosorbent (ELISA) techniques. In one study of 260 samples of spinal fluid from patients with tuberculous meningitis, the ELISA had a sensitivity of 72% and a specificity of 92%[18]. Bacterial cultures may or may not be positive. Diagnostic yield can be enhanced by guinea pig inoculation of the CSF and demonstration of disease in the animal.

If a diagnosis of tuberculous meningitis is suspected, treatment should begin immediately because bacteriological confirmation may take weeks, and prompt initiation of therapy is essential in order to limit mortality and morbidity.

The following combination is generally recommended:

INH 20 mg/kg/day in 2-3 divided doses orally for 18 months

Rifampin 15 mg/kg/day as a single daily oral dose for 18 months

Hepatic function should be monitored regularly during the course of treatment.

There is no proof that glucocorticoids significantly alter the course of the illness. Communicating hydrocephalus occurring as a complication of TB meningitis should initially be managed conservatively by medical measures to decrease

Table 4-4. CSF profile in Central Nervous System infections

	Cells	Protein	Glucose	Other
Bacterial meningitis	200-2000 WBC/cu mm, predominantly neutrophils	200-2000 mg/dl	0-20 mg/dl	Cultures positive Gram stain may be positive Bacterial antigen detectable by counter-current immunoelectro-phoresis, latex agglutination, or enzyme linked immunoassays
Partially treated bacterial meningitis	50-50 WBC/cu mm, predominantly neutrophils	200-1000 mg/dl	10-30 mg/dl	Cultures negative Gram stain generally negative Bacterial antigen detectable as above
Viral meningitis, meningo-encephalitis	5-200 WBC/cu mm, predominantly lymphocytes	50-200 mg/dl	Normal	Cultures positive or negative Elevated antibody index within 7-10 days and positive oligoclonal bands within 3-4 weeks seen in herpes encephalitis
Fungal meningitis	5-200 WBC/cu mm, predominantly lymphocytes	50-200 mg/dl	15-30 mg/dl	Cultures positive or negative Fungal antigen detectable India ink stain may be positive for fungus
Tuberculous meningitis	10-200 WBC/cu mm, predominantly lymphocytes	50-200 mg/dl	15-30 mg/dl	Cultures positive or negative Tubercular antigens may be detectable by ELISA

CSF formation (e.g., acetazolamide in a dose of 65-125 mg/day combined with furosemide 0.5-1.0 mg/kg/day). Ventriculo-peritoneal shunt placement should be considered only if the conservative treatment fails.

Despite appropriate therapy, the mortality still remains around 40%. Major neurological sequlae (cranial neuropathies, communicating hydrocephalus, hypothalamic dysfunction, seizures, cortical blindness, mental retardation, and spasticity) occur in approximately 24% of survivors.

CRYPTOCOCCAL MENINGITIS

The most common of central nervous system fungal infections, this disorder generally occurs in immune suppressed individuals. It may be associated with debilitating systemic illnesses (e.g., Hodgkin's disease), use of antimetabolites or steroids, and the Acquired Immune Deficiency Syndrome. Gradually worsening headache, apathy, memory loss, and cranial neuropathies evolving over 2-6 weeks.

The CSF demonstrates a lymphocytic cellular response, moderate reduction in glucose, and a moderate elevation in protein. The India ink stain may demonstrate the yeast-like organisms. Latex agglutination studies for cryptococcal antigen may at times be positive when the fungal cultures and India ink stain are negative. Fungal studies repeated on serial CSF samples enhance the diagnositc yield.

The treatment consists of a combination of amphotericin B and flucytosine. During an initial intravenous test dose of 1 mg of amphotericin administered over 6 hours, the patient should be monitored for chills, fever, and hypotension. If side effects are noted, it may be necessary to premedicate the patient with diphenhydramine or prochlorperazine and also add 25-50 mg of hydrocortisone sodium succinate to the intravenous amphotericin infusion. The test dose is followed by intravenous amphotericin administration of 0.25-0.5 mg/kg/day. Periodic monitoring of serum amphotericin B levels should ensure a level between 1-2 μg/ml. The medication may also require administration via the intrathecal route because it diffuses poorly across the blood-brain barrier. Hematocrit, serum potassium, blood urea nitrogen, serum creatinine, and urinalysis should be monitored twice a week during therapy with amphotericin B. Treatment should be continued for a period of 6-12 weeks. Flucytosine has excellent penetration across the blood-brain barrier, but development of resistance is a drawback, and therefore it should always be combined with amphotericin B. The dose is 150 mg/kg/day in four divided doses orally, with a reduction in dosage in the presence of renal dysfunction. The patient should also be monitored for hepatic and bone marrow toxicity; serum levels should be maintained between 50-75 μg/ml.

SUGGESTED READING

1. Kaplan SL, Fishman MA. Update on bacterial meningitis. J Child Neurol 3:82-93, 1988.

2. Bell WE and McGuiness GA. Current therapy of acute bacterial meningitis in children: Parts I and II. Pediatr Neurol 1:5-14, 201-209, 1985.

3. Beam TR and Allen JC. Assessment of antibiotic efficacy in acute bacterial meningitis. Clin Parmacol Ther 25:199-203, 1979.

4. Dodge PR and Swartz MN. Bacterial meningitis: A review of selected aspects. II. Special neurological problems, post meningitic complications and clinico-pathological correlations. N Engl J Med 272:954-960, 1965.

5. Feign RD, Stechenberg BW, Chang MG, Dunkle LM, Wong ML, Palkes H, Dodge PR and Davis H. Prospective evaluation of treatment of Hemophilus influenzae meningitis. J Pediatr 88:542-548, 1976.

6. Medoff G and Kobayashi GS. Strategies in the treatment of systemic fungal infections. N Engl J Med 302:145-154, 1980.

7. Johnson RT. The contribution of virological research to clinical Neurology. N Engl J Med 307:660-662, 1982.

8. Skoldenberg B, Forsgren M and Alestig K. Acyclovir versus vidarabine in herpes simplex enchephalitis. Randomized multicenter study in consecutive Swedish patients. Lancet 2:707-711, 1984.

9. Whitley JR, Soong S, Hirsch MS, Karchmer AW, Dolin R, Galasso G, Dunnick JK, Alford CA, and the NIAID Collaborative Antiviral Study Group. Herpes simplex encephalitis. Vidarabine therapy and diagnostic problems. N Engl J Med 304:313-318, 1981.

10. Whitley RJ, Soong S. Linneman C, Liu, Pazin G and Alford CA: Herpes simplex encephalitis: clinical assessment. JAMA 247:317-320, 1982.

11. Morawetz RB, Whitley RJ and Murphy DM. Experience with brain biopsy for suspected herpes encephalitis: A review of forty consecutive cases. Neurosurgery 12:654-657, 1983.

12. Nahmias AJ, Whitley RJ, Visintine AN, Takei Y and Alford CA. Herpes simplex virus encephalitis: Laboratory evaluations and their diagnositc significance. J Infec Dis 145:829-836, 1982.

13. Saito Y, Price RW, Rottenberg DA, Fox JJ, Su T, Watanabe KA and Philips PS. Quantitative autoradiographic mapping of herpes simplex virus encephalitis with radiolabelled antiviral drug. Science 217:1151-1153, 1982.

14. Sifontes JE. Rifampin in tuberculous meningitis. J Pediatr 87:1015-1017, 1975.

15. Steiner P and Portugaleza C. Tuberculous meningitis in children. Am Rev Respir Dis 107:22-29, 1973.

16. Ho DD, Pomerantz RJ and Kaplan JC. Pathogenesis of infection with human immunodeficiency virus. N Engl J Med 317(5):278-286, 1987.

17. Navia BA, Jordan BD and Price RW. The AIDS Dementia complex: clinical features. Ann Neurol 19(6):517-524, 1986.

18. Prabhakar S and Oommen AJ. ELISA using mycobacterial antigens as a diagnostic aid for tuberculous meningitis. J Neurol Sci 78:203-212, 1987.

19. Klein JO, and Feigin RD, McCracken GH. Report of the task force on diagnosis and management of meningitis. Pediatrics (Suppl) 78:959-982, 1986.

SEIZURE DISORDERS

PATHOPHYSIOLOGY

Clinical manifestations resulting from a paroxysmal, repetitive and excessive neuronal discharge constitute a seizure. Seizures originate at the level of the cerebral cortex, but neuronal pools in certain subcortical structures such as the thalamus play a role in modulation of the seizure activity. A combination of a variety of disturbances at the intracellular, neuronal membrane, axonal, and synaptic level is involved in pathogenesis of the seizure discharge. In neuronal pools not actively engaged in transmitting nerve impulses, the potential difference across the cell membrane is approximately 70 mV, with the interior of the cell being electronegative relative to the exterior. Flux of potassium into the extracellular space, antidromic transmission of neuronal impulses (from the axon towards the cell body), recurrent neuronal excitation, altered balance between excitatory and inhibitory neurotransmitters, and formation of giant excitatory post-synaptic potentials ultimately lead to the paroxysmal depolarization shift (PDS). This is the basic sub-unit of a seizure discharge. It correlates with the interictal spike on the electroencephalogram. Spatial and temporal summation of paroxysmal depolarization shifts eventually leads to a clinical seizure. As long as seizure discharges are localized to a small area of the cerebral cortex, consciousness is generally preserved (e.g., in partial simple seizures). Spread of the electrical discharge to a widespread area of the cerebral cortex (particularly bilaterally) or to the brainstem reticular formation results in loss of consciousness during the seizure. *Nonconvulsive* seizures (e.g., absence and complex partial) are frequently associated with staring and unresponsiveness. *Convulsive* seizures are usually accompanied by tonic, clonic, or tonic-clonic activity. Alterations in autonomic functions such as sweating, and tachycardia can be observed in a variety of seizure types.

INCIDENCE OF EPILEPSY

A tendency to develop recurrent seizures is termed epilepsy. It has worldwide prevalence, with no geographical, cultural, or sex predilection. Kurland has estimated the incidence of epilepsy in the United States as 0.331 per 1,000 persons per year and the prevalence as 3.7 per 1,000 per year. The incidence of epilepsy is highest in the first decade. Approximately 75% of all patients with epilepsy have onset of seizures prior to 20 years of age. A small, secondary peak in the incidence is also noted after age 60.

NOMENCLATURE

In the clinical account of a seizure, details about the following components should be elicited:

Prodrome. Features warning that an attack is imminent that are recognizable by the patient and close relatives for hours or even days in advance, usually by a subtle change in behavior; this term is, however, restricted to phenomena which do not form a part of the actual attack.

Aura. Subjective sensation perceived immediately upon onset of partial seizures; it is the very beginning of the attack and assumes great significance in localizing the anatomic focus (e.g., olfactory aura suggests onset of a seizure in the uncal portion of the hippocampus).

Ictus. The full-blown seizure; the manifestations may vary from behavioral automatisms to generalized convulsive activity and loss of consciousness.

Postictal State. A period of altered neurological function which immediately follows a seizure; it may consist of stupor, confusion, headache, vomiting, or transient paralysis.

CLASSIFICATION OF SEIZURES

In order to maintain uniformity of diagnostic features of seizure types amongst all physicians, the International Classification of Seizures was developed in 1969 (Table 5-1). It has subsequently undergone modifications and a revised classification is outlined here. This is a clinical classification, derived from historical information gathered from the patient and/or eyewitness.

Partial seizures are those whose origin can be localized to a certain anatomic or functional unit of the brain; they are likely to be associated with focal paroxysmal abnormalities on the electroencephalogram.

Generalized seizures, on the other hand, originate bilaterally and simultaneously from both hemispheres. **It is important not to confuse partial seizures with secondary generalization and seizures that are generalized from the very onset.**

Table 5-1. Revised International Classification of Seizures

  I. **Partial Simple** (consciousness preserved, focal EEG abnormality)
   a. with motor manifestations (e.g., Jacksonian march)
   b. with autonomic manifestations symptoms (e.g., epigastric sensation, pallor, sweating)
   c. with somatosensory or special sensory manifestations (e.g., tingling, light flashes, buzzing)
   d. with psychic manifestations (e.g., dysphasia, deja vu feelings—experiencing music, scenes)

Partial Complex (previous terminology: psychomotor or temporal lobe seizure—automatisms, consciousness impaired, EEG abnormalities generally focal)
   a. simple partial, evolving into complex partial
   b. consciousness impaired from the very onset

Partial Seizures with Secondary Generalization
   a. simple partial evolving into generalized tonic-clonic (GTC)
   b. complex partial evolving into generalized tonic-clonic
   c. simple partial evolving into complex partial evolving to generalized tonic-clonic

  II. **Generalized Seizures**
   a. absence
   b. atypical absence
   c. myoclonic seizures
   d. akinetic
   e. atonic
   f. generalized tonic
   g. generalized clonic
   h. generalized tonic-clonic

 III. **Unclassified** (neonatal seizures)

 IV. **Status epilepticus** (prolonged partial or generalized seizures without recovery of consciousness between attacks)

The history should carefully elicit the sequence of events from the very onset of the seizure, especially inquiring about aura, awareness by the patient of his/her surroundings during the event, adversive movements of the head and eyes, origin and spread of convulsive activity, and postictal features. If one adheres to meticulously outlining the sequence of events during a seizure, few errors will result in the classification process. Appropriate classification of seizures also helps in determining the etiology of the seizure. Partial seizures are more liable to be associated with focal cerebral dysfunction (trauma, infarction, sclerosis of the Ammon's horn of the hippocampus, neoplasm, etc.), whereas generalized seizures are more likely to be genetically determined (e.g., absence) or related to a diffuse metabolic, inflammatory, or toxic disturbance. The anticonvulsant of choice varies with the seizure type.

PARTIAL SIMPLE SEIZURES

Partial seizures associated with preservation of consciousness are termed as simple. Partial simple sensory seizures may be characterized by a contralateral sensory disturbance (e.g., numbness of face). Partial simple motor seizures are characterized by convulsive activity with preserved consciousness. The head and eyes generally deviate away from the hemisphere with the seizure focus and therefore have some localizing value. Todd's paralysis (transient postictal weakness) may follow a partial motor seizure and last up to 24 hours. Seizures originating in the perisylvian region of the hemisphere dominant for language are very often associated with ictal aphasia. Partial simple seizures may sometimes be related to focal structural central nervous system lesions (e.g., a-v malformation, porencephalic cyst, or head trauma). Carbamazepine and phenytoin are the anticonvulsants of choice for partial simple seizures.

Benign Rolandic Epilepsy of Childhood is a disorder characterized by irregular autosomal dominant transmission with age-dependent penetrance. It is manifest by predominantly nocturnal partial seizures, with onset usually between 5-15 years of age. It accounts for 11.5% to 20-25% of epilepsies in school-age children. Males outnumber females 60:40. Patients invariably have normal development and normal neurological examinations. The majority of the seizures are partial, commencing in the region of the face or upper limbs. Speech arrest during the course of the seizure is also common, with discharges originating from the dominant hemisphere. The paroxysmal EEG abnormalities are characteristically localized to the Rolandic sulcal or midtemporal regions (Fig. 3-3). Carbamazepine is the anticonvulsant of choice. The disorder has an excellent prognosis and almost always resolves by the end of the second decade.

PARTIAL COMPLEX SEIZURES

Previously termed psychomotor or temporal lobe seizures, partial complex seizures are *characterized by ictal impairment of consciousness and focal EEG abnormalities*. They constitute between 24 to 43% of all childhood epilepsies.

Type I complex partial seizures originate from the mesio-temporal region (e.g., uncus) and have an initial phase of motionless staring lasting 20-60 seconds, during which the patient is unresponsive to verbal commands or visual threat. This is followed by a period of "reactive automatisms," during which the patient becomes more aware of the environment and makes stereotyped eye blinking, lip smacking, or non-purposive limb movements.

Type II complex partial seizures usually have onset from an extratemporal focus, e.g, centro-partial or frontal regions, and are characterized by lack of an initial phase of motionless staring, with automatisms from the very onset.

Type III complex partial seizures are also termed temporal lobe syncope. They are associated with facial pallor, drop attacks, confusion, and amnesia.

Aura may precede about half of complex partial seizures. Postictal amnesia, confusion, drowsiness, or headache are common. Interictally, behavioural problems and learning disabilities develop in about a fourth of patients with complex partial seizures. Prolonged febrile seizures, hypoxia, hypoglycemia, central nervous system infections, and head trauma are some of the common etiological factors for complex partial seizures. Tissue from temporal lobectomy carried out for the surgical treatment of intractable complex seizures discloses sclerosis of the Ammon's horn in about 50% of cases, and occult tumors, hamartomas, and vascular malformations in approximately an additional 15%. The interictal EEG usually shows focal paroxysmal abnormalities localized to the anterior temporal or fronto-temporal regions. Sleep deprivation and the use of nasopharyngeal leads enhance the diagnostic yield of the EEG, which is generally abnormal in 60-70% of cases. Carbamazepine is the anticonvulsant of choice. Phenytoin is an alternate. Primidone (MYSOLINE) may be prescribed when carbamazepine and phenytoin are unsuccessful. For infants, phenobarbital is the most suitable anticonvulsant (See Table 5-3).

ABSENCE SEIZURES

Previously termed petit mal, this generalized paroxysmal disorder is associated with brief duration (5-20 seconds), periods of staring, and unresponsiveness. Automatisms (e.g., eye lid fluttering or chewing movements) frequently accompany seizure discharges of longer than 5-6 seconds duration. Body posture is generally preserved, although head dropping may sometimes be noted. There are generally no postictal manifestations. The usual age of onset is 5-15 years. It is slightly more prevalent in girls. Children with classical absence episodes usually have normal intelligence and neurological examinations. When the staring of absence seizures is accompanied by tonic-clonic or atonic components, or when the patient has an abnormal neurological examination, the disorder may be termed atypical absence. Generalized tonic-clonic seizures may accompany absence seizures in 38 to 59% of the patients. The frequency of absence episodes may be as high as a few dozen a day. The resulting inattentiveness may impair school performance. A family history of seizures is elicitable in approximately 40% of patients. The disorder is believed to be related to multiple genetic factors, some independent, other reinforcing or inhibitory to the trait. The diagnosis can be readily established by observing the classical attack, which sometimes can be precipitated in the examination room upon hyperventilating the patient for a period of three minutes or approximately 100 breaths. The EEG is confirmatory, demonstrating the characteristic 3 per second, generalized spike and wave discharges. Hyperventilating the patient during the EEG is especially useful in documenting the paroxysmal discharges. Absence seizures may be confused with complex partial seizures, as both present with staring and unresponsiveness. Table 5-2 outlines some distinctions between the two.

Ethosuxamide is the drug of choice for simple absence seizures. If there is a history of associated generalized tonic-clonic seizures, sodium valproate is recommended. Anticonvulsant therapy for absence seizures is continued for a seizure-free period of 3-4 years, by which time the disorder may spontaneously resolve. The overall remis-

sion rate is between 37-57%. Favorable prognostic indicators for resolution of absence seizures include a negative history of generalized tonic-clonic seizures, normal or above normal intelligence, a negative family history of other kinds of seizure disorders, and normal interictal EEG background activity. Nearly 90% of the patients who satisfy the above criteria ultimately outgrow the disorder.

Table 5-2. Differences between absence and complex partial seizures

	Absence	Complex Partial
Aura	none	frequently present
Duration of staring	5-20 seconds	20-120 seconds
Postictal drowsiness	none	frequently present
EEG pattern	generalized, 3/sec. spike-wave	focal spike, sharp or slow waves
Recommended anticonvulsants	ethosuxamide, sodium valproate	carbamazepine, phenytoin, phenobarbital

GENERALIZED TONIC-CLONIC SEIZURES

Also termed grand mal, this manifests with a sudden loss of consciousness, fall to the ground, an "epileptic" cry as a result of forceful contraction of the chest muscles, stiffening of the entire body with upward eye deviation, or extension of the trunk (tonic phase) followed by rhythmic jerking movements of the limbs, neck, and trunk (clonic phase). During the tonic or clonic phases, the patient may bite his tongue or lips. Urinary or fecal incontinence may also result. In the postictal period, drowsiness, stertorous respiration, and vomiting may occur. Some generalized tonic-clonic seizures are stimulus sensitive, being precipitated by flashing lights, visual patterns, or specific sounds. Tonic-clonic seizures that are generalized from the very onset should be distinguished from partial seizures which have undergone secondary generalization. The latter are frequently preceded by a focal signature like aura, or head and eye deviation to one side. Distinction also needs to be made between generalized tonic-clonic seizures which follow syncopal episodes and those which occur because of primary central nervous system dysfunction. In the former, facial pallor or palpitation are usually the initial manifestations, followed by the subject becoming limp and unconscious. Tonic-clonic movements usually develop a few seconds after onset of the syncope and are very brief in duration, merely a reflection of mild cerebral ischemia, and do not warrant therapy with anticonvulsants.

The electroencephalogram in patients with generalized tonic-clonic seizures usually discloses generalized spike/spike and wave discharges which vary in frequency between 2-12 Hertz (Fig. 3-5).

Valproic acid and phenytoin are the drugs of choice; phenobarbital is a third choice.

Presence of abnormalities on neurological examination, intellectual dysfunction, additional types of seizures, and interictal slowing on the EEG are unfavorable prognostic indicators for ultimately outgrowing the disorder.

INFANTILE SPASMS

Clinical Features

These seizures have onset in the first 12 months of life and are characterized by sudden, brief-duration muscular contractions which generally result in extension or flexion of the entire body for 5-10 seconds. They commonly occur in flurries at the sleep-wake interphase, and in numbers of between 50-100 per day. They are also termed "jack-knife" or "salaam" (respectful bowing) seizures owing to the sudden, forceful flexion of the lower extremities and trunk. Infantile spasms may be very subtle, and are frequently mistaken for normal movements of an infant or a Moro response (the latter always needs to be elicited by an examiner). They may frequently remain undiagnosed for weeks after onset owing to their subtle nature. It is therefore important to ask leading questions about the occurrence of such seizures in any infant who demonstrates significant neurological dysfunction.

Types, Etiology

Infantile spasms can be divided into the **idiopathic and symptomatic** forms. Patients with idiopathic infantile spasms frequently have had normal development prior to onset of the seizures and have a favorable prognosis. Symptomatic infantile spasms, on the other hand, are associated with severe central nervous system dysfunction even prior to onset of the seizures. Common etiologies in the symptomatic category include malformations of the central nervous system (e.g., hydranencephaly), congenital intrauterine infections, perinatal hypoxia and trauma, bacterial meningitis, inborn errors of metabolism, and heredofamilial disorders like tuberous sclerosis. In the idiopathic group, uncontrolled seizures may lead to progressive impairment of cellular and synaptic maturation and thereby further adversely impact development. In the symptomatic category, the infantile spasms probably constitute a mere epiphenomenon of the severe underlying cerebral dysfunction. There is no proof that vigorous anticonvulsant therapy modifies the outcome in symptomatic infantile spasms.

Investigations

The diagnosis of infantile spasms can be established on the basis of clinical and electroencephalographic features, especially when the patient has the charcteristic seizure events during the EEG recording session. The interictal EEG frequently displays hypsarrythmia—disorganzied background activity with generalized, high amplitude spike and wave discharges (Fig. 3-6) or multifocal spike and wave complexes. Administration of 50-100 mg of IV pyridoxine (vitamin B6) during the course of the test is recommended in order to exclude a rare but treatable disorder—pyridoxine dependency seizures. The recording should normalize in 15-20 minutes following pyridoxine administration in this condition. Computed cranial tomography is helpful in excluding some developmental malformations; periventricular calcification may also be seen on CT scans in tuberous sclerosis, congenital cytomegalovirus, and toxoplasmosis. Serum and urine metabolic screens for inborn errors of amino acid and carbohydrate metabolism, leukocyte lysosomal enzyme assays to exclude sphingolipidoses, and skin and conjunctival biopsies to exclude neuronal ceroid lipofuscinosis may also be necessary. Chromosomal analysis should be obtained whenever the child has multiple congenital anomalies so that partial deletion and trisomy syndromes can be ruled out.

Management

The treatment of infantile spasms calls for ACTH injections in a dose of 40-60 international units by the intramuscular route for a period about 4-6 weeks. Gradual tapering of the dose should be commenced after the initial 3-4 weeks. Side effects of ACTH include a cushingoid appearance, hypertension, peptic ulceration, and susceptibility to infection. Live virus immunizations should be avoided during the course of treatment. Clonazepam (0.1-0.2 mg/kg/day in 3 divided doses) or sodium valproate (10-50 mg/kg/day in 3 divided doses) are alternative medications for infantile spasms and may need to be substituted while ACTH is being tapered.

Prognosis

The less the interval of time between onset of seizures and commencement of therapy, the better the prognosis. This is especially true for patients with idiopathic infantile spasms, approximately 40% of whom revert to normal development. However, the outlook is dismal for patients with symptomatic infantile spasms, with 80-90% remaining severely mentally retarded despite prompt initiation of vigorous anticonvulsant therapy.

MINOR MOTOR SEIZURES

Myoclonic, akinetic, and atonic seizures as a group are also termed minor motor seizures. More than one of the above three types may occur in the same patient. The myoclonic jerks may involve only a small segment of the body or be massive and generalized, often resulting in forceful, sudden flexion of the head, or a fall to the floor with injuries. The akinetic seizures are usually accompanied by sudden, brief cessation of body movement. Drop attacks are common in the atonic seizures, with falls resulting from sudden loss of tone in the lower extremity extensor musculature. Most minor motor seizures last 5-15 seconds, and can occur in flurries of up to 50-100 times a day. They are frequently clustered around the sleep-wake interphase. The usual age of onset is between 2-15 years.

Children with minor motor seizures are a heterogenous population, being composed of a number of distinct syndromes. Some may have significant preexisting neurological dysfunction. On other occasions, the myoclonic-akinetic seizures develop in a previously well child, in which case the prognosis is more favorable.

Lennox-Gastaut syndrome is characterized by onset of myoclonic/astatic/atonic seizures between the ages of 2 and 5 years. The patient can have scores of seizures in a day. Intellectual dysfunction is common, in particular, regression of language skills. This may be secondary to the excessive number of seizures or partly a side effect of the multiple anticonvulsants prescribed for treatment. The patients may also develop generalized tonic-clonic seizures. The EEG demonstrates generalized, 2-2.5 Hertz or slow spike and wave complexes.

Sodium valproate is the drug of choice when minor motor seizures occur along with generalized tonic-clonic seizures (see Table 5-3 for dose). Anticonvulsant dosage should be gradually increased every 3-5 days, with monitoring of serum sodium valproate levels, SGOT, and SGPT until adequate seizure control is achieved. Clonazepam is an alternative anticonvulsant for minor-motor seizures, but does not have any protective effect against any accompanying generalized tonic-clonic seizures. A ketogenic (medium chain triglyceride) diet is also helpful in patients with refractory seizures. In most patients with minor motor seizures, it is likely that concurrent use of more than two anticonvulsants will induce cumulative side effects (e.g., drowsiness, slurred speech, ataxia and impaired cognition) but not a cumulative therapeutic affect. The urge to indulge in polypharmacy should therefore be resisted.

JUVENILE MYOCLONIC EPILEPSY

This disorder usally has onset in adolescents or young adults. It is equally prevalent in males and females and is most likely transmitted in an autosomal dominant pattern with variable penetrance.

It is characterized by the occurence of myoclonic seizures upon awakening from sleep, along with generalized tonic-clonic seizures. The latter typically develop during wakefulness. Rarely, absence seizures may also coexist. Alcohol ingestion and sleep deprivation are common precipitants of seizures. The patient is of normal intelligence. The neurological examination is generally normal.

The EEG demonstrates generalized 3.5-6 Hz spike and wave discharges in th interictal period and generalized 10-16 Hz spike and wave discharges ictally that are superimposed over a normal background rhythm.

Valproic acid is the anticonvulsant of choice. Patients generally have a very favorable response to valproate and function as completely normal adults. However, regardless of how long they have remained seizure free, 75-100% of patients have relapse of seizures whenever anticonvulsant therapy is withdrawn. Treatment should therefore be lifelong.

BENIGN EPILEPSY WITH OCCIPITAL PAROXYSMS

Patients with this disorder generally have onset of symptons between 5-10 years of age. It is more prevalent in girls. The seizures are usually partial simple with sensory symptomatology, e.g., transient blindness or seeing flashes of light. On some occasions, they may evolve into complex partial or generalized tonic-clonic seizures. A family history of seizures is present in approximately 50% of the patients, and migraine in approximately 20%. The patients have normal intelligence and a normal neurological examination. The sleep EEG is characterized by the presence of characteristic spikes and sharp waves in one or both occipital regions that are abolished by eye opening and awakening and are not activiated by photic stimulation. Carbamazepine is the anticonvulsant of choice. The prognosis is excellent, and approximately 90% have resolution of the seizure disorder by the age of 19 years.

FEBRILE SEIZURES

Clinical Features

Between 2-5% of children develop seizures with febrile illnesses. They are most common between the ages of 6 months to 3 years, with a peak age at occurrence of between 18 to 22 months. They rarely have onset after the age of 5 years. Febrile seizures are either transmitted as an autosomal dominant trait with age-dependent penetrance, or have a polygenic inheritance. Both the absolute level of rise in body temperature and the rate of elevation play a role in precipitating the seizure. Acute otitis media, upper respiratory tract infections, pneumonia, gastroenteritis, and roseola are frequently associated with febrile convulsions.

Classification

A distinction should be made between simple and complex febrile seizures. The former occur in a child who has had normal prior development, with no family history of afebrile seizures. The convulsion is usually generalized and of brief duration, lasting less than 15 minutes. There does not appear to be a stastically significant risk of developing intellectual dysfunction or subsequent afebrile seizures in this category. Complex febrile seizures. however, may occur in children with delayed development or a family history of epilepsy. The febrile seizure in such instances may have a focal onset and be prolonged, lasting usually more than 15 minutes. In this group the risk of developing afebrile seizures is approximately 13 times that in the general population. Onset in the first year of life, in particular in the 6-9 month age group, is also associated with a greater likelihood of developing subsequent afebrile seizures.

Investigations

The medical evaluation of a child with the first febrile seizures should include lumbar puncture to exclude central nervous system infection (meningitis or meningoencephalitis). Serum electrolytes and blood glucose should also be checked, as hypernatremic dehydration and ketotic hypoglycemia may occasionally present with fever and seizures. Electroencephalographic investigation of patients with febrile seizures is best carried out 10-14 days after the seizure, by which time any postictal slowing of background frequency should have resolved and the study is normal.

Management

Only approximately 40% of patients who have suffered a febrile seizure have recurrent episodes. It is therefore generally not necessary to prescribe anticonvulsants following the first simple febrile seizures. After the second simple febrile seizure, prophylaxis with daily phenobarbital may be commenced and continued for a seizure-free period of 12-18 months. With complex febrile seizures, therapy for the same duration should be commenced after the first seizure. Serum phenobarbital levels should be checked periodically and maintained between 15 and 20 ug/ml. In patients who develop hyperactivity or cutaneous hypersensitivity reactions to phenobarbital, treatment with sodium valproate is an alternative. There is no clear proof that antipyretic measures prevent febrile seizures or that prophylaxis of febrile seizures with anticonvulsants prevents the development of epilepsy in the later years.

GENERAL PRINCIPLES IN EPILEPSY TREATMENT

1. Only approximately 50% of children who have had their first afebrile seizure go on to have recurrent seizures. Anticonvulsant therapy should therefore be withheld until occurrence of a second seizure.

2. When a decision to commence anticonvulsant therapy has been made, a drug appropriate for the seizure type should be selected. (See Table 5-3).

3. The dosing frequency should depend upon the elimination half-life of the drug (See Table 5-3).

4. Periodic monitoring of serum anticonvulsant levels is essential, particularly when the seizure control is suboptimal or if anticonvulsant intoxication is suspected.

5. Periodic monitoring for adverse effects such as hepatic dysfunction, or anemia is also called for.

6. As far as possible, use of multiple anticonvulsants (more than two) should be kept to a minimum.

7. A clear and simple explanation to the patient and the parents as to the potential benefits and side effects of the anticonvulsant enhances compliance in the long run. One should also indicate that it takes a few weeks following initiation of therapy to achieve the optimum anticonvulsant effect.

8. Parents of children with epilepsy are frequently anxious about how to manage the child in case he/she goes on to develop seizures at home. It is imperative, therefore, that first aid measures for seizures be discussed with them and that they be made to feel as comfortable as possible in handling such situations.

9. Parents should also be informed about the length of time that the child will require anticonvulsant therapy. As a general rule, assuming that the child has been seizure free for a period of 2-3 years, approximately 70% of the children can be withdrawn from anticonvulsants without seizure recurrence. Children with poorly controlled seizures, fixed neurological deficits (e.g., microcephaly, hemiplegia, mental retardation, etc.) are more likely to have relapse of seizures when anticonvulsants are withdrawn.

10. Rehabilitation for the intellectual, emotional, and motor handicaps that accompany epilepsy is crucial. Psychometric evaluation and provision of assistance at school in areas of academic weakness, play-therapy, supportive psychotherapy, and group therapy with peers should be arranged as and when indicated.

ROLE OF THE ELECTROENCEPHALOGRAM IN PATIENTS WITH SEIZURES

The electroencephalogram is a measure of cortical synaptic function, reflects maturational changes, and also helps determine focal or diffuse, paroxysmal or non-paroxysmal brain dysfunction. In the neonate, the EEG is helpful in diagnosing occult seizures and in establishing a long-term prognosis. In febrile seizures, the EEG is usually normal when carried out 10-12 days following the seizure.

Sampling of the electroencephalogram during sleep is essential because of the enhanced yield of paroxysmal abnormalities (spikes, spike and wave, and sharp wave discharges). Sleep deprivation for 4-6 hours is probably the best method of inducing sleep in a child for the purpose of obtaining the EEG recording. Sedative-hypnotic medications to induce sleep for the study should be used only as a last resort, as drug induced changes may mask underlying paroxysmal abnormalities. The diagnostic yield is greatly enhanced when serial EEG's are carried out over a period of weeks or months.

Table 5-3. Common anticonvulsant agents

Drug	Indications	Elimination Half Time	Oral Maintenance Dosage	Plasma Therapeutic Levels	Common Side Effects	Toxic Effects	How Available
Phenobarbital	Generalized tonic, clonic, tonic-clonic seizures in neonates and infants	60-90 hours	Infants and young children: 3-5 mg/kg/day in one dose Adolescents: 1-2 mg/kg/day in one dose	10-25 μg/mL	Drowsiness	Hyperactivity Stupor Ataxia Steven's-Johnson syndrome	Elixir 20mg/5mL Tablets of 15, 30, 60, and 100 mg
Phenytoin (DILANTIN)	Partial simple seizures Generalized tonic-clonic seizures	7-18 hours	Under 20 kg; 5-15 mg/kg/day in 3 divided doses Between 20-40 kg; 5-7 mg/kg/day in 3 divided doses Over 40 kg; 4-6 mg/kg/day in 3 divided doses	10-20 μg/mL	Gingival hyperplasia Hirsutism Thickening of facial features Nystagmus	Ataxia Stupor Paradoxical increase in seizures Steven's-Johnson syndrome	Suspension 30mg/mL and 125mg/5mL Tablets of 50 mg Capsules of 30 and 100 mg
Ethosuxamide (ZARONTIN)	Absence seizures Adjunct for myoclonic, atonic	22-68 hours	20-30 mg/kg/day in 2 divided doses	50-100 μg/mL	Nausea Anorexia	Drowsiness Abdominal pain Irritability	Syrup 250 mg/5mL Capsules 250 mg
Clonazepam (CLONOPIN)	Myoclonic, atonic, and atypical absence seizures	16-40 hours	0.01-0.02 mg/kg/day to a maximum of 0.1-0.2 mg/kg/day	15-64 ng/mL	Tolerance Drowsiness Excessive bronchial secretions Irritability	Ataxia Excessive weight gain Stupor	Tablets of 0.5, 1.0, and 2.0 mg
Sodium Valproate (DEPAKENE) or Divalproex Sodium (DEPAKOTE)	Absence combined with generalized tonic-clonic seizures Myoclonic, akinetic and atonic seizures Generalized tonic-clonic seizures	8-12 hours Depakote has slower absorption and longer half-life	10-40 mg/kg/day in 3 divided doses (Depakene) or 2 divided doses (Depakote)	50-100 μg/mL; upper limit variable	Drowsiness Behavioral change Nausea, vomiting Weight gain	Stupor (may raise levels of concurrently administered phenobarbital) Hepatocellular injury (sometimes fatal) Thrombocytopenia Impaired platelet aggregation Hyperammonemia	Syrup 250 mg/5mL Tablets, 125, 250, and 500 mg Sprinkles, 125 mg
Carbamazepine (TEGRETOL)	Complex partial seizures, partial simple seizures	12-26 hours	10-30 mg/kg/day in 3 divided doses	6-14 μg/mL	Drowsiness Dizziness Double vision	Bone marrow suppression Hepatocelluar and renal dysfunction	Tablets of 100 and 200 mg Suspension of 100mg/5mL

BRAIN IMAGING STUDIES
IN PATIENTS WITH SEIZURES

Computed tomographic (CT) scan, Magnetic Resonance Imaging (MRI), radionuclide brain scan, or cranial ultrasound studies are called for in the evaluation of patients with seizures in whom structural abnormalities are suspected. As a generalization, it can be stated that with the exception of neonates and infants, patients with well-controlled seizures who have normal neurological examinations and normal interictal EEGs require such studies infrequently. On the other hand, poorly controlled seizures, presence of focal abnormalities on neurological examination, and of focal slow wave abnormalities on EEG may be suggestive of an underlying structural CNS lesion (infarct, contusion, etc.), warranting a contrast CT scan. Computed tomographic, Magnetic Resonance, and ultrasound studies are also helpful in the diagnosis of neurocutaneous syndromes like tuberous sclerosis and Sturge-Weber syndrome. The MRI scan may detect small lesions that could be missed on CT scans. Positron Emission and Single Photon Emission Tomographic studies are helpful in the evaluation of patients for surgical treatment of epilepsy. They demonstrate ictal hypermetabolism and interictal hypometabolism in most seizure foci. One needs to maintain a low threshold for obtaining brain imaging studies in neonates and infants because their neurological examination has a limited yield.

SURGICAL TREATMENT OF EPILEPSY

Indications

1. Seizures for more than 4 years despite appropriate anticonvulsant therapy.

2. The patient is 10 years of age or older; younger children are unsuitable candidates owing to the likelihood of spontaneous resolution of seizure disorders with time as well as the inconstant location of some seizure foci at a young age. Sturge Weber syndrome is an exception, as such patients benefit most when hemispherectomy is carried out prior to 2 years of age.

3. In instances where a lateralized hemispheric ablative procedure is being contemplated, the remaining hemisphere should be capable of sustaining language and memory functions. Intracarotid injection of amytal sodium is used in determining this, as it induces a transient unilateral suppression of hemispheric function (Wada test).

Surgical Procedures

1. Hemispherectomy; for patients with intractable seizure originating in one hemisphere with the presence of contralateral hemiplegia, e.g., Sturge-Weber syndrome.

2. Anterior temporal lobectomy, including resection of the amygdala and hippocampus; for patients with intractable complex partial seizures. This is the most common surgical procedure.

3. Limited extratemporal cortical resections.

4. Corpus callosotomy; especially useful for patients with atonic, generalized tonic, tonic-clonic, and partial complex seizures.

Investigative Methods Used in Evaluating Patients for Surgical Treatment

1. Long-term Video-EEG or subdural electrode recording.

2. Nasopharyngeal, sphenoidal leads; help localize mesiotemporal seizure foci.

3. PET/SPECT; interictal hypometabolism and ictal hypermetabolism are seen with seizure foci.

4. MRI, CT scans; to determine presence of foci focal structural lesions.

5. Neuropsychological testing, including the Wada test; patterns of derangement in neuropsychological function help localize the seizure focus and also determine whether lateralized ablative procedures will impair language and memory.

Results

Anterior temporal lobectomy results in complete cessation of seizure activity in 42-79% of patients and significant reduction in seizure frequency in another 18-33%.

Corpus callosotomy is especially useful in patients with intractable atonic seizures. Seventy-five to 100% of patients demonstrate either complete resolution or significant reduction in seizure frequency.

Cognitive function and behavior may also improve steadily following surgical treatment. This is in part related to improvement in seizure control and in part to lowering in the requirement for anticonvulsants.

SUGGESTED READING

1. Pedley TA. The pathophysiology of focal epilepsy: Neurophysiological considerations. Ann Neurol 3:2-9, 1978.

2. Dreifuss FE. Classification of seizures and the epilepsies. In: Dreifuss FE, ed. Pediatric Epileptology. John Wright Publishers, Boston, 1983; 1-13.

3. Dodson WE. Special pharmacokinetic considerations in children. Epilepsia 28(Suppl 1):S56-S70, 1987.

4. Shinnar S, Vining E, Mellits E, et al. Discontinuing antiepileptic medication in children with epilepsy after two years without seizures. N Engl J Med 313:976-980, 1985.

5. Sato S, Dreifuss F, Penry J, et al. Long-term follow up of absence seizures. Neurology 33:1590-1595, 1983.

6. Gomez MR and Klass DW. Epilepsies of infancy and childhood. Ann Neurol 13(2):113-124, 1983.

7. Delgado-Escueta AV, Treiman DM and Walsh GO. The treatable epilepsies, parts I and II. N Engl J Med 308(25):1508-1514, 1983 and 308(26):1576-1584, 1983.

8. Schomer DL. Partial epilepsy. N Engl J Med 309(9): 536-539, 1983.

9. Hirtz DG and Nelson KG. The natural history of febrile seizures. Annu Rev Med 34:453-471, 1983.

10. Mizrahi EM. Neonatal seizures: problems in diagnosis and classification. Epilepsia 28(Suppl 1):S46-S55, 1987.

11. Neonatal Seizures. Dehkharghani F and Sarnat HB, In: Sarnat HB, ed. Topics in Neonatal Neurology, Grune and Stratton, Orlando, 1984; 209-232.

12. Tharp BR. An overview of pediatric seizure disorders and epileptic syndromes. Epilepsia 28(Suppl 1):S 36-45, 1987.

13. Kotagal P and Rothner DA. Complex partial seizures in children: diagnosis and management. Int Pediatr 2:182-188, 1987.

CHAPTER VI

PAROXYSMAL, NON-EPILEPTIC DISORDERS

Syncope

Night Terrors and Sleep Walking (Refer to Chapter XIII)

Breath-Holding Spells

Near-Miss Sudden Infant Death Syndrome

Paroxysmal Choreoathetosis (Refer to Chapter VIII)

SYNCOPE

Pathophysiology, Clinical Features

A transient loss of consciousness due to reduction in blood or glucose supplies to the brain below levels critical to maintaining consciousness is defined as syncope.

It is usually characterized by an abrupt loss of consciousness and generalized decrease in muscle tone, lasting a few seconds to 1-2 minutes. Twitching movements of the face or fingers may accompany the longer duration episodes. Nausea, palpitation, sweating, generalized weakness, a feeling of "blacking out," or excessive warmth commonly precede the event.

Etiology

I. Metabolic disturbances
   Hypoglycemia
   Hypoxia

II. Primary disturbances of cardiac function
   Congenital cyanotic heart disease (e.g., Fallot's tetralogy)
   3rd degree heart block
   Syndrome of QT interval prolongation
   Subaortic stenosis
   Pulmonic stenosis
   Stokes-Adams syndrome
   Mitral valve prolapse

III. Vaso-vagal disturbances with secondary impairment of cardiac output (in response to pain, fright, stimulation of hypersensitive carotid sinus, etc.)

IV. Orthostatic hypotension

Differential Diagnosis

Seizures. These are usually characterized by a greater degree of convulsive activity, bowel and bladder incontinence, and a postictal period lasting at least 10-15 minutes. The interictal EEG may disclose paroxysmal discharges. Facial pallor at the onset is common in syncope, but infrequent in seizures.

Basilar Migraine. Occasionally, ischemia from a migrainous event may involve the brainstem reticular formation, resulting in loss of consciousness. The constellation of accompanying diplopia, dizziness, visual disturbances, nausea, and headache helps distinguish migraine from syncope.

Suggested Investigations for Syncope

I. EKG

II. 24-hour Holter monitor

III. EEG (to rule out complex partial or atonic seizures)

IV. Echocardiogram (if indicated on the basis of clinical exam and EKG)

V. Glucose tolerance test (if sweating, tremor and restlessness precede syncopal episodes and if episodes can be aborted by ingestion of food)

Management

This varies with the mechanism underlying syncope. Vasovagal syncope, the commonest form, usually peaks around adolescence and resolves spontaneously with time.

BREATH-HOLDING SPELLS

Definition

Breath-holding spells are defined as transient episodes of loss of consciousness in which crying is the initial, sentinel manifestation. There may be associated convulsive activity, but evidence of a primary seizure disorder is lacking.

Clinical Manifestations

Pallid breath-holding spells are common in infants of 3-9 months of age. They are characterized by facial pallor in response to crying, followed by generalized loss of muscle tone and unconsciousness. Each episode may last 30-60 seconds, following which the patient returns to normal. These attacks may be a reflection of immature cardiorespiratory reflexes triggered by crying.

The *cyanotic* breath-holding spells usually occur in children between the ages of 1-3 years. The child starts crying in response to a noxious stimulus or after being emotionally upset and is unconsolable. A few seconds later, the child may hold the breath in inspiration, turn cyanotic, and loose consciousness because of cerebral hypoxia, and on some occasions, go on to have a brief generalized convulsion.

Over indulgence on the part of the parents and altered parent-child interaction have been erroneously suggested as the pathogenetic basis underlying breath-holding spells. However, a fair number of children with breathing-holding spells (pallid or cyanotic types) probably have an immature autonomic nervous system.

Investigations

The electroencephalogram is normal. An ocular compression test performed during the electroencephalogram with simultaneous monitoring of the electrocardiogram may, however, be abnormal. The test is usually carried out by carefully compressing one or both eyeballs of the patient for 10 seconds. Patients with a hypersensitive vagal system develop asystole of three or more seconds during this maneuver.

Management

a. Reassurance to the parents that the child does not have epilepsy, that the disorder is maturational, and almost always resolves spontaneously by 4-5 years of age.

b. Positive (e.g., praise) and negative reinforcement (e.g., ignoring) of behavior helps the child improve his tolerance of frustration, cry less often, and thereby become less liable to develop breath-holding syncope.

c. In rare instances, in children with a strong predilection for bradycardia or asystole (following documentation upon the ocular compression test), a trial of vagolytic agents (e.g., atropine 0.06 mg/kg/day in two divided doses orally) may be of benefit.

NEAR-MISS
SUDDEN INFANT DEATH SYNDROME

Definition

Sudden infant death syndrome (SIDS) occurs in 2-5/1000 live births per year in the United States. It occurs in apparently previously well children, usually between 0-6 months of life. There is sometimes a history of upper respiratory tract infections preceding the near-miss SIDS event by a few days.

The term "near-miss" Sudden Infant Death Syndrome characterizes those patients in whom the apnea was detected in a timely manner

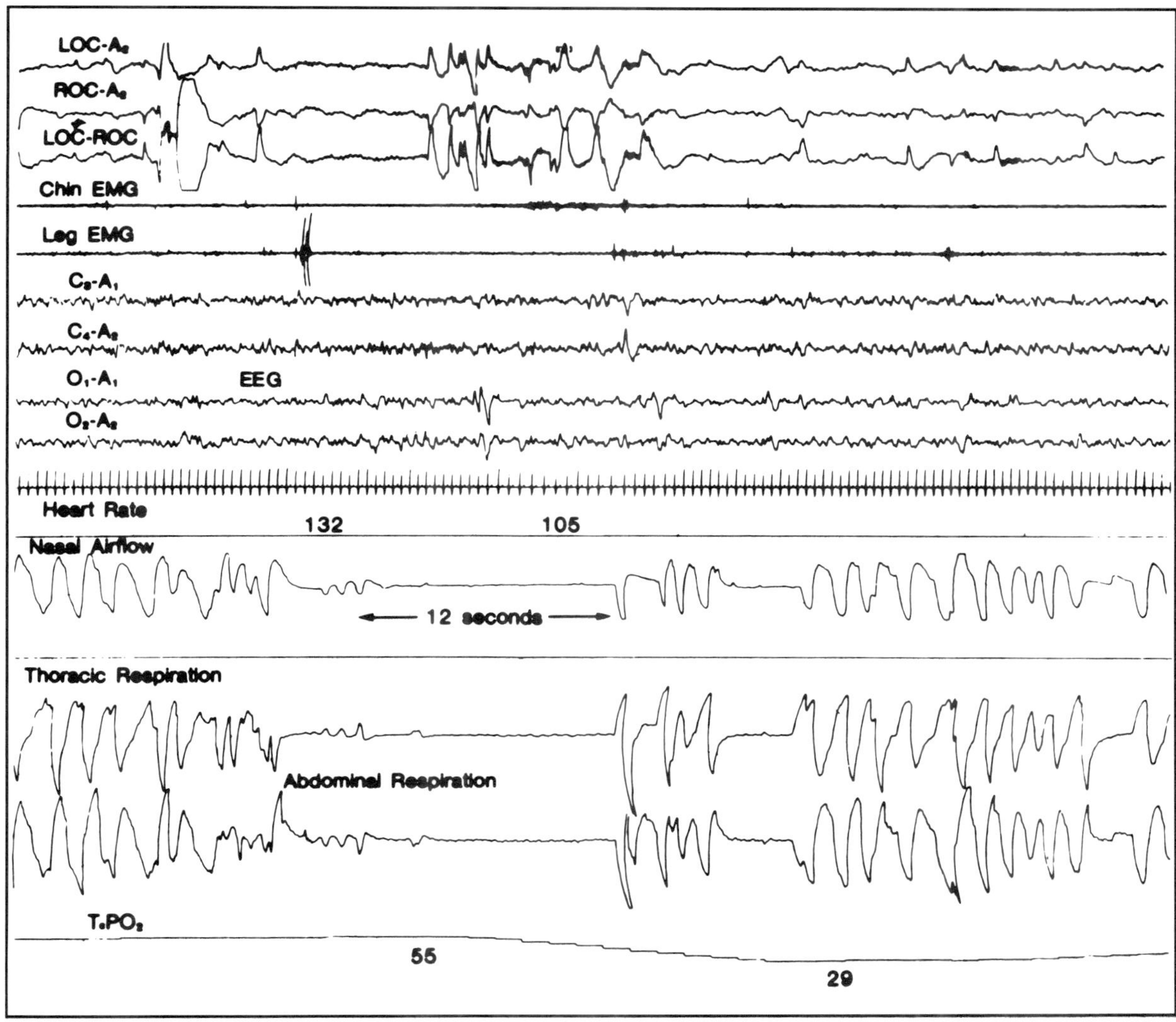

Fig. 6-1. Polysomnogram on three-month-old infant with recurrent apneic episodes, demonstrating a 12 second episode of central apnea that is associated with hypoxemia and bradycardia. The top three channels denote eye movement recording, channels 4 and 5 represent electromyographic activity, channels 6 through 9 EEG activity, channel 10 heart rate, channels 12, 14, 15 respiration, and channel 16 transcutaneous pO_2 values; channel 11 and 13 are blank. Oximetry is preferred over monitoring of transcutaneous pO_2.

and cardiorespiratory resuscitation was successful. While SIDS and near-miss SIDS are sometimes considered expressions of a common underlying disturbance, this assumption may or may not be correct.

Pathogenesis

Infants who die suddenly, unexpectedly, and without a sufficient cause detectable at postmortem examination probably share an abnormality in the autonomic regulation either of cardiovascular functions, respiratory functions, or both. The abnormality may be triggered or exaggerated by an exogenous stimulus, e.g., inflammation of the respiratory tract. (Shannon DC and Kelly DH, N Engl J Med 306:959-965, 1982).

In some patients with near-miss SIDS, a high incidence of sleep-related respiratory disturbances (mixed or obstructive apnea, periodic breathing, hypoxemia, hypoventilation) has been found. In others, no definite respiratory abnormalities have been noted and a primary disturbance of cardiac function has been postulated.

Risk Factors for SIDS

Prematurity and low birthweight for age

Low Apgar scores

Need for neonatal resuscitative efforts and oxygen

Male infants

Prior history of SIDS in family

Apnea of prematurity

Management of Near-Miss SIDS

1. EKG for detection of any treatable cardiac etiology (e.g., QT interval prolongation).

2. Teaching parents cardio-pulmonary resuscitative techniques.

3. Home apnea monitoring for a period of 4-6 months, by the end of which time the risk for SIDS has abated in most infants.

4. If apnea is recurrent and the episodes are long enough (20-30 seconds) that resuscitation is required, polygraphic studies of sleep and respiration are recommended in studying the disorder, but may not necessarily alter the management plan.

5. Some infants with polygraphically documented central hypoventilation (Fig. 6-1) may benefit from central nervous system respiratory stimulants like theophylline or acetazolamide. Diaphragmatic pacing can be used as an adjunct in assisting respiration in older infants and toddlers. However, the technique cannot be relied upon to adequately sustain ventilatory function by itself.

SUGGESTED READING

1. Wright FS. Recurrent paroxysmal nonepileptic disorders. In: Swaiman KF and Wright FS, eds. Practice of Pediatric Neurology, C.V. Mosby, St. Louis, 1982; 1074-1077.

2. Rendle-Short J. The pathophysiology of breath-holding attacks: a hypothesis. Aust Pediatr 8:92, 1972.

3. Rabe EF. Recurrent, paroxysmal nonepileptic disorders. Curr Probl Pediatr 4(8):3-31, 1974.

4. Guilleminault C and Anders TF. Sleep disorders in children. Recent Advances in Pediatrics 22:151-174, 1976.

5. Shannon DC and Kelly DH. SIDS and near-SIDS. Parts I and II. 306(16):959-965; 306(17):1021-1028, 1982.

HEADACHES

Introduction

Headache is a frequently encountered disorder. It may be related to organic or non-organic factors. The exact incidence is difficult to estimate, as severity of the symptom varies, and not every child with headache is brought forth for medical evaluation. Based upon a questionnaire survey, Bille in Sweden[1] noted that by age 7 years 2.5% of the children had frequent non-migrainous headache, 1.4% true migraine, and 35% infrequent headache of other varieties. In another Swedish study, Vahlquist[2] found an 18% incidence of headache in children of 10-12 years, with 5% having migraine and 13% having other forms of headache. By far the most common cause of headache in the United States in children of school-going age is emotional tension.

Classification

I. Headache related to increased intracranial pressure.

    Neoplasm

    Subdural hematoma

    Pseudotumor cerebri

    Hydrocephalus

II. Inflammatory disorders

    Aseptic meningitis

    Bacterial meningitis

    Cerebral vasculitis

III. Vascular disorders

    Migraine

    Arterio-venous malformation

    Subarachnoid hemorrhage

    Hypertension

    Cerebrovascular insufficiency

IV. Pain referred from adjacent extracerebral structures

    Acute sinusitis

    Glaucoma, optic neuritis, iridocyclitis

    Dental, gingival or mandibular disorders

    Otitis media

    Cervical arthritis

V. Tension or psychogenic headache

VI. Miscellaneous

Post-lumbar puncture headache
Epileptic headaches
Post-traumatic headache.

HISTORY TAKING IN
A PATIENT WITH HEADACHE

A carefully obtained history forms the basis of evaluation. If by the end of the history-taking session, the examiner is unclear about the etiology of the headache, it is unlikely that the neurological examination will be of any additional help. The emphasis should be on determining events in the family, school, and social circles which could cause unhappiness in the child or lead to emotional tension or anxiety. Some points which should be addressed in the history include:

1. **Frequency of headache.** Migraine headaches vary in frequency from 2-3 per year to 2-3 per week. However, they rarely occur every day, as is generally noted with tension headache, sinusitis, or in advanced stages of increased intracranial pressure.

2. **Duration of illness.** Migraine may commence as early as 3-5 years, last for a period of 5-10 years, then gradually subside and disappear by adulthood. Tension headaches may also continue for quite some years. Depending upon whether or not the underlying emotional conflict is resolved, tension headaches may persist into adulthood or disappear. Headaches related to increased intracranial pressure and referred pain rarely continue for more than a few weeks before presentation to the physician. Acute onset (within hours) of excruciating pain is usually seen in migraines, aseptic and bacterial meningitis, or subarachnoid hemorrhage.

3. **Time of onset.** Headaches from increased intracranial pressure are generally worse in the early morning and late evening hours, whereas those from acute sinusitis are most severe towards mid-day; tension headaches also worsen as the day goes by. In children with school phobia, the headache complaint may be voiced only when separational anxiety is maximal, i.e., on school-going days but not during weekends and vacation.

4. **Exacerbating factors.** Headache associated with increased intracranial pressure is made worse by coughing, bending, or sneezing. Birth control pills, stress, and menstrual periods may worsen migraine to variable degrees.

5. **Relieving factors.** Analgesics are of little value in relieving headache from increased intracranial pressure. Common non-narcotic analgesics (acetaminophen and aspirin) fairly readily relieve childhood migraine, as does lying down in a dark and quiet room. Nasal decongestants and antibiotics may relieve pain associated with acute sinusitis. Tension headache is relieved to some extent by non-narcotic analgesics and relaxation techniques.

6. **Associated symptoms.** Vomiting is frequently associated with headache of increased intracranial pressure and acute meningeal inflammation. Nausea alone or nausea combined with vomiting suggest migraine. Visual symptoms (diplopia, flashes of light, scotomata) and dizziness may also accompany migraine. Lack of interest in social and family activities, declining academic performance, behavioral disorders, change in appetite and sleep-wake function may point to depression or emotional tension as cause for the headache.

CLINICAL EXAMINATION

Neoplasms originating in the hypothalamic region may be associated with emaciation or obesity. Patients with pseudotumor cerebri may also be obese.

It is important to exclude meningitis or meningoencephalitis in any patient with acute onset of headache associated with presence of non-focal neurological findings, normal fundii, fever, and signs of meningeal irritation (neck stiffness, Kernig's or Brudzinski's signs). Tenderness over the paranasal sinuses may be noted in acute sinusitis. Scalp tenderness is usually indicative of tension headache. An asymmetric bruit over the eyeball or head may be audible with arterio-venous malformations. Attention should also be directed towards the cervical spine, ears, mandible, teeth, and gums for pathology that could lead to pain referred to the head.

Careful examination of the ocular fundus is a must. If the patient is uncooperative, pupillary dilatation with 2-3% neosynephrine is recommended prior to repeating the fundoscopy. Papilledema is characteristic of disorders associated with increased intracranial pressure. Loss of venous pulsations is the initial change in papilledema. However, approximately 30% of normal individuals may also have physiologic absence of venous pulsations. Therefore, by itself, lack of venous pulsations becomes significant only if such pulsations were present at an earlier examination or if they are asymmetric. The retinal vessels become progressively tortuous as papilledema evolves. The optic disc margins become blurred from edema in the retinal nerve fiber layer due to dampening of axoplasmic flow. Visual acuity is preserved into the late stages of papilledema. Long standing increase in intracranial pressure may, however, lead to ischemic optic atrophy, in which case the optic discs assume a pale white color instead of the normal pink. The pupillary response to light may then become poor and unsustained, and there may be significant deterioration in visual acuity. Retinal vasospasm and pallor may be seen during migraine attacks. Refractive errors rarely lead to headaches.

Paresis of upward gaze may be noted with pressure on the pretectal region of the midbrain from a midline mass. Lateral gaze paresis due to 6th cranial nerve paresis, exaggerated tendon reflexes, and extensor plantar responses are false localizing signs that may develop from traction on lone tracts and cranial nerves from increased intracranial pressure.

Macrocephaly is indicative of long-standing expansion in intracranial volume, usually due to a neoplasm, hydrocephalus, subdural collection of fluid, or megalencephaly.

The patient's mood, affect, and volume of speech are sometimes clues to an underlying emotional disturbance.

MIGRAINE

Definition

The Research Group on Headaches of the World Federation of Neurology has defined migraine as a "familial disorder characterized by recurrent attacks of headache widely variable in intensity, frequency, and duration. Attacks are commonly unilateral and are usually associated with neurological and mood disturbances. All of the above characteristics are not necessarily present in each attack or in each patient." It should be stressed that migraine headaches in children are very often diffuse, poorly localized, and do not possess the hemicranial distribution characteristically observed in adults.

Pathogenesis

It has been generally felt that there is an initial phase of intracranial vasoconstriction followed by vasodilatation of the intracranial and extracranial blood vessels. The vasoconstriction could be regional or global, and if regional, manifest as aura which correlates clinically with ischemic symptoms from the area of the brain that is involved (e.g., flashes of light or scotomata with visual cortical ischemia). This is followed by a period of dilatation of the extra and intracranial vessels. Stretching of pain sensitive nerve endings in the extracranial vessels may lead to the pulsatile headache.

Recent studies of regional cerebral blood flow using intracarotid injection of radioactive xenon, however, indicate diminished perfusion both during the aura and acute headache phase of classical migraine. No definite hemodynamic changes have been noted in common migraine. The origin of migraine headache could primarily be on a neurohumoral basis. Substance P, which is a vasoactive peptide, prostaglandin E1, serotonin, and bradykinin have all been postulated to play a role in triggering neural mechanisms subserving pain.

Classification

1. Common migraine (no aura)
2. Classical migraine (aura preceding onset of headache)
3. Complicated migraine (enduring neurological deficit after migraine attack)
   hemiplegic
   ophthalmoplegic
   central retinal artery occlusion with visual impairment
4. Basilar migraine (at least two clear-cut symptoms of brainstem dysfunction present)
5. Migraine variants (headache non-existent or only minimal)

benign paroxysmal vertigo

cyclic vomiting

stupor

6. Cluster headaches (frequent in adults, rare in children)

Clinical Features

As with most other episodic disturbances of brain function, a good history is diagnostic. The patient may give a typical history of a pounding or pulsatile headache which is associated with nausea, vomiting, photophobia, and visual manifestations (scotomata, bright flashes of light, zig-zag lines, visual field deficits). Diplopia may be secondary to cranial neuropathies or ischemia of the medial longitudinal fasiculus in the brainstem that regulates conjugate gaze. Dizziness may occur from ischemia of the vestibular nuclei or the labyrinth. The nausea and vomiting commonly seen in migraine are probably a consequence of an ischemic or neurochemical disturbance in the area postrema of the medulla, the hypothalamus, or labyrinth.

In between the attacks, the neurological examination is usually normal, unless the child has residual deficit from an attack of complicated migraine.

Management

Acute Attack. Aspirin and acetaminophen are quite effective in controlling childhood migraine, provided they are taken promptly at the onset of symptoms and combined with some general measures for relaxation (e.g., lying down in a quiet, dark room). There is no proof that two "extra strength" acetaminophen tablets (each 500 mg) necessarily confer any more pain relief in adolescents than two regular strength tablets (each 300 mg). If the headache is not relieved, acetaminophen combined with codeine might be tried. Ergot-containing preparations (CAFER-GOT) are useful only in older adolescents, to whom they may be administered as one tablet every 30-60 minutes to a maximum of 3-4 tablets per day.

Migraine Prophylaxis. This becomes necessary when headaches become frequent enough (2-3 times/week) that the child's emotional health, school and social activities begin to suffer. All prophylactic agents are only of moderate efficacy and breakthrough headaches may still occur periodically. Prophylactic agents should be administered on a daily basis for a period of 6-8 months, then tapered and discontinued, and the patient observed for spontaneous remission. Some of the common agents used for migraine prophylaxis are:

Propranolol. Fatigue is a common dose-related side effect. Complete heart block and history of bronchial asthma are contraindications to use of propranolol. The dosage varies between 20-80 mg/day, administered in 2-3 divided doses.

Phenytoin. Most effective in migraine patients with EEG abnormalities; 2-4 mg/kg/day in 2 divided doses.

Cyproheptadine. This antiserotonin and antihistamine agent may be administered in a dosage of 0.25 mg/kg/day in 2-3 divided doses; bronchial asthma is a contraindication. Drowsiness is a common side effect.

Biofeedback. When emotional tension is compounding the situation and playing a triggering role, biofeedback therapy may be useful in teaching the patient how to relax and better handle stress.

TENSION HEADACHE

Clinical Characteristics

1. Very often daily, generalized, dull, or causing a band-like compression around the head.

2. Worsens as the day goes by or following stressful events.

3. Normal neurological examination except for abnormal affect (the patient may be anxious or depressed).

4. Tenderness may be elicited over the frontalis and temporalis muscles because of excessive muscle contraction.

5. A history of declining school performance, changes in the home environment, loss of a loved one, school phobia, declining appetite, apathy, and poor socialization with peers may also be present.

Management

1. Reassurance that the disorder is benign. The

patient should be encouraged to maintain a positive attitude.

2. Helping the patient handle underlying stress with supportive psychotherapy and/or biofeedback.

3. Amitryptiline, 25-100 mg/ day is also a useful adjunct.

POST-TRAUMATIC HEADACHE

This is a diffuse pain which is sometimes accompanied by dizziness. It generally develops a few weeks following cerebral concussion, persists for a few months, and then resolves spontaneously. It is most likely multifactorial, resulting from a combination of a pre-existing personality disturbance, depression, litigation neurosis, and perhaps, altered neurotransmitter functions in the brain. In an uncontrolled clinical trial, amitryptiline was found to be beneficial in relieving post-traumatic headache[3].

"EPILEPTIC" HEADACHES

Patients with suboptimally controlled seizures may develop a generalized dull, non-pulsatile headache, sometimes associated with nausea. The EEG usually discloses paroxysmal changes. Placement on anticonvulsants or optimizing the dosage of the anticonvulsant that the child is already receiving may abolish the headache.

INVESTIGATION OF PATIENTS WITH HEADACHE

CT Head Scan. This is by far the most useful test. When performed with intravenous contrast administration, it helps exclude structural lesions, especially arterio-venous malformation, neoplasm, hydrocephalus, subdural hematoma, and brain abcess. A CT scan is indicated when the headache is consistently localized to the same region of the head, is occurring daily, or if the neurological examination is abnormal.

Magnetic Resonance Imaging (MRI). This non-invasive technique is superior to CT in visualizing posterior fossa and suprasellar lesions and is particularly indicated in assessing for neoplastic and inflammatory disorders.

Electroencephalogram. Non-specific abnormalities (e.g., generalized or focal slowing, focal spike, or sharp wave discharges) may be noted in migraine. They may persist for up to two weeks after the attack. Continuous polymorphous focal delta slow wave abnormality may be associated with an underlying structural lesion.

Lumbar puncture. In a febrile patient with acute headache and neck stiffness, aseptic and bacterial meningitis or subarachnoid hemorrhage should be suspected and cerebrospinal fluid assessed for color, WBC and RBC counts, protein, glucose, and bacterial cultures. In patients with pseudo-tumor cerebri, the spinal fluid opening pressure (adequate sedation prior to LP is recommended in young children) is elevated above 200 mm. The protein is usually normal to low normal, while glucose and cell counts are invariably normal.

X-rays of the paranasal sinuses, cervical spine, mastoids, or mandible. Indicated when referred pain from any of these structures is suspected. Skull x-rays are of limited value and are not recommended if CT or MRI studies are available.

Psychologic evaluation. Psychometric and projective tests are indicated in tension headaches to determine the underlying cause for stress.

REFERENCES

1. Bille BS. Migraine in school children. Acta Paediatr 51(Suppl 136):1-151, 1962.

2. Vahlquist B. Migraine in children. Internat Arch Allergy 7:348-355, 1955.

3. Tyler SG, McNeely HE and Dick LM. Treatment of post-traumatic headache with amitryptiline. Headache 20:213-216, 1980.

SUGGESTED READING

1. Rose CF. The pathogenesis of a migraine attack. Trends in Neuro Sci 6:247-248, 1983.

2. Moskowitz MA. The neurobiology of vascular head pain. Ann Neurol 16:247-248, 1983.

3. Kriel RL Headache. In: Swaiman KF and Wright FS, eds. Practice of Pediatric Neurology. C.V. Mosby, St. Louis, 2nd edition; 215-221, 1982.

4. Rothner AD. Headaches in children: a review. Headache 19:156-162, 1979.

5. Rothner AD. The migraine syndrome in children and adolescents. Pediatr Neurol 2:121-126, 1986.

CHAPTER VIII

MOVEMENT DISORDERS

Tourette Syndrome

Sydenham's Chorea, Benign Familial Chorea, Paroxysmal Choreoathetosis

Dystonia Musculorum Deformans

Myoclonus

Essential Tremor

Athetosis

Spasmus Nutans

Bobble-head Doll Syndrome

Comparison of Some Movement Disorders (Table)

TOURETTE SYNDROME

First described by Gilles de la Tourette in 1885, this disorder is characterized by onset in childhood of a variety of involuntary tics and a behavioral disturbance. Increasing awareness of the ailment over the past two decades is now leading to early diagnosis and treatment.

Pathophysiology

Decreased CSF homovanillic acid (a dopamine metabolite) in Tourette syndrome suggests primary hypofunction in the central nervous system dopaminergic pathways. Tic development is probably a reflection of consequent dopamine receptor hypersensitivity, as tics are ameliorated by the dopamine receptor blocking agent haloperidol. Genetic factors are also operant.

Clinical Features

Onset of motor and vocal tics is generally between the ages of 5 and 10 years. The motor tics seen most frequently consist of stereotyped and repetitive head jerking, shrugging of shoulders, twisting motions of the trunk and body, or skipping. Vocal tics generally consist of repeated sniffing (sometimes erroneously leading to refer-ral to an allergist), grunting or barking noises. Tics characterized by foul utterances (coprolalia) are relatively infrequent in children, but may develop by adulthood. Characteristically, all forms of tics are worsened by anxiety or emotional disturbances, with a tendency towards periodic (generally once in 6 weeks to 6 months) remission and relapse. This disorder is chronic (more than 6 months duration).

There is a greater predilection for males to females (ratio 4:1 to 3:1). Tourette syndrome is most likely transmitted as an autosomal dominant trait with variable penetrance. Questioning and examination of other family members may unearth affected relatives.

Behavioral disorder includes hyperactivity; and acting out can develop either as a direct consequence of the primary neurochemical disturbance, secondary to the social pressures encountered by the child on account of the tics, or from a combination of these factors.

Sleep disturbances commonly observed in Tourette syndrome include disturbed, restless sleep with increased body movements and parasomnias, as well as suppression of slow wave (stages III and IV NREM) sleep.

Differential Diagnosis

Simple tics. The age of onset is not necessarily restricted to the 5-10 year age group characteristically seen with Tourette syndrome. Also, the tendency for frequent remissions and relapse is absent and the disorder is transient.

Chorea. The semipurposive movements of chorea are generally proximal, and in contrast to tics, non-stereotyped and more complex.

Myoclonus. This term applies to brief, involuntary muscle jerks affecting any segment of the body. Unlike tics, they may be non-stereotyped. While some forms of myoclonus are physiological (e.g., hiccups and sleep-onset myoclonus), other varieties may be related to central nervous system dysfunction at cerebral cortical or subcortical levels.

Treatment

The management of a patient with Tourette syndrome calls for a close, long-term working relationship between the physician, patient, and his family.

Pharmacotherapy for tics should be commenced if tics begin to affect the child's emotional health and interpersonal relationships. Haloperidol, generally commenced at a dosage of 0.25-0.5 mg twice a day is the drug of choice. The dosage can be increased to a maximum of 4-5 mg per day. As the natural history of tics in Tourette syndrome is one of periodic remission and relapse, the family should be taught to exercise flexibility in adjusting the dose according to the severity of the tics at a given time. Efforts at complete control of tics usually lead to overmedication; 80-90% control of tics is quite adequate. Side effects of haloperidol include dry mouth, restlessness, depression, and tardive dyskinesia. Clonidine, a central or adrenergic agonist, is an alternate medication in the treatment of Tourette syndrome (dose 0.025 mg twice a day, with dose being increased every 7-10 days to a maximum of 0.15 mg/day). Pimozide and fluphenazine are also effective.

Supportive psychotherapy may be necessary of adolescents. It can be provided through a counselor, voluntary support organizations, or other family members.

Prognosis

The tics in most patients can be satisfactorily controlled using a rotation of the various pharmacological agents, permitting normal day-to-day function. Early studies suggested that Tourette syndrome was a lifelong disorder, with a tendency to periodic remission and relapse. It now appears that the prognosis may be more favorable than previously anticipated. Ehrenberg et al.[4] recently documented that 73% of their 58 subjects had a marked decrease or almost complete disappearance in their tics by adolescence or early adulthood. The likelihood of improvement was not related to severity of the tics, response to therapy, or other identifiable factors.

SYDENHAM'S CHOREA

Described initially in 1684, Sydenham's or rheumatic chorea is the principal neurological manifestation of rheumatic fever. Chorea is an involuntary movement disorder, characterized by rapid, quasi-purposive, non-rhythmic body movements that predominantly affect the head segment, trunk, and proximal extremities. Sydenham's chorea is more common in girls and usually has onset between 3-13 years of age.

Pathophysiology

The disorder is secondary to an immunological disturbance in the central nervous system, triggered by a circulating IgG antibody in response to a Group A streptococcal infection. The reaction is maximal in the regions of the basal ganglia, cerebral, and cerebellar cortices. The cerebral pathology consists of arteritis with cellular degeneration. While a majority of patients have a history of a preceding streptococcal infection, evidence of such infection is absent in approximately a third of the patients at the time of initial presentation. These patients may develop carditis and other manifestations of acute rheumatic fever subsequent to onset of the chorea.

Clinical Features

Rheumatic chorea has insidious onset over days, interrupts voluntary movements, is worsened by apprehension, and subsides during sleep. The choreic movements may sometimes begin unilaterally. The child appears restless and fidgety. Facial grimacing, lizard-like tongue protrusion and retraction, as well as non-rhythmic movements of the shoulders and trunk are common. Inability to sustain muscle contractions leads to indistinct, explosive speech with fluctuations in pitch, and also to rhythmic fist contractions when asked to grasp the examiner's finger ("milkmaid's grip").

Moderate to severe hypotonia results in hyper-extensibility of joints and a tendency to pronate both hands when they are raised above the head, palms facing. In some cases, profound generalized weakness may precede onset of choreic movements, subsiding gradually as the latter become more prominent (chorea malis).

Emotional lability and inappropriate behavior are seen in approximately 60% of the patients.

An elevated serum anti-streptolysin 0 titre, positive throat culture for group A streptococcus, and clinical or electro-cardiographic evidence of carditis (e.g., prolonged PR interval, tachycardia, aortic or mitral insufficiency) are frequently present along with chorea.

Natural History

In about 75% of patients, the chorea resolves spontaneously within six months. A third of the patients may have recurrences, especially along with subsequent streptococcal throat infections and pregnancy.

Differential Diagnosis

Sydenham's chorea should be differentiated from other causes of chorea, which include:

1. **Juvenile Huntington's disease.** Chorea in this progressive disorder is generally associated with dementia. Seizures and rigidity may also be present. In contrast to the sporadic transmission of Sydenham's chorea, Huntington's disease has autosomal dominant transmission. The CT scan may show atrophy of the caudate nuclei.

2. **Cerebral vasculitis secondary to systemic lupus erythematosus** is generally associated with evidence of multisystem involvement and sero-

logical evidence of the disease (positive antinuclear antibody tests with a speckled pattern).

3. **Acute viral encephalitis.** Fever and decreased sensorium are usually also present.

4. **Hematological disorders.** Henoch-Schonlein purpura and polycythemia.

5. **Acute, drug-induced extrapyramidal reaction** secondary to phenothiazines, insoniazid, and phenytoin. Withdrawal of the drug, and additionally in the case of phenothiazines, administration of Benadryl should result in prompt amelioration of the extrapyramidal reaction.

6. **Metabolic and toxic disturbances.** Hypocalcemia, hypomagnesemia and hyperthyroidism; kernicterus, carbon monoxide poisoning and Wilson's disease.

7. **Inborn errors of metabolism.** Lesch-Nyhan syndrome and hyperalaninemia.

8. **Degenerative neurologic disorders.** Ataxia telengiectasia and neuronal ceroid lipofuscinosis.

9. **Benign familial chorea.** This dominantly transmitted disorder has onset generally in infancy or early childhood, is not associated with intellectual dysfunction, is non-progressive, and persists for years.

10. **Choreiform syndrome associated with Attentional Deficit Disorder.** This is most prominent in the distal extremities; impulsivity and poor concentration are also present.

11. **Familial paroxysmal choreoathetosis.** In between episodes of involuntary movements, patients with this disorder are completely normal. Two forms have been described: one precipitated by movements, with dominant or recessive transmission and favorable response to phenytoin; the other being non-kinesigenic, autosomal recessive, and refractory to anticonvulsant therapy.

Management

a. Bedrest is helpful in ameliorating the chorea.

b. Haloperidol in an initial dosage of 0.5-1.0 mg/day, or phenobarbital in a dose of 2-4 mg/kg/day are useful in controlling the movement disorder. The treatment should be continued for a period of 4-6 months, following which it may be gradually tapered and discontinued.

c. If an active streptococcal throat infection is present, treatment with oral penicillin (200-250 mg four times a day for 10 days) or an intramuscular form (benzathine penicillin, single dose of 1.2 million units) is recommended. Lifelong prophylaxis for streptococcal infections is recommended using monthly intramuscular benzathine penicillin injections. Prophylactic intramuscular penicillin should also be administered prior to contemplation of any surgical procedure.

DYSTONIA MUSCULORUM DEFORMANS

Introduction

The term dystonia refers to faulty muscle tone and posture without pyramidal deficit. Oppenheim (1911) was the first to introduce the term dystonia musculorum deformans (DMD) for a distinct, genetically transmitted organic disease that is often misdiagnosed as hysteria.

Epidemiology

The condition is prevalent worldwide, but the highest concentration has been found in Southern Lithuania, adjacent parts of Belorussia and Poland. Patients originating from this region account for approximately one half of the total documented cases in world literature. The disorder is transmitted in an autosomal dominant form with variable expressivity. It is most common amongst the Ashkenazi Jewish population. The male:female ratio for DMD is 1.4:1. The gene has just recently been localized to the long arm of chromosome 9(9q32-q34).[1]

Pathophysiology

The basic electrophysiological abnormality in dystonia consists of simultaneous contraction of agonist and antagonistic muscles upon attempted voluntary movement. While involvement of the putamen, globus pallidus, dentate nucleus, and thalamus has been implied in the causation of DMD, the results cannot be confirmed owing to lack of any single definite pathological finding. A depletion of norepinephrine from the posterior hypothalamus and the locus ceruleus has been documented.[2]

Clinical Features

1. The age of onset may vary, but approximately 60% become symptomatic prior to 15 years of age.

2. The most common dystonic abnormalities consist of difficulty in walking or in use of one or both arms owing to involuntary twisting and turning of body parts during voluntary movement. Walking on the toes or on the lateral aspects of the feet are common early manifestations in children. Dystonic contortions or spasms may be maintained for periods varying from a minute to hours, and are frequently painful. Dystonic involvement of muscles of the face, trunk, tongue, and pharynx may also occur. Blepharospasm, writer's cramp, and torticollis are formes frustes of the disorder.

3. In spite of the grotesque dystonic hyperkinesia, the patient may be able to execute some skilled motor tasks with finesse.

4. The muscle tone may fluctuate between hypertonia and hypotonia. Intellectual and sensory functions, as well as tendon reflexes, are invariably normal.

5. Progression of the disease is not so much by way of aggravation of the initial difficulty as it is by gradual spread to other parts of the body. The life span is generally not altered. Spontaneous remissions may occur in a minority, usually early in the course of the disease. Approximately 50% of patients in whom the disease does not remit progress to generalized dystonia, and the rest continue to have segmental dystonia. Onset in the lower extremities and prior to age 11 years is highly indicative of progression to generalized dystonia.

6. A subgroup of patients who have dystonia combined with resting tremor and a diurnal fluctuation in the severity of the dystonia and a favourable response to L-Dopa has also been reported.[3]

Diagnostic Prerequisites

1. Normal perinatal history and early development.

2. No history of a precipitating illness or drug use.

3. No evidence of pyramidal, intellectual, cerebellar, or sensory deficit.

4. Exclusion of symptomatic dystonia (e.g., Wilson's disease, see differential diagnosis).

Differential Diagnosis

To begin with, **dystonia** must be distinguished from **athetosis**, which is also characterized by twisting body movements. In contrast to athetosis, dystonic movements are more powerful and sustained for longer periods of time. Denny-Brown however, equated the two by stating that "the beginning of dystonia musculorum deformans is essentially athetoid in character."

Chorea. This movement disorder is more rapid and associated with normal or decreased muscle tone.

Symptomatic dystonia. The causes are varied and include perinatal hypoxia, kernicterus, head trauma, viral encephalitis, drugs (phenytoin, phenothiazines), carbon monoxide poisoning, Wilson's disease, and GM_2 gangliosidosis.

Treatment

Pharmacological measures generally do not lead to resolution of the disorder, but may suppress dystonia to the point of making the patient comfortable and able to handle activities related to daily living.

Trihexiphenidyl (ARTANE) in a starting dosage of 1-2 mg/day that is gradually increased to 25-30 mg/day, carbamazepine, diazepam, bromocriptine, and tetrabenazine have all been used with variable success. In a variant characterized by association with tremor and rigidity, the carbidopa/levo dopa combination, administered as SINEMET, 1-2 tablets of 10/100 mg/day is also helpful.

Cryothalamectomy may induce a remission in patients with hemidystonia. Owing to the high incidence of relapse, the status of this modality of treatment remains controversial.

Physical and occupational therapy are of value in helping the patient cope with activities of daily living and in preventing contractures.

MYOCLONUS

Myoclonus is a nonspecific term that describes quick muscle jerks generally affecting a segment of the body. If repetitive, they are usually arrythmic. When involving the upper extremities, myoclonus may result in flinging of objects held in the hand; when the trunk or lower extremities are involved, there may be sudden forceful trunk flexion or fall to the floor. It may occur spontaneously or in response to auditory, visual, and tactile stimuli (stimulus-sensitive myoclonus).

Classification[4]

I. **Epileptic myoclonus** (muscles contracting in the same jerk are activated synchronously; simultaneous EEG paroxysmal correlates can be identified), e.g., myoclonic seizures and epilepsia partialis continua.

II. **Non-epileptic myoclonus** (asynchronous contraction of muscles, no simultaneous paroxysmal EEG correlate).

a. Dystonic myoclonus (fragment of an involuntary movement disorder with basal ganglionic origin).

b. Ballism (large amplitude flinging movements, usually involving the upper extremities due to subthalamic nuclear involvement).

c. Startle response to auditory, visual or tactile stimuli.

d. Physiological myoclonus (hiccups, sneezing, sleep-onset body jerks).

e. Periodic movements in sleep (nocturnal myoclonus).

f. Segmental, including spinal and palatal myoclonus.

g. Benign myoclonus of infancy (a maturational disturbance of subcortical origin which mimics myoclonic seizures; the development, neurological exam, and EEG are completely normal; spontaneous resolution is seen within months).

h. Opsoclonus-myoclonus syndrome (opsoclonus is a disorder characterized by irregular, chaotic involuntary eye movements; the myoclonus generally affects the distal parts of the extremities). The disorder usually develops as an immune response to a systemic viral infection or occult neuroblastoma. Spinal fluid immunoglobulins may be elevated. Most patients have a favorable response to corticosteroid therapy (4-6 week course).

Etiology

Pathological forms of myoclonus may result from central nervous dysfunction at the cortical or subcortical levels. Some common etiological factors include hypoxic encephalopathy, kernicterus, fluid and electrolyte imbalance, hepatic encephalopathy, lysosomal storage diseases such as sialidosis, myoclonic epilepsies, and degenerative neurological illnesses, e.g., subacute sclerosing panencephalitis. The opsoclonus-myoclonus syndrome may be a non-metastic manifestation of an occult neuroblastoma or post-infectious (viral) autoimmune central nervous system disturbance. Spinal fluid immunoglobulins may be elevated in this disorder.

Management

This varies with the underlying cause. In some instances the myoclonus abates spontaneously, along with resolution of the underlying metabolic encephalopathy, e.g., flapping tremor of hepatic coma. Anticonvulsants like sodium valproate and clonazepam are indicated in the treatment of epileptic myoclonus. An alteration in serotonergic functions at the level of the brainstem and cerebellum probably underlies post-anoxic intention myoclonus and nocturnal myoclonus. A favorable response is therefore observed in both following treatment with clonazepam, a serotonergic agonist. Corticosteroids may be useful in the treatment of the opsoclonus-myoclonus syndrome.

ESSENTIAL TREMOR

Clinical Features

Tremor is an involuntary movement caused by rapid, alternating, to and fro contraction of opposing groups of muscles. Essential tremor is transmitted as an autosomal dominant trait, or may develop de novo following a mutation. The age of onset is usually between 5 and 15 years.

Unlike the tremor of Parkinson's disease, essential tremor is characteristically absent at rest and worse in the terminal phase of a voluntary movement. It is coarse, rhythmic, and most commonly affects muscles of the hands and neck. It may adversely affect the quality of the child's handwriting. Intelligence, sensation, coordination, reflexes, and gait remain unimpaired. Examination of other family members may disclose affected relatives. Essential tremor is lifelong, but does not progress beyond a certain degree.

Differential Diagnosis

Wilson's disease. The tremor is more coarse and also present at rest. The muscle tone is usually increased. Kayser-Fleischer rings are invariably present, the serum ceruloplasmin is low, and plasma copper levels are elevated.

Tremor associated with hyperthyroidism is fine in amplitude. Tremor associated with drug withdrawal states, e.g., alcohol, has a brief history and may be associated with alteration in mental status and autonomic dysfunction, e.g., sweating, tachycardia.

Physiological tremor. Normal individuals may experience tremor under stressful situations such as fright and apprehension. It is generally transient.

Treatment

Essential tremor responds favorably to treatment with the beta adrenergic blocker, propranolol. An initial dosage of 10 mg twice a day is recommended. It may be increased to a total of 60-80 mg per day. The therapy may be required life-long; periodic drug holidays (e.g., during the summer vacations) are therefore advisable in order to maximize drug effect when prolonged use is necessary. Primidone (MYSOLINE) in a dose of 125-250 mg/day is also effective.

ATHETOSIS

This abnormal posture is characterized by predominantly distal, slow, snake-like twisting combined with flexion, extension, and pronation at the distal joints, particularly in the upper extremi-

Table 8-1. Comparison of common movement disorders

	Athetosis	Chorea	Tremor	Tics	Myoclonus
Description	Distal, snake-like, twisting	Proximal semipurposive	Proximal or distal, rhythmic, fine oscillations	Proximal or distal, stereotypic contraction of groups of muscles	Proximal or distal, non-stereotyped/ stereotyped contraction of muscle groups
Speed	Slow	Rapid	Rapid	Rapid	Rapid
Amplitude	Large	Large	Small	Intermediate	Intermediate to large
Rhythmicity	Absent	Absent	Present	Present	Absent
Common etiological factors	Perinatal hypoxia, kernicterus, viral encephalitis, head trauma, drug reaction (e.g., to phenothiazines)	Rheumatic fever, benign familial, drugs (e.g., phenytoin), Huntington's disease	Familial, anxiety, drug withdrawal, Wilson's disease	Idiopathic (simple tics) Tourette syndrome	Physiologic (e.g., hiccups), metabolic encephalopathies, degenerative diseases (e.g., SSPE)

ties. The movements are slower than chorea, but frequently combined with it (choreoathetosis). Basal ganglionic dysfunction, especially involving the putamen, has been implicated. Common etiological factors include kernicterus, perinatal hypoxia, central nervous system infections, and phenothiazine ingestion.

SPASMUS NUTANS

This disorder has onset between 3 and 12 months of age and is characterized by a triad of repetitive head nodding, head tilt, and nystagmus. The development and neurological examination are otherwise completely normal. Viral encephalitis may precede the onset of spasmus nutans in some instances, but no definite etiology can be identified in the majority of patients. The disorder is benign, self-limiting, and almost always resolves spontaneously by the age of 3 years.

BOBBLE-HEAD DOLL SYNDROME

Repetitive head nodding movements in infants may sometimes be associated with a third ven

tricular mass and obstructive hydrocephalus. In contrast to spasmus nutans, developmental delay, bulging anterior fontanelle, lethargy, vomiting, macrocephaly, and abnormal tendon reflexes are frequently present along with the head nodding. The diagnosis of an intraventricular mass can be readily established using a CT scan.

MOVEMENT DISORDERS

Table 8-1 lists and compares various aspects of the common movement disorders.

REFERENCES

1. Ozelius l, Kramer P, Moskowitz C, et al. Human gene for torsion dystonia located on chromosome 9q32-q34. Neuron 1989; in press.

2. Hornykiewcz O, Kish SJ, Becker LE, et al. Brain neurotransmitters in dystonia musculorum deformans. N Eng J Med 315:347-353, 1986.

3. Nygaard TC, Duvoisin RC. Hereditary dystonia-parkinsonism syndrome of juvenile onset. Neurology 36:1424-1428, 1986.

4. Hallett M. Myoclonus: relation to epilepsy. Epilepsia 26(Suppl 1):67-77, 1985

SUGGESTED READING

1. Butler IJ. Tourette syndrome. Some new concepts. Neurologic Clinics 2(3):571-579, 1984.

2. Singer HS, Butler IJ, Tune LE, Seifert WE and Coyle JT. Dopaminergic dysfunction in Tourette Syndrome. Ann Neurol 12(4):361-366, 1982.

3. Nee LE, Caine ED, Polinsky RJ, Eldredge R. and Ebert MH. Gilles de la Tourette syndrome: clinical and family study of 50 cases. Ann Neurol 7:41-49, 1980.

4. Erenberg G, et al. The natural history of Tourette syndrome: a follow up study. Ann Neurol 22:383-385, 1987.

5. Aaron AM, Freeman JM and Garter S. The natural history of Sydenham's Chorea. Am J Med 38:83-93, 1965.

6. Chun RWM, Daly RF, Mansheim BJ and Wolcott GJ. Benign familial chorea. J Amer Med Assoc 225(13):1603-1607, 1973.

7. Goodenough DJ, Fariello RG, Annis BL and Chun RWM, Familial and acquired paroxysmal dyskinesias. Arch Neurol 35:827-831, 1978.

8. Cartwright GE, Diagnosis of treatable Wilson's Disease. N Engl J Med 298(24):1347-1350, 1978.

9. Marsden CD and Harrison MJG, Idiopathic torsion dystonia. A review of 42 patients. Brain 97:793-810, 1974.

10. Marsden CD, Marion MH, Quinn N. The treatment of severe dystonia in children and adults. J Neurol Neurosurg Psychiatry 47:1166-1173, 1984.

11. Fahn S. The varied clinical expressions of dystonia. Neurol Clin 2(3):541-554, 1984.

12. Burke RE, Fahn S and Marsden CD. Torsion dystonia: a double-blind, prospective trial of high-dosage trihexyphenidyl. Neurology 36(2):160-164, 1986.

13. Chadwick D, Hallett M, Harris R, Jenner P, Reynolds EH and Marsden CD. Clinical biochemical and physiological features distinguishing myoclonus responsive to 5-hydroxytroptophan, tryptophan with a monoamine oxidase inhibitor and clonazepam. Brain 100:455-487, 1977.

14. Coleman RM, Pollak CP, Weitzman ED. Periodic movements in sleep (nocturnal myoclonus): relation to sleep disorders. Ann Neurol 8:416-421, 1980.

15. Keepers GA and Casey DE. Clinical management of acute neuroleptic-induced extrapyramidal syndromes. Curr Psychiatr Ther 23:139-157, 1986.

MICROCEPHALY

DEFINITION

Microcephaly is defined as presence of occipito-frontal circumference that is below two standard deviations for age, sex, and gestational age. For infants born prematurely, correction needs to be made throughout the first year of life for the abbreviated gestational period in order to ensure accurate plotting of head size. Myelination, neuronal and glial cell proliferation, cerebellar growth and synaptognesis are important physiologic correlates of enlargement in brain size. There is little, if any, inter-racial difference in the rate of head growth.

HISTORICAL ASSESSMENT

The history should address insults during pregnancy (exposure to drugs or radiation, viral infections, and maternal diseases such as diabetes or hypertension that could lead to uteroplacental insufficiency), perinatal insults (hypoxia, hypoglycemia, hyperbilirubinemia, status epilepticus, bacterial meningitis, trauma) and encephalopathies in infancy (e.g., inborn errors of aminoacid or carbohydrate metabolism, trauma, or central nervous system infections). Microcephaly apparent at birth may be associated with other congenital malformations or congenital intrauterine infections (toxoplasmosis, cytomegalovirus, herpes simplex, rubella, or syphilis) or cerebrovascular accidents. On some occasions, however, microcephaly at birth is not associated with any other disorder and is autosomal recessive; in such instances it is termed microcephaly vera or primary microcephaly. The physician should also inquire about commonly associated manifestations such as seizures, motor and intellectual developmental delay, feeding difficulties, strabismus, hearing and visual function.

MICROCEPHALY AND INTELLIGENCE

In an unselected group of 9379 children studied under the NIH Collaborative Project on Cerebral Palsy, head circumference of less than 43 cm in a boy or less than 42 cm in a girl at one year of age was associated with an approximately 50% chance of I.Q. being less than 80 at age four years.[1] The association between microcephaly and intellectual dysfunction is, however, by no means invariable, and some microcephalic children have normal intelligence. Intellectual dysfunction is more likely to be present when there is associated retardation in linear growth and when the head circumference is below three, rather than two, standard deviations for age.

SUGGESTED INVESTIGATIONS

1. **Chromosome studies** to exclude trisomy and partial deletion syndromes.

2. **Serum IgM and titers** on mother and patient (or umbilical cord) blood for toxoplasmosis,

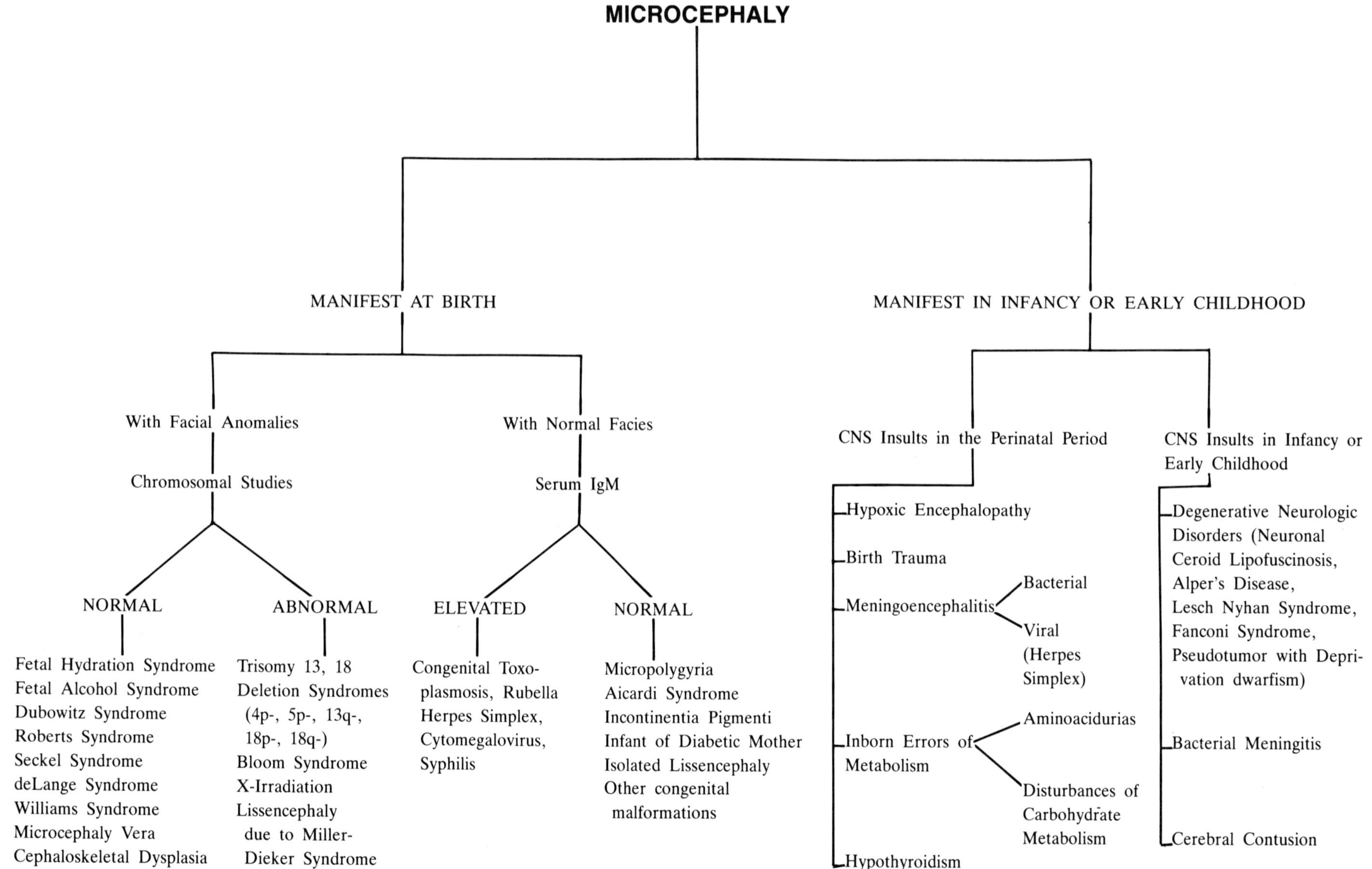

MICROCEPHALY
MANIFEST AT BIRTH
With Facial Anomalies
Chromosomal Studies
NORMAL
Fetal Hydration Syndrome
Fetal Alcohol Syndrome
Dubowitz Syndrome
Roberts Syndrome
Seckel Syndrome
deLange Syndrome
Williams Syndrome
Microcephaly Vera
Cephaloskeletal Dysplasia
ABNORMAL
Trisomy 13, 18
Deletion Syndromes (4p-, 5p-, 13q-, 18p-, 18q-)
Bloom Syndrome
X-Irradiation
Lissencephaly due to Miller-Dieker Syndrome
With Normal Facies
Serum IgM
ELEVATED
Congenital Toxoplasmosis, Rubella Herpes Simplex, Cytomegalovirus, Syphilis
NORMAL
Micropolygyria
Aicardi Syndrome
Incontinentia Pigmenti
Infant of Diabetic Mother
Isolated Lissencephaly
Other congenital malformations
MANIFEST IN INFANCY OR EARLY CHILDHOOD
CNS Insults in the Perinatal Period
Hypoxic Encephalopathy
Birth Trauma
Meningoencephalitis
Bacterial
Viral (Herpes Simplex)
Inborn Errors of Metabolism
Aminoacidurias
Disturbances of Carbohydrate Metabolism
Hypothyroidism
CNS Insults in Infancy or Early Childhood
Degenerative Neurologic Disorders (Neuronal Ceroid Lipofuscinosis, Alper's Disease, Lesch Nyhan Syndrome, Fanconi Syndrome, Pseudotumor with Deprivation dwarfism)
Bacterial Meningitis
Cerebral Contusion

rubella, cytomegalovirus, herpes simplex, and syphilis (TORCHS) to exclude, intrauterine infections.

3. **Blood and urine aminoacid screens, blood ammonia** to rule out inborn errors of metabolism such as phenylketonuria. If these qualitative screens are abnormal, quantitative 24-hour urine amino acid chromatography should be carried out.

4. **Blood sugar, serum lactate and pyruvate levels, urinary reducing substances assay** are helpful in screening for inborn errors of carbohydrate metabolism. If abnormal, consideration should be given towards obtaining specific tissue assays (e.g., red cell galactose-1-phosphate uridyl transferase assay for galactosemia, or liver biopsy to diagnose glycogen storage diseases, fructose 1, 6-diphosphate deficiency, and disorders affecting the pyruvate dehydrogenase complex).

5. **Serum thyroxine, thyroid stimulating hormone** to exclude hypothyroidism.

6. **Electroencephalogram.** Abnormalities noted on the EEG are generally not specific for any neurologic disorder, but do indicate whether the abnormality of cortical function is focal or diffuse, paroxysmal, or non-paroxysmal as well as its severity.

7. **Conjunctival and skin biopsy** are helpful in establishing a diagnosis of certain degenerative neurological disorders like neuronal ceroid lipofuscinosis in which characteristic inclusions are seen upon electronmicroscopy.

8. **Computed Cranial Tomography (CT).** This is useful in determining congenital malformations such as porencephaly, holoprosencephaly, and agenesis of the corpus callosum. Intracranial calcification associated with congenital intrauterine infections can be seen far more readily with CT than on skull x-rays. Ventricular dilatation secondary to atrophy of the periventricular white matter and prominent cortical sulci and gyri (indicating cortical atrophy) can also be easily visualized using CT.

9. **Brainstem Auditory Evoked Potentials and behavioral audiometry** are indicated for assessing hearing and brainstem function in children who have suffered congenital intrauterine infections, bacterial meningitis, or neonatal bilirubin encephalopathy (kernicterus).

10. **Urine culture** for cytomegalovirus.

SUGGESTED READING

1. Nelson KB and Deutschberger J. Head size at one year as a predictor of four-year I.Q. Develop Med Chil Neurol 12:487-495, 1970.

2. Martin H. Microcephaly and mental retardation. Am J Dis Child 119:128, 1970.

3. Jones KL, ed. Smith's Recognizable Patterns of Human Malformation. W.B. Saunders, Philadelphia, 4th edition, 1988.

CHAPTER X

MACROCEPHALY

NORMAL GROWTH IN HEAD SIZE

Under normal circumstances, brain growth is the most important correlate of growth in size of the head. Neuronal and glial cell proliferation, synaptogenesis, myelination, and cerebellar growth contribute to increase in brain size. Serial measurements of the occipito-frontal circumference (OFC) form an accurate index of intracranial volume and help follow the course of the disorder. The rate of head growth in healthy premature infants in the first and second extrauterine months is roughly double that of healthy full-term infants and averages approximately 1.1 cm/week. In premature infants recovering from a non-neurological illness (e.g., respiratory distress syndrome), head growth may go through three separate phases: for the initial 2-4 weeks after birth coinciding with the period of acute systemic illness, there may be little or no increase in head size. The second phase is of approximately 6-8 weeks duration, during which head growth parallels the normal curve. The third phase occurs around 38-40 weeks post-conceptional age and is characterized by a period of catch-up growth. Intracranial pathology should be suspected when catch-up growth occurs earlier than age 2-10 weeks after birth, if it is too little, or delayed. In uncomplicated infants born at full-term, the rate of head growth in the first three months is 2 cm/month, in the second three months 1 cm/month, and 0.5 cm/month in the subsequent six months.

CLINICAL ASSESSMENT

1. Occipito-frontal circumference should be carefully obtained and plotted on growth grids appropriate for preterm and term infants. Correction should be made for abbreviated gestation in premature infants whenever the head circumference is plotted on a standard head growth chart after the first 10-12 weeks of life.

2. Transillumination of the skull should be routinely carried out in a dark room using a standard light source (Chun gun). Transillumination is a valuable bedside aid in the diagnosis of cystic, fluid-filled intracranial lesions such as hydrocephalus or chronic subdural effusion. The normal zone of transillumination varies between 1-2 cm from the center of the light source in the occipital regions to 2-3 cm in the frontal regions. Transillumination is normally dependent upon a number of factors, including skull thickness, diameter of the subarachnoid space, and water content of the cortex and white matter. The zones of transillumination may be increased in patients with chronic subdural fluid collections, hydrocephalus, and intracranial cystic lesions like hydranencephaly and porencephaly. Transillumination may be attenuated in the presence of excessive skull thickness and should not be relied upon exclusively beyond the first year of life to evaluate for fluid-filled intracranial lesions. It may be increased spuriously in the presence of scalp edema or an excessively thin skull.

3. Depression in the level of consciousness, palpable splitting of sutures, a tense, bulging anterior fontanelle, neck stiffness, the "sunset" sign (tonic downward deviation of the eyes together with retraction of the upper eyelid) indicate increased intracranial pressure.

4. Examination of the fundus may disclose cherry red macular lesions in some of the gray matter storage diseases such as GM_2 gangliosidosis. In the leukodystrophies, optic disc pallor and a poorly sustained pupillary light reaction may be seen.

5. In the initial phase of hydrocephalus, ventricular dilatation is directed supero-laterally, resulting in an altitudinal change in pyramidal system function. As pyramidal fibers subserving the lower extremities closely approximate the supero-lateral aspect of the lateral ventricles, they are the first to be affected by the ventricular dilatation, leading to lower extremity spasticity and hyperreflexia.

6. The patient should be examined for cutaneous lesions suggestive of neurofibromatosis or tuberous sclerosis. Family history in these patients is usually positive for epilepsy or mental retardation. Familial megalencephaly may be autosomal recessive or autosomal dominant. OFC measurements of family members and examination of their childhood photographs may also help establish this diagnosis.

7. With the exception of pseudotumor cerebri, most megalencephalic disorders are associated with variable degrees of intellectual dysfunction. Motor, intellectual, and social developmental milestones should be elicited during history taking. If pseudotumor cerebri is suspected, the physician should inquire about ingestion by both the infant and the mother (if she is breast feeding) of medications which could precipitate this condition.

ASSOCIATED DISORDERS

Hydrocephalus

Ventricular dilatation owing to an increase in size of the pool of cerebrospinal fluid constitutes hydrocephalus. With the exception of choroid plexus papilloma, which may cause overproduction of CSF, hydrocephalus is generally related to obstruction in the drainage of CSF. Cerebrospinal fluid is normally formed by the choroid plexus and in the interstitium of the cerebral white matter. The normal rate of formation is 0.3 ml/minute. The CSF drains caudally from the lateral ventricles under the influence of gravity as well as pulsations of the choroid plexus vessels. It emerges from the fourth ventricle through the foramina of Luschka, enters the superficial subarachnoid space, and from there drains across the parasagittal arachnoid villi into the venous sinuses.

Hydrocephalus apparent at birth in a full-term infant is usually of the **non-communicating** type (i.e., there is an impediment in communication between the ventricular system and the superficial subarachnoid spaces). It may be secondary to congenital aqueductal stenosis, Dandy Walker syndrome, or the Arnold Chiari malformation. Non-communicating hydrocephalus may develop postnatally in premature infants following intraventricular hemorrhage. Owing to the extremely soft consistency of the periventricular white matter in preterm infants, ventricular enlargement may lag behind cranial enlargement by 7 to 10 days.

Communicating hydrocephalus is usually related to obliteration of the superficial subarachnoid spaces following subarachnoid hemorrhage or bacterial meningitis and is almost always of postnatal onset.

Brain dysfunction in hydrocephalus is partly related to increased intracranial pressure. In the acute or subacute stages of hydrocephalus there may also be a secondary reduction in cerebral blood flow. Transependymal seepage of cerebrospinal fluid also leads to demyelination of the adjacent white matter.

Chronic Subdural Hematoma of Infancy

Direct or indirect trauma, as in whip-lash type shaking of infants, may result in venous hemorrhage into the subdural space. With time, a semipermeable membrane forms around the localized area of hemorrhage. A local increase in osmotic pressure relative to the intravascular space leads to further accumulation of fluid within the subdural space, ultimately causing macrocephaly, increased intracranial pressure, and increased transillumination. A high index of suspicion for child abuse should always be kept in this disorder. Tell-tale, flame-shaped retinal hemorrhages (seen frequently after vigorous shaking of infants) or fractures in varying stages of healing on a skeletal X-ray survey help establish the diagnosis of the battered child syndrome. On other occasions, chronic subdural hematoma may be a consequence of birth trauma. The management involves serial, daily taps of the subdural space through the open anterior fontanelle using a short bevelled, wide bore subdural needle. If the effusion does not resolve completely in about two weeks with repeated subdural taps, consideration may need to be given to placement of a subdural-peritoneal shunt.

Post-meningitic Subdural Effusion

Bacterial meningitis (particularly of the Hemophilus influenzae type) may be associated with a sterile effusion in the subdural space, manifesting with increase in head size and transillumination. Most such effusions resolve spontaneously in 7-10 days coincident with resolution of the meningeal inflammatory process. However, development of subdural empyema should be suspected when resolution of the meningitis is delayed. It is usually associated with signs of increased intracranial pressure, locally increased transillumination, stupor, rapidly enlarging head size, and persistent fever. Management requires periodic aspiration of the subdural fluid, as well as ensuring adequate antibiotic coverage.

Pseudotumor Cerebri

This condition usually results in brain swelling due to increase in brain water content from impaired absorption of CSF at the level of arachnoid granulations. Pseudotumor cerebri is usually seen in male infants and obese adolescent females. It may be associated with hypoparathyroidism, pseudohypoparathyroidism, use of steroids, tetracycline, nalidixic acid, hypervitaminosis A and D, steroid withdrawal, and intracranial venous sinus thrombosis. Papilledema is generally present in older children, but may be absent in infants. The diagnosis can be established by the presence of subacute evolution of manifestations of increased intracranial pressure, i.e., macrocephaly, suture splitting, papilledema, tense bulging anterior fontanelle, occasional compression of ventricles on cranial CT, and normal or low CSF protein. The management consists of removal of the precipitating agent e.g., hypervitaminosis, and daily withdrawal of CSF (10-15 ml) by serial lumbar punctures for 10-14 days. Weight reduction is useful in obese adolescents and the use, if necessary, of oral hyperosmolar agents like glycerol also lowers intracranial pressure. The disorder is self-limiting in most children, resolving spontaneously in 3-6 months.

Tuberous Sclerosis and Neurofibromatosis

These neurocutaneous syndromes are associated with postnatal megalencephaly. Histologically, this correlates with excessive proliferation of glial and neuronal cells. Patients with neurofibromatosis may also occasionally develop aqueductal stenosis leading to hydrocephalus. Central nervous system neoplasms (e.g., astrocytoma) may also evolve in either condition. Family history, examination for the characteristic skin lesions, and CT scan help establish the diagnosis (Refer to Chapter XI).

Familial Megalencephaly

This is a relatively common, benign disorder with either autosomal dominant or recessive transmission. Involvement of other family members can be established by inspection of family pictures and measurement of head size of all family members. There are no signs of increased intracranial pressure. The CT head scan is normal. Most individuals are either of normal or low normal intelligence.

Metabolic Megalencephaly

Lysosmal enzyme deficiencies resulting in central nervous system lipid storage are sometimes associated with megalencephaly and signs of increased intracranial pressure (e.g., split sutures). Patients with gray matter storage diseases may additionally manifest dementia, seizures, macular degeneration, and hypotonia. Those with white matter storage diseases may have spasticity, hyperreflexia, and ataxia.

INVESTIGATIONS

Skull X-Rays

Suture splitting secondary to increased intracranial pressure may occur anytime during the first 12-13 years, in particular in children of less than 3-4 years of age. With long standing increase in intracranial pressure, there may be an increase in the cranio-facial ratio, which is normally 3:1 to 4:1. Erosion of the clinoid processes and a "beaten silver" appearance of the calvarium are other radiologic markers of increased intracranial pressure. Macrocephalic patients with hydrocephalus, chronic subdural hematoma, intracranial mass lesions, and metabolic megalencephaly usually demonstrate x-ray evidence of increased intracranial pressure.

Computed Tomography

Contrast computed tomography will readily help establish the presence of structural central nervous system disease and the specific diagnosis.

Lumbar Puncture

The spinal fluid opening pressure is elevated over 200 mm in pseudotumor cerebri. Care must be taken to minimize spurious elevations in the opening pressure from agitation or from external compression of the venous system in the neck or abdomen. Thorough sedation of the child prior to obtaining the lumbar puncture is essential; some patients with pseudotumor cerebri may also have a low CSF protein content (5-10 mg/dl), which is a dilutional change due to increase in the overall size of the CSF pool. Patients with leukodystrophy generally have a mild elevation in CSF protein and presence of myelin basic protein in the spinal fluid. Children with chronic subdural effusion may also have a mild to moderate increase in spinal fluid protein. Obtaining a cranial CT scan prior to lumbar puncture in macrocephalic children is recommended in order to exclude mass lesions, e.g., neoplasm.

Lysosomal Enzyme Assays

These assays are carried on circulating leukocytes using 5-10 ml of heparinized blood on cultured fibroblasts. They help to establish the nature of the lysosomal storage disease, particularly of disorders commonly associated with macrocephaly (GM_2 gangliosidosis, mucopolysaccharidoses, metachromatic leukodystrophy).

Conjunctival and Rectal Biopsy

Certain neuronal storage diseases such as GM_2 gangliosidosis may be associated with characteristic membranous-cytoplasmic bodies upon electron microscopic examination of the conjunctiva. Distended neurons with eccentrically placed nuclei may be seen upon light microscopy of the rectal submucosal parasympathetic plexus.

A scheme for evaluation of the common disorders associated with macrocephaly is outlined in the algorithm.

MACROCEPHALY

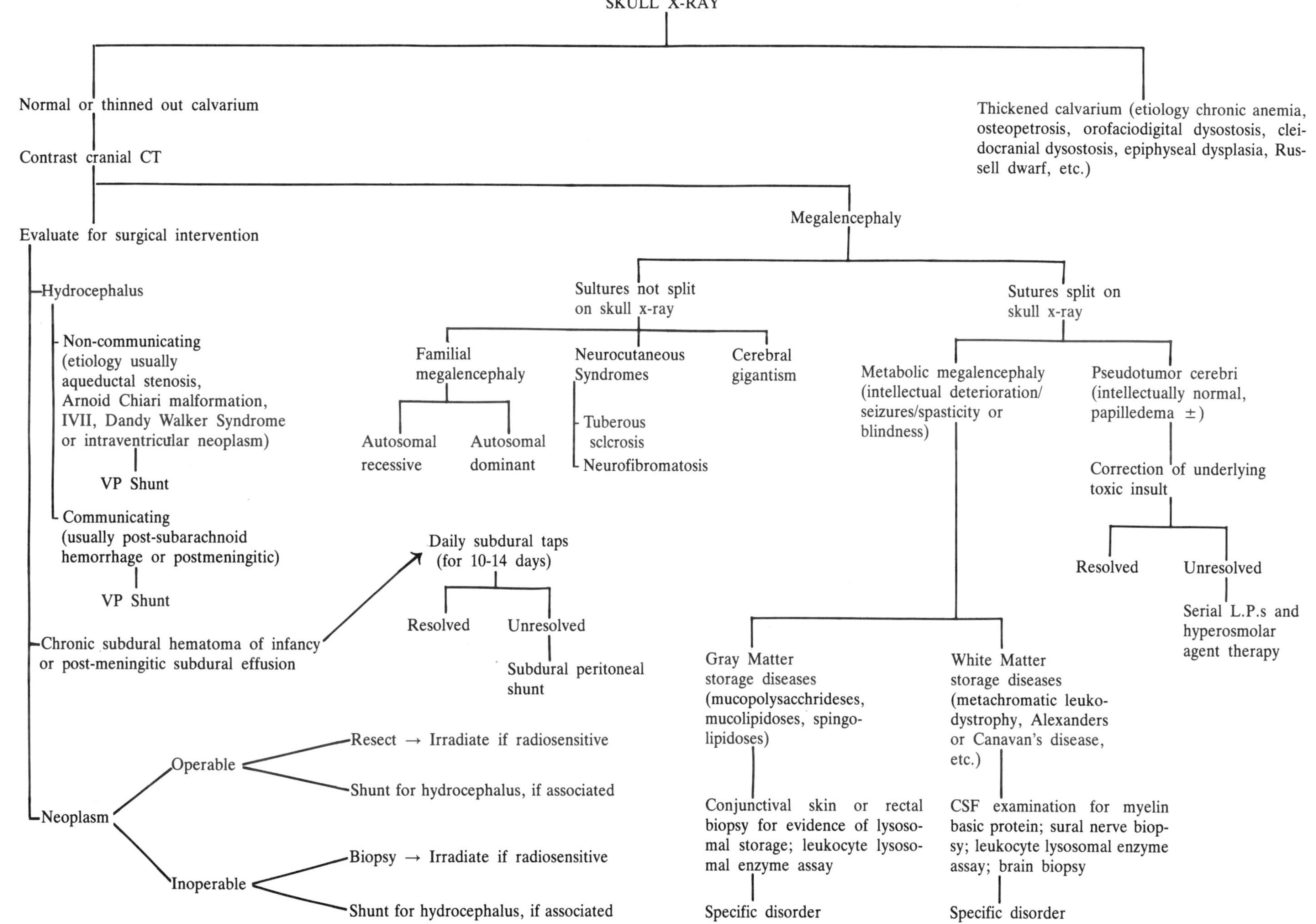

SUGGESTED READING

1. DeMyer W. Megalencephaly in children. Neurology 22:634-643, 1972.

2. Bray PF, Shields WD, Wolcott GJ, et al. Occipito-frontal circumference — an accurate measurement of intracranial volume. J Pediatr 75:303-305, 1969.

3. Brown S, Sher PK, and Wright F. In: Swaiman KF and Wright FS, eds. Practice of Pediatric Neurology. C.V. Mosby Company, St. Louis, 2nd Edition; 9-51, 1982.

4. Rosman NP. Increased intracranial pressure in childhood. Pediatr Clin North Am 21:483, 1974.

5. Marks KH, Maisels MJ, Moore E, et al. Head growth in sick premature infants: a longitudinal study. J Pediatr 94:282-285, 1979.

6. Gaab MR and Koos WT. Hydrocephalus in infancy and childhood: diagnosis and indication for operation. Neuropediatrics 15:173-179, 1984.

7. Barlow CF. CSF dynamics in hydrocephalus — with special attention to external hydrocephalus. Brain and Dev 6:119-127, 1984.

CHAPTER XI

NEUROCUTANEOUS SYNDROMES

Neurofibromatosis

Tuberous Sclerosis

Sturge Weber Syndrome

Ataxia-telangiectasia

von Hippel-Lindau Disease

Incontinentia Pigmenti

Hypomelanosis of Ito

Neurocutaneous syndromes or phakomatoses are a group of unrelated disorders, all characterized by abnormal proliferation, singly or in combination, of ecto, meso, or endodermal elements. The skin and nervous system are most commonly affected. Defective cell migration and proliferation or neoplastic change form the basis for the clinical manifestations. The mode of transmission may be sporadic, autosomal dominant, or recessive. Only the more common of approximately forty documented neurocutaneous syndromes are discussed in this chapter.

NEUROFIBROMATOSIS

These are progressive, dominantly inherited disorders that affect growth of neural tissues. It is currently felt that the eponyms used in the past to describe this group of illnesses should be discarded.

NF-1

Previously known as von Recklinghausen's disease, NF-1 affects about 1 in 4000 individuals. Its transmission has been localized to the nerve growth factor receptor gene on chromosome 17.[1] The disorder is inherited in an autosomal dominant manner with variable penetrance, but may also develop following a spontaneous mutation.

Diagnostic Criteria

Two of the following categories of findings must be present to establish the diagnosis of NF-1.

1. Five or more **cafe-au-lait spots** of over 5 mm in prepubertal children and over 15 mm in postpubertal individuals. In children below the age of three years, the presence of three or more cafe-au-lait lesions of more than 15 mm is also diagnostic.[2]

2. Two or more **neurofibromata** of any type or one **plexiform neurofibroma**. Most neurofibromata are sessile, soft nodules which become apparent in the 2nd or 3rd decade. The patient ultimately develops scores of such lesions. Malignant transformation is a potential complication and is usually heralded by a sudden increase in size, local pain, and fixation to the underlying tissue. The plexiform neurofibroma usually leads to hypertrophy of a limb.

3. **Freckling** in the axillary or inguinal regions.

4. **Optic glioma**. The incidence of such tumors in children with neurofibromatosis may be as high as 15%, some of them being asymptomatic.

5. Two or more **Lisch (iris) nodules**. These are yellowish brown hamartomas which become evident around the limbus and are pathognomic of the disorder. Lewis and Ricardi[3]

found that 92%of a series of 77 patients with NF above the age of six years had iris lesions. Retinal hamartomas, usually of a "mulberry" shape, may also be visible.

6. **Distinctive osseous lesion**, such as sphenoid dysplasia or thinning of long bone cortex, with or without pseudarthrosis.

7. **Presence of a first degree relative** with similar lesions also helps to establish the diagnosis.

Central nervous system lesions in NF-1

Postnatal megalencephaly characterized by excessive cranial enlargement in the first 3 to 4 years is common, with 27 to 69% of children having a head circumference above the 97th percentile. It is usually related to abnormal and excessive proliferation of glial elements.

Seizures of the partial or generalized type may occur as a consequence of abnormal function of glial and nerve cells. The incidence of seizures in children with neurofibromatosis is approximately three to four-fold higher than in the general population.

Mental retardation. Approximately 40% of patients with neurofibromatosis manifest intellectual deficit of some degree or another, with the incidence of mental retardation approaching 5% (2% in the general population).

Neoplasms. Formation of low grade astrocytomas may occur at any age. Optic nerve glioma is the most common neoplasm in children with neurofibromatosis.

Hydrocephalus. Periaqeuductal glial proliferation may lead to aqueductal stenosis and obstructive hydrocephalus.

Miscellaneous Lesions

Orbital dysplasia, hypertension (from pheochromocytoma or renal artery stenosis), rhabdomyosarcoma, scoliosis, visceral neurofibromata, and pruritus are other common manifestations. Failure to thrive is frequently seen in infants and young children. Magnetic resonance imaging studies of the brain may demonstrate focal areas of increased signal intensity on gadolinium enhanced T_1 images, which most likely represent hamartomatous change.

NEUROFIBROMATOSIS-2

Previously termed central neurofibromatosis, this dominant disorder occurs with a frequency of 1 in 50,000, and is transmitted by a gene on chromosome 22. It is most often characterized by the presence of bilateral acoustic neuromas. Alternatively, such patients may have meningiomas, dumbbell-shaped neurofibromata within the spinal canal, and schwannomas. Intellectual function is usually normal. The bilateral eighth nerve tumors are best detected using temporal bone CT scans, gadolinium enhanced MRI, and brainstem auditory evoked potentials.

Suggested Work-Up for Patients with Neurofibromatosis

1. CT head scan or magnetic resonance imaging in case of macrocephaly to exclude hydrocephalus or mass lesions.

2. Gadolinium enhanced magnetic resonance imaging or x-rays of the spine in patients with scoliosis to exclude intraspinal neurofibromata.

3. Psychometric evaluation in children of the preschool and school-going age with a view to making modifications in the school program, when necessary.

4. EEG in patients suspected to have seizures.

5. Skeletal survey in patients with suspected bony lesions.

6. Genetic counselling for all familial cases.

7. Brainstem auditory evoked responses and audiology evaluation in patients with suspected hearing deficits or acoustic neuroma.

8. Periodic monitoring of blood pressure, somatic growth, head circumference, intellectual function, and for neoplastic transformation. This is best carried out through multi-disciplinary clinics dedicated to the follow-up of patients with neurofibromatosis.

TUBEROUS SCLEROSIS

This disorder is also transmitted as an autosomal dominant trait with variable penetrance and occurs with a frequency of 1 in 30,000. It is characterized by involvement mainly of the skin and central nervous system. However, cardiac, renal, and bony abnormalities may also occur. The disorder is gradually progressive over a period of years.

Clinical Manifestations

Cutaneous lesions consist of three types:

Hypopigmented skin patches, sometimes of an ash leaf configuration, are the most common cutaneous manifestation and may become apparent during infancy. Their visualization in fair-skinned children can be enhanced using an ultraviolet light source like the Wood's lamp in a dark room, whereupon the patches can be seen to stand out better in contrast to the adjacent normal skin.

Adenoma sebaceum. These are actually punctate angiofibromata that are raised, reddish and discrete, first becoming visible over the malar region of the face by age 5 years. The lesions should not be mistaken as acne, which has a uniform distribution over the entire face (Fig. 11-1).

Shagreen patches. These raised, irregular skin lesions are commonly seen over the lower back, once again being more prominent in older children.

Neurological manifestations

The incidence of seizures is high, reaching 85 to 93% of the affected inidividuals. Myoclonic and atonic seizures are a common presentation in infancy and early childhood. Generalized tonic-clonic and partial complex seizures may also occur.

Mental retardation. The incidence is estimated at between 40 to 60% of all affected patients. Poorly controlled seizures and sedation from anticonvulsants may further impair intellect.

Neoplastic transformation. Abnormal proliferation of astrocytes may lead to the formation of astrocytomas, in either the supra or infratentorial compartments. This should be suspected anytime there is progressive deterioration in neurological status.

Other organs

Retinal hamartomas (Fig. 11-2), angiolipomas in the kidney, rhabdomyosarcoma in the heart, and subungual fibroma are additional manifestations.

Suggested Work-Up in Patients with Tuberous Sclerosis

1. CT head scan, with and without contrast. The typical periventricular calcification or hypodense parenchymal lesions may be readily seen. CT studies should also be repeated periodically in order to monitor for neoplastic transformation of hamartomas.

2. EEG in patients suspected of having seizures.

3. Psychometric assessment in patients with intellectual impairment to help formulate an appropriate educational program.

4. Genetic counselling.

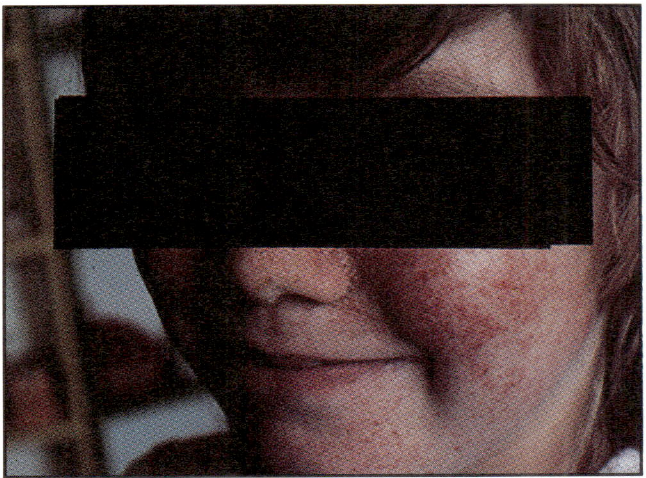

Fig. 11-1. Adenoma sebaceum in a patient with tuberous sclerosis.

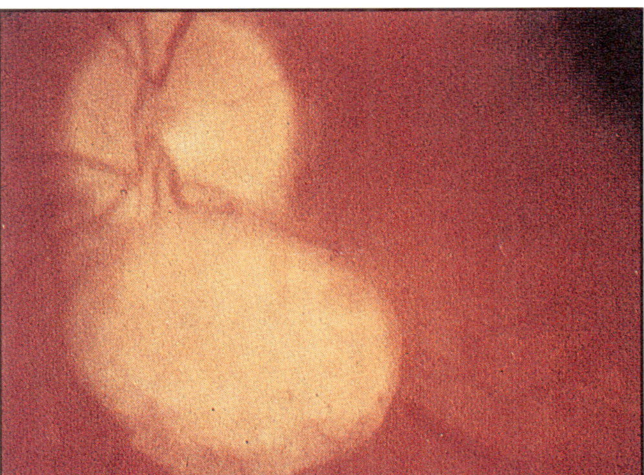

Fig. 11-2. Retinal hamartoma in a patient with tuberous sclerosis.

STURGE WEBER SYNDROME

This disorder is characterized by a port-wine stain facial nevus and an ipsilateral leptomeningeal angiomatous malformation which results in ischemic injury to the underlying cerebral cortex, thereby leading to focal seizures, hemiparesis, hemiatrophy, and variable degrees of intellectual deficit. The condition is transmitted sporadically. Neurological symptoms become manifest usually in infancy or early childhood. The facial nevus invariably involves the region of distribution of the ophthalmic division of the trigeminal nerve; if more extensive, the maxillary and mandibular areas may also be affected. Involvement of the inner canthus of the eye is frequently associated with a defect in formation of the canal of Schlemm. Consequently, about 25% of patients develop congenital glaucoma.

Diagnosis

The diagnosis of Sturge Weber syndrome can be readily established by the presence of the facial nevus combined with CT scan findings consisting of gyral calcification and cortical atrophy ipsilateral to the facial hemangioma (Fig. 11-3). The calcification, which has a serpentine "railroad" configuration, may also be seen on skull x-rays when it is dense.

Management

Management includes prescription of an appropriate anticonvulsant for the seizures. They may be particularly difficult to control in the first two to three years of life. Resection of the involved cerebral cortex should be considered when a child of less than 12-18 months has seizures refractory to

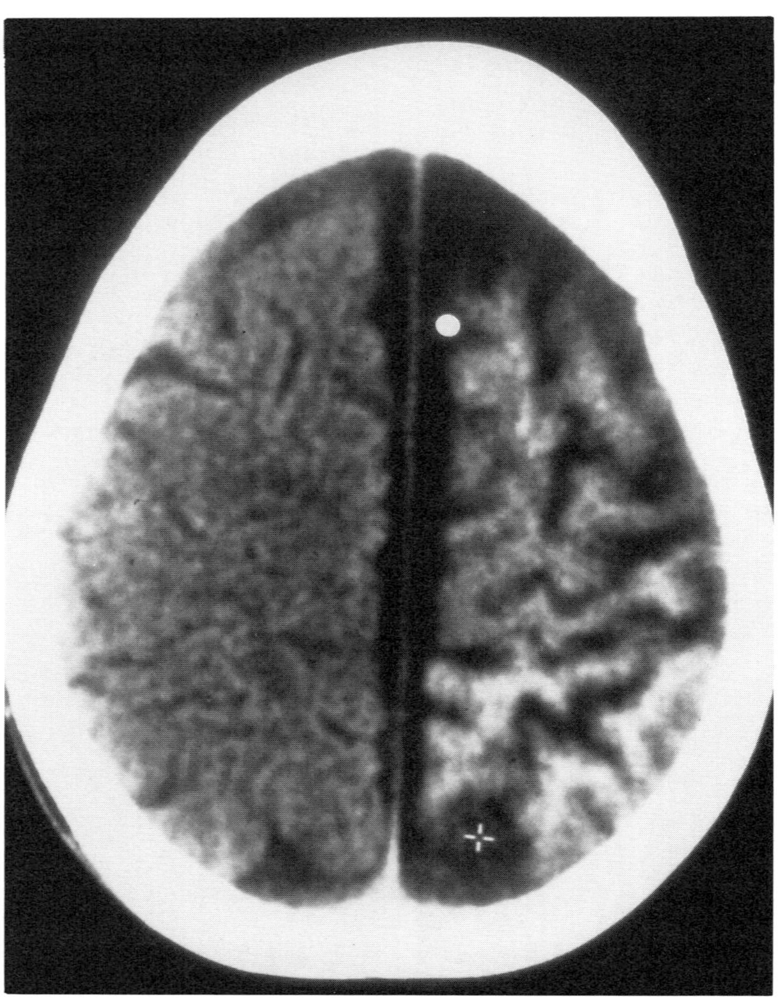

Fig. 11-3. CT scan of patient with Sturge-Weber syndrome, demonstrating gyral calcification and atrophy.

anticonvulsant therapy. Psychometric evaluation and placement in a preschool program at the earliest are also called for in all patients in order to compensate for the intellectual deficit. As the child becomes older, orthopedic consultation may be necessary to assist in managing scoliosis resulting from asymmetry in length of the lower extremities, as well as from asymmetric paraspinal muscle contraction.

ATAXIA TELANGIECTASIA

This disorder is characterized by telangiectatic conjunctival and skin lesions, progressive cerebellar degeneration, and immunological disturbances, as well as a propensity to develop neoplasms. It is generally sporadic, but autosomal recessive transmission has also been documented.

Clinical Manifestations

Myoclonus and choreoathetoid movements are the early manifestations, becoming apparent by 5 years. Subsequently, progressive ataxia becomes evident. It is secondary to a combination of degeneration of the cerebellar parenchyma and sensory tracts in the spinal cord. Hypotonia from cerebellar or anterior horn cell degeneration is another manifestation.

Telangiectatic lesions develop on the bulbar conjunctiva by the age of 5-6 years. Similar lesions may be subsequently seen over the pinnae and malar regions of the face.

Both **cell mediated and humoral immunity** are impaired, the former characterized by a decrease in the population of T cells, the latter be decreased IgA and IgE levels. The immunological disorder leads to a tendency to increased sinopulmonary infections in early childhood and a high incidence of reticuloendothelial malignancies in the 2nd and 3rd decades of life.

Diagnosis

a. The presence immunological abnormalities in a child with cerebellar ataxia is highly suggestive of the disorder.

b. An elevated serum alpha fetoprotein level is also considered diagnostic and can be applied in establishing a prenatal diagnosis.

Management

Management is essentially symptomatic, consisting of treatment of systemic infections and provision of radiotherapy and chemotherapy for malignant complications. While antibiotics and immunoglobulin transfusion may help combat systemic infections, no therapy is available for the central nervous system manifestations, which are steadily progressive.

von HIPPEL-LINDAU SYNDROME

Retinal hemangioma and cerebellar hemangioblastoma characterize this disorder, which usually becomes symptomatic in the second decade. The retinal lesion may give an appearance of clumps of abnormally dilated vessels. The cerebellar hemangioblastoma may produce ataxia or signs of increased intracranial pressure. Polycythemia may develop from a tendency of the hemangioblastoma to occasionally produce erythropoeitin. Pancreatic and renal cysts may also develop. It is transmitted in an autosomal dominant manner with variable penetrance. The diagnosis can be readily established by fundoscopy combined with CT scanning of the posterior fossa.

INCONTINENTIA PIGMENTI

Also known as **Block-Sulzberger Syndrome**, this neurocutaneous syndrome can be diagnosed in early infancy or the neonatal period. It is believed to be transmitted by a mutant X-linked gene which is lethal to male offspring in utero. Consequently, the disorder is seen exclusively in females. Cutaneous lesions in the neonatal period consist of vesicles and bullae with an erythematous base. They subsequently progress to hyperkeratosis and hyperpigmentation and form linear streaks or whorls. Patients with this disorder may also have mental retardation, seizures, and focal or bilateral motor deficits. Patchy alopecia, delayed eruption of teeth, microphthalmia and corneal opacities have also been described.

The management is entirely symptomatic and should address the educational, psychological, and social needs of the mentally handicapped child, as well as prescription of an appropriate anticonvulsant for the seizure disorder.

HYPOMELANOSIS OF ITO

This disorder is also know as **incontinentia pigmenti achromians**. It is characterized by whorled hypopigmented skin lesions, central nervous system and musculo-skeletal abnormalities. No clear genetic pattern of transmission or sex predilection are seen. The cutaneous changes usually become apparent in early childhood, but in contrast to those of incontinentia pigmenti, are rarely seen in the neonatal period and are almost a negative image of skin lesions of the latter—*hypo*pigmented whorls and streaks present over the limbs and trunk. Central nervous system manifestations are seen in approximately half the children/seizures, mild mental retardation and macrocephaly being the most frequent. Discrepancy in leg length, scoliosis, and iris heterochromia are other common manifestations.

REFERENCES

1. Seizinger BR, Roleau GA, Ozelius LJ, et al. Genetic linkage of von Recklinghausen's Neurofibromatosis to the nerve growth factor receptor gene. Cell 49:589-594, 1987.

2. Whitehouse D. Diagnostic value of the cafe-au-lait spot in children. Arch Dis Child 41:316-319, 1966

3. Lewis AR and Ricardi VM. Neurofibromatosis: incidence of iris hamartomata. Ophthalmology 88:348-354, 1981

SUGGESTED READING

1. Ricardi VM. von Recklinghausen Neurofibromatosis. N Engl J Med 305:1617-1626, 1981.

2. Neurofibromatosis. National Institutes of Health Consensus Development Conference Statement. 6(12), July 13-15, 1986.

3. Hoffman HJ, Hendrik BE, Dennis M and Armstrong D. Hemispherectomy for Sturge-Weber syndrome. Child's Brain 5:233-248, 1979.

4. Chalub EG. Neurocutaneous syndromes in children. Pediatr Clin North Am 23(3):499-516, 1976.

5. Schwartz MF, Easterly NB, Fretzin DF, Pergament E and Rozenfeld IH. Hypomelanosis of Ito (incontinentia pigmenti achromians): a neurocutaneous syndrome. J Pediatr 90:236-240, 1977.

6. Ross DL, Boleslaw HL, Chun RWM and Gilbert E. Hypomelanosis of Ito (incontinentia pigmenti achromians)—a clinico-pathological study: macrocephaly and gray matter heterotopias. Neurology 32:1013-1016, 1982.

7. O'Doherty NJ and Norman RM. Incontinentia pigmenti (Bloch-Sulzberger syndrome) with cerebral malformation. Dev Med Child Neurol 10:168-174, 1968.

8. MacFarlin DE, Strober D and Waldmann TA. Ataxia-telengiectasia. Medicine 51:281-314, 1972.

9. Gomez MR, Kuntz NL and Westmoreland BF. Tuberous sclerosis, early onset of seizures and mental subnormality: study of discordant, homozygous twins. Neurology 32:604-611, 1982.

10. Neurofibromatosis. National Institutes of Health Consensus Development Conference Statement. vol. 6(12), July 13-15, 1987.

CHAPTER XII

NEUROMUSCULAR DISORDERS

CLINICAL MANIFESTATIONS OF NEUROMUSCULAR DISEASE

Weakness. This is defined as inability to carry out a motor function due to lack of power, and is the hallmark of diseases of the motor unit (anterior horn cell, peripheral nerve, neuromuscular junction, and muscle). Peripheral neuropathy is generally accompanied by distal, symmetric, or asymmetric weakness. This weakness may cause frequent stumbling or falls, interfere with activities like buttoning and zipping clothes, or grasping a crayon or pencil firmly with the fingers.

Myopathies, on the other hand, are usually associated with proximal and symmetric weakness. Myopathic disorders affecting the lower extremities may hinder climbing stairs without holding onto the bannister, or running and hopping. The Gower's sign, a manifestation of hip extensor muscle weakness, is characterized by the patient having to stoop forward and brace his hands against the knees for additional leverage when coming to an erect stance from the supine or sitting position.

Proximal weakness in the shoulder girdle can lead to difficulty in brushing the teeth, combing the hair, or reaching for objects located above the level of the chest. The sternomastoid muscles (neck flexors) are invariably involved in myopathies. Facial muscle weakness can cause difficulty smiling or drinking from a straw. Patients with masseter weakness may have difficulty chewing meat; those with extraocular weakness may develop ptosis or diplopia. A nasal quality to speech, pooling of saliva in the mouth, and dysphagia are indicative of palatal and oropharyngeal muscle dysfunction.

A diurnal fluctuation in severity of the weakness, with worsening towards the evening, is seen in myasthenia gravis, a neuromuscular junction disorder.

Hypotonia, with resultant hyperextensible joints, occurs in most motor unit diseases. However, as the patient starts to become inactive with progression of the disease, contractures may develop around the joints and limit local mobility.

Atrophy. Decrease in muscle mass and consequent prominence of adjacent bony landmarks can occur with any motor unit disease, but is the least prominent in neuromuscular junction disorders.

Fasiculations. These are ripple-like movements of groups of muscle fibers which may become apparent only upon gentle muscle percussion. They accompany active degeneration of anterior horn cells or peripheral nerves.

Muscle tenderness. This may be seen in viral myositis or polymyositis, but absence of pain does not necessarily exclude inflammatory myopathies. Painful cramps, along with myoglobinuria, can occur in metabolic myopathies (McArdle's or type V glycogen storage disease). Pain may also accompany acute denervation in poliomyelitis and infectious polyneuritis.

Abnormal muscle consistency. Normal muscle is firm upon palpation and in individuals with little subcutaneous fat, ridges separating bundles of muscle fibers can be felt when fingers are run lightly across a muscle belly. In Duchenne's muscular dystrophy, the muscles become pseudohypertrophic (large, bulky, but weak, with replacement of muscle fibers by fibro-fatty connective tissue). This confers a doughy feel upon palpation. Denervated muscle may feel soft and flabby.

Myotonia. Delayed relaxation of the muscle, which becomes apparent spontaneously or upon local percussion, is termed myotonia. It is generally demonstrable on an electromyogram. The phenomenon occurs in a variety of myopathies, including myotonic dystrophy, phosphofructokinase deficiency, myotonia congenita, and the Schwartz-Jampel syndrome (dwarfism, diffuse bone disease, ocular and facial abnormalities). Myotonia may become clinically apparent only in mid or late childhood. Percussion myotonia is best elicited over the thenar eminence or tip of the tongue using a reflex hammer. While normal muscle may also show some degree of contraction with this maneuver, patients with myotonia

demonstrate sustained adduction of the thumb onto the palm.

Tendon reflex changes. With both neuropathic and myopathic disorders, tendon reflexes become hypoactive and at times absent. The change is more significant in myopathies and involves both proximal and distal reflexes. In peripheral neuropathy, the reflexes are initially lost distally. It may be hard to identify the distal to proximal evolution of reflex abnormality in infants and when there is extensive or rapid progression in peripheral neuropathies.

Sensory disturbances. Neuropathies may be accompanied by feelings of numbness, burning, pins and needles, or pain. Impairment of joint and vibratory sensation correlates with dysfunction in the large diameter myelinated nerve fibers, whereas impaired pain and thermal sensation indicate involvement of small diameter unmyelinated and myelinated nerve fibers. Trophic ulcers may be noted over anesthetic segments of the body in hereditary sensory neuropathies.

Gait abnormalities. A waddling, lordotic gait is generally seen in myopathies due to weakness of the hip musculature. Patients with peripheral neuropathy may have difficulty clearing the foot off the floor, thereby causing it to drag and manifest foot drop. Toe walking may be seen in Duchenne's muscular dystrophy owing to contracture formation in the Achilles tendon.

Skeletal deformities. Kyphoscoliosis and lumbar lordosis may develop as a consequence of defective vertebral column bracing from paraspinal muscle weakness in patients with myopathies and certain hereditary neuropathies. Hip dislocation, genu recurvatum, and high-arched feet are other common orthopedic changes secondary to weakness.

Altered cardio-pulmonary function. Myopathies may involve the striated cardiac musculature, and this can be easily documented using electrocardiography and echocardiography. Also, restrictive lung disease, pulmonary insufficiency, and chronic cor pulmonale may evolve in the late stages of myopathies and lead to a fatal outcome.

Functional assessment. The evaluation is not complete without documentation of physical activities that the patient can and cannot carry out in the daily living routine and of those circumstances perceived by the patient as the most disabling.

THE HYPOTONIC INFANT

Introduction

The resistance felt upon movement of muscles is termed tone. The muscle spindle (which lies in parallel with skeletal muscle fibers), its gamma afferent and efferent connections with the spinal cord, and the alpha motor neuron and its efferent connection with the skeletal muscle form the feedback loop which regulates muscle tone. This system is constantly under facilitatory and inhibitory influences from various levels of the brain: cerebral cortex, basal ganglia, reticular formation, vestibular nuclei, and the cerebellar system. A reduction in the suprasegmental facilitatory input to the spinal cord or development of disease intrinsic to the lower motor unit (anterior horn cell, peripheral nerve fiber, neuromuscular junction and muscle) can both cause hypotonia. However, in the former category (cerebral, brainstem, or cerebellar disease), the muscle power remains normal. However, weakness is an essential feature of motor unit disease. The diagnostic approach and outcome are quite different in the two major categories of disease causing hypotonia in infancy. The clinical evaluation should aim at accurate localization as the essential first step.

Common Causes of Hypotonia in Infancy

I. **Central Nervous System Disorders**

Cerebral and cerebellar malformations

Neonatal hypoxia, hypoglycemia and hyperbilirubinemia

Congenital intrauterine infections

Inborn errors of metabolism (e.g. nonketotic hyperglycinemia)

II. **Lower Motor Unit Disease**

Infantile spinal muscular atrophy (Werdnig-Hoffman disease), poliomyelitis

Acute infectious polyneuritis (Guillain-Barre syndrome) Hereditary motor-sensory neuropathies

Botulism

Transient neonatal myasthenia gravis

Congenital myasthenia gravis

Myopathies (dystrophies, metabolic, inflammatory and congenital "non-progressive")

III. **Combined Upper and Lower Motor Unit Disease**

Prader Willi syndrome

Zellweger (cerebrohepatorenal) syndrome

Metachromatic leukodystrophy (late stages)

Clinical Assessment

The history should focus upon prenatal and perinatal central nervous system insults, motor and intellectual developmental milestones, and presence of easy fatigability while sucking and swallowing. An inquiry should be made regarding family history of neuromuscular diseases or mental retardation.

The muscle tone should be assessed in the prone, supine, and erect positions. The degree of head lag is estimated by pulling the infant to a sitting position from supine. When the baby is suspended in the prone position over the examiner's palm, a 6 week infant should be able to raise the head above the horizontal plane. Hyperextensibility around joints is another indication of hypotonia.

Fasiculations indicate active denervation of the muscle, generally from anterior horn cell disease or peripheral neuropathy, and are most frequently seen in Werdnig Hoffmann disease. As limb muscles in infants are covered generously with subcutaneous fat, the most suitable site for observing fasiculations is the lateral aspect of the tongue while the child is asleep with the mouth partially open.

The presence of microcephaly, delay in intellectual development, and seizures are indications of central nervous system origin of the hypotonia.

Tendon reflexes are generally exaggerated in hypotonia of central nervous system origin; they are normal or hypoactive in diseases of the motor unit.

Presence of facial anomalies may indicate cerebral dysgenesis. **Zellweger syndrome**, for example, is associated with a prominent forehead, wide open anterior fontanelle, hypotelorism, epicanthal folds, and malrotated ears. Hepatomegaly can be seen in hypotonic infants with the Zellweger syndrome or glycogen storage diseases.

An assessment for hypotonia in infancy is not complete without examination of other family members. Neonatal myotonic dystrophy generally has dominant transmission through the mother, who may display the characteristic myopathic facies and percussion myotonia in the thenar eminence or tongue. Transient neonatal myasthenia gravis due to transplacental transfer of antibody to the acetylcholine receptor is associated with typical features of myasthenia gravis in the mother. Hereditary neuropathies may be manifest in other family members with pes cavus, scoliosis, deafness, impaired proprioception, or absent tendon reflexes—sometimes with the affected individual being unaware of the neurological deficit.

Investigations

Hypotonia of central nervous system origin. The head CT scan helps in determining presence of major structural lesions such as porencephaly, intracranial calcification, and cerebellar hypoplasia. Serological studies for toxoplasmosis, rubella, cytomegalovirus, herpes simplex, syphilis, blood and urine amino acid screens, and EEG are also indicated. Hyperammonemia, hypercalcemia, and hypermagnesemia should also be excluded with appropriate serum analyses. In patients with facial features suggestive of the Zellweger syndrome, a plasma assay for elevated very long chain fatty acids (C24 through 26) is recommended. Chromosomal studies should be carried out when dysmorphic facial features are present in order to exclude trisomy and partial deletion syndromes.

Hypotonia secondary to lower motor unit disease:

1. Serum creatine kinase is elevated in dermatomyositis, certain congenital "non-progressive" myopathies, and in the preclinical stages of Duchenne's dystrophy.

2. Motor and sensory nerve conduction studies help exclude peripheral neuropathies.

3. The electromyogram (EMG—a study of muscle action potentials carried out by insertion of needle electrodes into the muscle) helps identify neuropathic and myopathic patterns, as well as neuromuscular junction disorders such as botulism and myasthenia gravis.

4. A skeletal muscle biopsy is the single most useful diagnostic test in infants with suspected lower motor unit disease. Generally obtained from a muscle of intermediate weakness, the biopsy specimen is processed at a minimum for histochemistry. If necessary, additional studies such as electron microscopy may be carried out. The biopsy helps determine myogenic or neurogenic origin of muscle atrophy; further categorization of the neurogenic pattern into anterior horn cell or peripheral nerve lesion is also possible.

5. In patients with peripheral neuropathy, teased fiber preparations from a sural nerve biopsy specimen help to differentiate axonal degeneration from segmental demyelination and detect the presence of lipid storage, e.g., in metachromatic leukodystrophy, or the onion-bulb configuration of myelin hypertrophy (in certain hereditary motor-sensory neuropathies).

6. If the muscle biopsy is inconclusive despite strong suspicion of neuromuscular disease, the patient should be evaluated for myasthenia gravis and botulism. Patients with myasthenia gravis demonstrate progressive decrease in amplitude of the muscle action potentials upon repetitive nerve stimulation (see under myasthenia gravis, this chapter). A pharmacological test for exclusion of myasthenia gravis in infancy consists of intramuscluar administration of neostigmine (see under myasthenia gravis, this chapter). Botulism is associated with characteristic electromyographic findings (brief duration, small amplitude polyphasic action potentials) and positive stool cultures for clostridium botulinum.

NOTE: An important cause of hypotonia in infancy, acute **Werdnig Hoffmann disease**, is transmitted as an autosomal recessive trait and characterized by progressive degeneration of alpha motor neurons in the spinal cord and brainstem. Onset of the illness may occur in utero, with the mother giving a history of decrease in fetal movements in the final trimester. The disorder generally develops at the latest by the age of 6 months. Delay in motor development, a weak cry, dysphagia, fasiculations on the tongue, profound generalized weakness, hypotonia (Fig. 12-1), and hyporeflexia are common. Higher functions are spared and the child remains alert until the very end. Most afflicted patients die from respiratory insufficiency by 2 to 3 years of age. The diagnosis can be readily established by a skeletal muscle

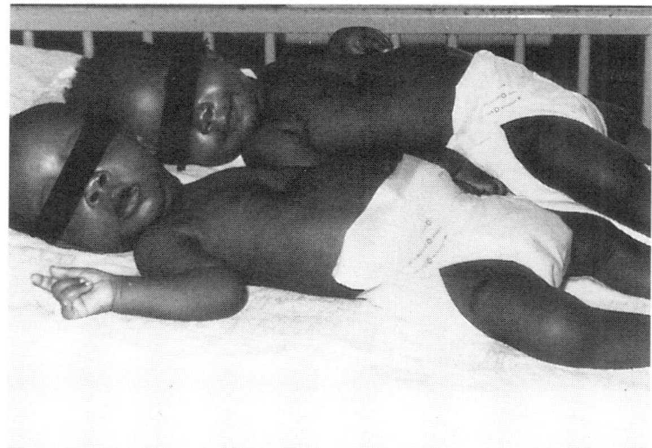

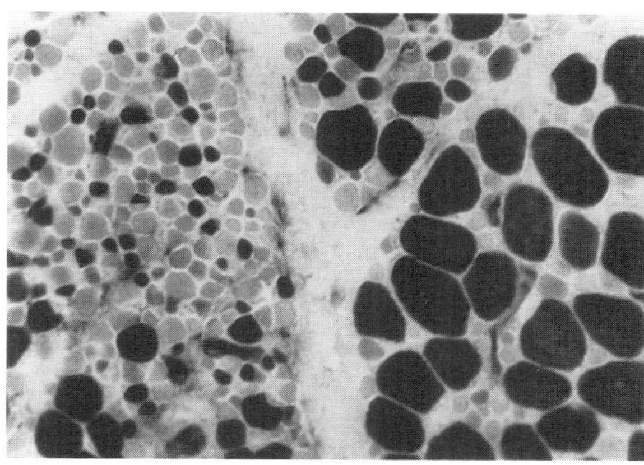

Fig. 12-1. Monozygotic twins with Werdnig Hoffmann disease, demonstrating abduction at the hips and substernal retraction secondary to muscle weakness and hypotonia.

Fig. 12-2. ATPase stain on a muscle biopsy specimen from a patient with Werdnig Hoffmann disease, demonstrating grouped muscle fiber atrophy in the top left corner. Type I fibers appear dark and Type II fibers appear lighter in shade.

biopsy, which discloses sheets of atrophic fibers of the same histochemical type (grouped atrophy), among which are interspersed groups of giant, hypertrophic fibers (Fig. 12-2).

ACUTE ONSET OF WEAKNESS IN CHILDHOOD

Differential diagnosis for this condition must include the following possibilities: acute poliomyelitis (See Chapter IV), acute infectious polyneuritis (Guillain-Barré syndrome), myasthenia gravis, botulism, tick paralysis, and periodic paralysis.

ACUTE INFECTIOUS POLYNEURITIS

This is also known as Guillain-Barré Syndrome. Viral gastrointestinal or upper respiratory infections, immunization, or surgery usually precede this illness by 1-2 weeks and serve as trigger factors in initiating an immunological disturbance characterized mainly by segmental demyelination and occasionally by axonal degeneration. Paresthesia and numbness may be felt over the distal extremities. An ascending, symmetric paralysis with onset in the lower extremities is common. It is frequently accompanied by bilateral facial weakness. Decreased joint and vibration sense, and hypoactive or absent tendon reflexes indicate involvement of the large diameter myelinated fibers. Respiratory insufficiency may develop in

the first 7-10 days. Autonomic dysfunction characterized by hypotension or hypertension is another serious life-threatening complication.

The diagnosis can be confirmed by the presence of albumino-cytological dissociation in the CSF, i.e., disproportionately greater increase in CSF protein relative to the cell count. The protein concentration may vary between 50-200 mg/dl; the cell count is usually less than 10-12 WBC/c mm (predominantly lymphocytes), but on some occasions may be as high as 50/cubic mm.

Nerve conduction studies with attention to the study of proximal segments may demonstrate decreased velocity. The illness gradually commences spontaneous resolution after the second or third week. Full recovery occurs in approximately 80% of children, but may take between 6 to 12 months. The remaining 20% have residual weakness.

Management in the Acute Stage

1. Daily monitoring of respiratory function for the first two weeks; a rough, bedside measure of vital capacity is having the patient take a deep breath and count rapidly—most children can count between 30-40 in one breath. Formal tidal volume, vital capacity, and blood gas determinations will also detect evolving respiratory insufficiency.

2. Endotracheal intubation and respiratory support should be provided if the patient is unable to sustain adequate ventilation on his/her own.

3. Excessive lengthening of flaccid, paralyzed muscles and contracture formation can be prevented by regular, passive range of motion exercises and judicious use of splints.

4. If the muscle weakness and respiratory insufficiency are severe, with no sign of resolution by 7-10 days, continuous plasmapharesis is recommended to alleviate weakness.

5. Since glucocorticoids are not of any benefit in the management; their prescription is not recommended.

MYASTHENIA GRAVIS

This disorder usually has a subacute or chronic course; but it may sometimes present with acute weakness, as a direct consequence of over-treatment (cholinergic crisis), worsening of the disease on its own, or following inadvertant administration of agents that impair neuromuscular transmission (curare for dental procedures, aminoglycosides, Ringer's lactate, bolus of steroids, phenothiazines, phenytoin, lithium, or propranolol).

Myasthenia gravis (MG) is a disease of the neuromuscular junction, characterized by destruction of the post-synaptic acetylcholine receptors (AChR) by a circulating antibody. Thymic hyperplasia or thymomas are seen in over 80% of patients and the thymus may very well be the site of anti-AChR antibody production. The disease has a prevalence of 2-10/100,000. About 20% of patients have onset prior to age 20 years.

Classification

I. Immune Etiology

Neonatal MG	Due to passive transfer of anti-AChR antibody from a myasthenic mother.
Juvenile MG	Similar to adult form; thymic hyperplasia frequent.
Adult MG	Onset < 40 years: thymoma infrequent; onset > 40 years: thymoma frequently present.
Ocular MG	Symptoms restricted to extra-ocular muscles, not progressing to generalized disease; low anti-AChR antibody titre.
Drug-induced MG	Usually penicillamine induced, during treatment of rheumatoid arthritis.

II. Non-immune etiology

Congenital MG	Heterogenous group, high familial incidence, not associated with anti-AChR antibody; probably due to congenital or genetic defects at the neuromuscular junction.

Clinical Features

1. Weakness and fatigue upon sustained muscle contraction, becoming more prominent towards the evening. Extraocular muscle weakness may cause diplopia and ptosis. Oropharyngeal weakness may result in dysphagia or dysphonia. Difficulty in brushing teeth, combing hair, or dressing can occur from shoulder girdle weakness.

2. A circulating antibody to the acetylcholine receptor can be detected in the serum of approximately 85% of patients with myasthenia gravis.

3. The bedside pharmacological test for diagnosis consists of demonstrating reversal of weakness following administration of intravenous edrophonium (TENSILON), an ultra-short-acting cholinesterase inhibitor. Muscle weakness is quantified prior to edrophonium administration (measuring width of palpebral fissures, range of ocular movement, deltoid strength, etc). A test dose of 1 mg of edrophonium is then administered intravenously, monitoring for hypersensitivity reactions such as cramps and bradycardia. If there is no hypersensitivity, up to an additional 9 mg is slowly administered intravenously. The dosage should be appropriately decreased in infants and young children. Patients with myasthenia gravis demonstrate an immediate, though transient, improvement in muscle power. Atropine (0.01 mg/kg for intramuscular or intravenous use) should be kept at hand in case the patient develops signs of cholinergic toxicity (e.g., bradycardia, hypotension, abdominal cramps).

In infants and young children with myasthenia gravis, the improvement in muscle strength after edrophonium administration may be difficult to assess owing to the transient nature of the improvement and difficulty in evaluating muscle strength at a young age. A longer acting cholinesterase inhibitor (neostigmine bromide 0.1 mg IM) may be administered in such instances immediately prior to feeds in order to determine whether sucking and swallowing functions are improved by the drug.

4. Electrophysiological studies used in the diagnosis of myasthenia gravis consist mainly of recording the amplitude of muscle action potentials upon repetitive nerve (ulnar/median) stimulation. Patients with the disease demonstrate an amplitude decrement of 10% or more by the 4th or 5th pulsed nerve stimulus. This decrement can be reversed by administration of parenteral edrophonium or neostigmine. Single-fiber EMG studies are also abnormal, with presence of the "jitter" phenomenon (variability in consecutive discharges of the time interval between origin of action potentials from two muscle fibers of the same motor unit).

Management

Transient neonatal myasthenia gravis requires provision of respiratory and nutritional support and neostigmine bromide 0.1 mg IM every 6-8 hours, especially immediately prior to feeds. Complete recovery may take 2-3 months.

Congenital myasthenia gravis is best managed with cholinesterase inhibitors, but the response is far from satisfactory in a number of patients. Pyridostigmine (MESTINON) is one such agent which may increase muscle strength in a dosage of 15-60 mg every 4-6 hours orally. Neostigmine bromide (15 mg every 3-4 hours orally) may also be effective, though with a shorter duration of action. In acute situations, neostigmine can be administered by the intramuscular route. The cholinergic effect achieved by intramuscular administration of 1.5 mg of neostigmine is equivalent to that of an oral dose of 15 mg of neostigmine, which in turn is equal to that produced by 60 mg of oral pyridostigmine.

Juvenile myasthenia gravis is best treated by commencing the patient on oral anticholinesterase medication and following up within 6 weeks with total thymectomy, using a midline, sternum-splitting approach. The beneficial effect of thymectomy upon myasthenia gravis may become evident only 6-12 months postoperatively. The longterm outlook in juvenile myasthenics who undergo early thymectomy is quite favorable. In one series, improvement in muscle strength was noted in 67.8% of the subjects, with full remission in 42.8%. On longterm follow-up in another study, 80% of juvenile myasthenics who had undergone thymectomy were alive at 40 years of age, i.e, about 90% of what would be expected in the general population.

Ocular myasthenia gravis. When weakness is restricted to the extraocular muscles, cholinesterase inhibitors and thymectomy seem to be of limited therapeutic value. Such patients may respond favorably to a gradually increasing oral dose of glucocorticoids—prednisone 10 mg every other day increased slowly over 3-6 months to 2 mg/kg/day is recommended. Initiation of therapy at high doses in an ambulatory setting should be avoided as it may lead to a sudden worsening in severity of the muscle weakness.

Myasthenic crisis. An acute increase in muscle weakness can be precipitated by intercurrent infections and may manifest with acute respiratory insufficiency and dysphagia. This is associated with an increase in the need for anticholinesterase agents. The diagnosis of myasthenic crisis can be established by the intravenous edrophonium test, which should produce an immediate, though transient, improvement in muscle power. Respiratory support and intramuscular neostigmine in a dose of 0.5-1.5 mg every 3-4 hours may be administered until the patient improves. When available, plasmapheresis should also be carried out every 2-3 days until there is adequate improvement in muscle strength.

Cholinergic crisis. Overdosage of anticholinesterase agents may lead to an acute exacerbation of muscle weakness. The intravenous Tensilon test helps confirm the diagnosis, since it causes a further increase in weakness. The treatment is essentially supportive.

TICK PARALYSIS

This disorder usually occurs in the summer

and fall seasons and is secondary to a neurotoxin secreted by the wood tick (*Dermacentor andersoni*) or the dog tick (*Dermacentor variabilis*). The gravid tick attaches itself to the skin surface. The exotoxin produced by the tick interferes with release of acetylcholine from the presynaptic terminals of neuromuscular junctions and may also affect cerebellar function.

The incubation period is 5-6 days. Irritability, paresthesia, an acute ascending flaccid paralysis, hyporeflexia, occasional distal sensory deficit, and cerebellar ataxia are common clinical manifestations. In contrast to Guillain Barré syndrome or poliomyelitis, the cerebrospinal fluid examination is normal. The gravid tick can be found attached to the skin, usually around the scalp and neck regions. The management consists of removal of the tick and support of vital functions.

HYPOKALEMIC PERIODIC PARALYSIS

This dominantly transmitted disorder usually has its onset in the second decade and is characterized by attacks of abrupt skeletal muscle paralysis lasting 12-24 hours. The weakness generally commences in the lower extremities and spreads rostrally to involve the trunk and upper limb musculature. Respiratory muscle involvement is generally mild. Facial and extraocular muscles are usually spared; there is no associated sensory deficit. The muscle is mechanically and electrically inexcitable during the attack and tendon reflexes are absent. Rest following a period of vigorous exercise, exposure to cold, and consumption of alcohol or a high carbohydrate diet are frequent precipitants of the attack.

Diagnosis. This is established by documenting hypokalemia during the acute event. A provocative test, designed to induce hypokalemia and thereby muscle weakness, consists of intravenous infusion of 10% dextrose combined with 20 units of insulin. The serum potassium and electrocardiogram should be monitored closely during the procedure.

Treatment. The acute attack is treated by administration of an oral potassium supplement. Spironolactone and acetazolamide are of some value in prophylaxis. The disorder peaks in severity by the 3rd and 4th decade, and then shows gradual, spontaneous resolution.

HYPERKALEMIC PERIODIC PARALYSIS

This dominantly inherited disorder has its onset in infancy and early childhood. The periods of weakness are more brief than in the hypokalemic form and last 30-60 minutes. The muscle is electrically and mechanically inexcitable during the acute attack and tendon reflexes are temporarily absent. Eyelid myotonia may accompany the disorder, causing an inability to suddenly look down after a period of upward gaze. The diagnosis can be established by serum potassium determinations during the acute attack. Acetazolamide and chlorthiazide are effective in prophylaxis.

NONMOKALEMIC PERIODIC PARALYSIS

The disorder is clinically quite similar to the hyperkalemic form, but serum potassium values are within the normal range during an acute attack.

BOTULISM

The exotoxin that is produced by *Clostridium botulinum* can induce acute skeletal muscle paralysis by interfering with release of acetylcholine from the presynaptic terminals of the neuromuscular junctions. The toxin may be ingested preformed in contaminated foods, elaborated in the gastrointestinal tract following a clostridial bowel infection, or spread into the systemic circulation from a clostridial wound infection. Constipation frequently heralds the onset of the disease in infancy. The acute, generalized muscle weakness may be accompanied by such symptoms as dysphagia and respiratory insufficiency. The diagnosis can be confirmed by the presence of characteristic brief-duration, small amplitude polyphasic action potentials on the electromyogram. The stool culture may yield a growth of the causative organism. The management is essentially supportive, and complete recovery may take as long as two to three months.

CHRONIC NEUROMUSCULAR DISORDERS OF CHILDREN

Table 12-1 lists the various chronic neuromuscular disorders of children.

Table 12-1. Chronic Neuromuscular Disorders of Children

Anterior Horn Cell Diseases

1. Chronic Werdnig Hoffmann disease
2. Juvenile spinal muscular atrophy

Peripheral Neuropathies

1. Hereditary sensory neuropathies (Types I-IV, Table 12-2)
2. Hereditary motor-sensory neuropathies (Types I-VI, Table 12-3)
3. Spinocerebellar degeneration
4. Chronic, relapsing polyneuropathy
5. Metabolic neuropathies (diabetes mellitus, porphyria, primary amyloidosis, uremia)
6. Nutritional neuropathies (mixed vitamin deficiency, B6 deficiency or intoxication, B1 and B12 deficiency)
7. Toxic neuropathies (arsenic, thallium, lead, mercury, nitrofurantoin, isoniazid, phenytoin, vinca alkaloids, organic solvents and clioquinol)
8. Collagen vascular diseases (polyarteritis nodosa, systemic lupus erythematosus and rheumatoid arthritis and sarcoidsosis)
9. Infectious and inflammatory diseases (diptheria, leprosy, infectious mononeucleosis, Bell's palsy)
10. Entrapment or traction neuropathies

Myopathies

1. Muscular dystrophies (myotonic, Duchenne's, Becker's, facio-scapulo humeral and limb-girdle type)
2. Metabolic myopathies (glycogenoses types II, III, IV and V; systemic carnitine deficiency and carnitine palmityl transferase deficiency; hypothyroidism)
3. Congenital "non-progressive" myopathies (nemaline rod disease, central core disease, myotubular myopathy and muscle fibre type disproportion)
4. Inflammatory (dermatomyositis, polymyositis, trichinosis and viral myositis)
5. Drug induced (steroids, alcohol, etc.)

ANTERIOR HORN CELL DISEASES

Chronic Werdnig Hoffmann Disease

Also termed type II spinal muscular atrophy, this autosomal recessive disorder has onset between 6 months and 3 years of age. As in the acute infantile form, there is progressive degeneration of motor neurons of the spinal cord. Brainstem cranial nerve nuclei are minimally involved and the rate of progression is slow, i.e., over years, with the disease burning itself out over time in some patients. Hypotonia, delayed motor development, fasiculations, hyporeflexia, and kyphoscoliosis are common. Sensory functions are preserved. The diagnosis can be confirmed by muscle biopsy that shows changes identical to the acute infantile form of the illness.

Juvenile Spinal Muscular Atrophy

This condition is also known as Kugelberg-Welander disease. It is generally transmitted as an autosomal recessive trait, but dominant and X-linked forms have also been described. Onset of the illness usually occurs between 5-15 years. There is progressive degeneration of spinal alpha motor neurons, with preservation of sensory and higher functions. The distribution of weakness is initially proximal, particularly involving the sternomastoids and shoulder girdle muscle, thereby mimicking muscle disease. Fasiculations may be noted over limb muscles in one half of the patients. Tendon reflexes are often depressed. The diagnosis can be established by muscle biopsy, which shows grouped atrophy. The electromyogram is also abnormal, demonstrating giant amplitude, polyphasic action potentials (owing to muscle denervation from anterior horn cell disease followed by reinnervation from adjacent healthy motor neurons). Kugelberg-Welander disease is gradually progressive over years and patients may become wheelchair-bound by the third decade. It is now becoming apparent that the syndrome is heterogenous, and that at least in some individuals, the primary abnormality is hexosaminidase A deficiency, with the resultant anterior horn cell GM_2 ganglioside storage leading to neuronal degeneration and weakness.

PERIPHERAL NEUROPATHIES
Spinocerebellar Degeneration

Friedreich's ataxia is the most common form of spinocerebellar degeneration in childhood, characterized by "dying back" of sensory axons in a distal to proximal progression. Mitochondrial malic acid deficiency has been suggested as the primary metabolic defect. The condition is transmitted as an autosomal recessive trait, with onset of symptoms in the first or second decade. The gene is localized to chromosome 9. Proprioceptive

and cerebellar function and tendon reflexes are severely impaired. Unsteadiness of gait, truncal titubation, positive Romberg's sign, dysmetria on finger to nose testing, loss of tendon reflexes distally, pes cavus with hammer toes and scoliosis are some of the common manifestations. Nystagmus is infrequent, but ocular square wave jerks may be present. A cardiomyopathy characterized by subaortic hypertrophic stenosis, low voltage QRS complexes, deep Q waves, and ST segment elevation or depression may also occur. The neurologic syndrome is steadily progressive, with the patient becoming confined to bed by the end of the second decade, and death occurring by the end of the third decade from cardiac or respiratory complications. The other peripheral neuropathies are listed in Tables 12-1 through 3. Hexosamidase A deficiency may cause an identical clinical syndrome.

MYOPATHIES
Myotonic Dystrophy

This autosomal dominant disorder may become apparent in infancy, or mid or late childhood. When the patient is an infant, transmission is

Table 12-2. Hereditary sensory neuropathies (HSN)

Disorder	Transmission	Age at Onset of Symptoms	Clinical Features	Nerve Conduction Studies	Management
Type I	Autosomal dominant	2nd or later decades	Impairment of pain, thermal sensation, greatest in distal lower extremities; mild to moderate distal muscle weakness; absent ankle reflexes	Normal motor conduction; absent sensory action potentials	Symptomatic (prevention of foot ulcers by wearing comfortable shoes; avoiding weight bearing when trophic foot ulcers develop)
Type II	Autosomal recessive	Infancy or early childhood	All modalities of sensation impaired in both upper and lower extremities; generalized hyporeflexia; sweating absent over limbs; stress fractures; mutilating acropathy characterized by paronychia, ulcers of fingers and toes	Absent sensory action potentials	Symptomatic (prevention of acral mutilation by splinting; antibiotics for infected ulcers
Type III (Familial dysautonomia)	Autosomal recessive, in Jewish population	Infancy or early childhood	Poor feeding, repeated episodes of vomiting and bronchospasm, hypertension, blotchy skin rash, defective thermoregulation, excessive sweating, insensitivity to pain, absent fungiform papillae on tongue, absent flare response to intradermal histamine injections; high incidence of sudden death in infancy and early childhood	Motor velocity slightly decreased; absent sensory action potentials	Symptomatic
Type IV	Autosomal dominant	Infancy	Insensitivity to pain; anhidrosis with episodic hyperthermia; mental retardation	Absent sensory action potentials	Symptomatic

generally via an affected mother, examination of whom may disclose facial weakness and percussion myotonia. Hypotonia, delayed development, and poor sucking and swallowing are commonly seen in infants with myotonic dystrophy. There may be decompensation of pulmonary function with respiratory tract infections. Older children with myotonic dystrophy generally display ptosis, as well as elongated facies with atrophy of the masseter and temporalis muscles. Cataracts, mild to moderate intellectual impairment, testicular atrophy, baldness, and myotonia upon percussion of thenar and tongue muscles may also be seen in young adults. The diagnosis can be confirmed by muscle biopsy, which discloses atrophy of Type I (oxidative) muscle fibers and presence of internal nuclei. The electromyogram may disclose myopathic action potentials. Myotonic discharges become electromyographically apparent by mid-childhood. The disorder may progress gradually over decades, but survival into the fourth and fifth decades is common.

Duchenne's Dystrophy

This disorder is transmitted as an X-linked recessive trait. However, approximately one third of the cases are due to spontaneous mutations. It has a prevalence of approximately 3 per 100,000. Onset of symptoms is usually noted in the second or third year of life, with a clumsy, waddling gait, frequent falls, and inability to run or climb stairs without holding onto the the bannister. A lumbar lordosis and protuberant abdomen may be seen. Some children manifest pseudohypertrophy of the calf muscles. Progressive difficulty in arising from the floor, necessitating use of the hands for support (Gower's sign), is common. Patients may be mildly mentally retarded or of borderline intelligence. Tendon reflexes disappear early in the course of the illness. Sensory functions are fully preserved. Cardiomyopathy and respiratory insufficiency evolve over time. The disorder is steadily progressive, with most patients becoming

Table 12-3. Hereditary motor-sensory neuropathies (HMSN)

Disorder	Genetics	Clinical Features	Nerve Conduction Velocity	Pathology
Type I	Autosomal dominant	Onset in 2nd-4th decade; weakness, atrophy of mainly small muscles of feet and pernei; sensation normal to mildly impaired; absent tendon reflexes; palpable thickening of peripheral nerves	Markedly decreased (motor and sensory)	Axonal atrophy; segmental demyelination and hypermyelination with "onion bulb" formation
Type II	Autosomal dominant	Onset in 3rd-4th decade; weakness, mainly restricted to the lower extremities; peripheral nerves not palpably thickened	Mildly decreased (motor and sensory)	Neuronal atrophy with secondary segmental demyelination
Type III (Hypertrophic neuropathy of Dejerine and Sottas)	Autosomal	Onset in infancy with delayed motor development, especially walking, running; club feet; kyphoscoliosis; generalized muscle weakness and atrophy; generalized hyporeflexia; markedly palpable thickening of peripheral nerves; moderate elevation of CSF protein	Markedly decreased (motor and sensory)	Axonal atrophy with secondary segmental demyelination and hypermyelination with "onion bulb" formation
Type IV (Refsum's disease)	Autosomal recessive	Onset in 1st-3rd decade; retinitis pigmentosa, motor and sensory neuropathy, generalized hyporeflexia, nerve deafness, skeletal anomalies and ichthyosis; elevated CSF protein and serum phytanic acid levels; dietary restriction of phytanic acid is therapeutic	Markedly decreased (motor and sensory)	Demyelination and hypermyelination with "onion bulb" formation
Type V (with spastc extremities)	Autosomal dominant	Onset in 2nd or later decades; predominantly motor neuropathy with spastic paraplegia	Usually normal in upper extremities, slightly decreased	Decrease in number of myelinated nerve fibers
Type VI (with optic atrophy)	Autosomal dominant	Onset in 2nd-5th decades; motor and sensory symptoms with lancinating pains in limbs, visual loss, weakness and atrophy of muscles in the lower extremities; tendon reflexes normal to slightly decreased	Slightly decreased	Segmental demyelination

wheelchair-bound by the middle of the second decade and dying by the end of the second decade.

Serum creatine kinase, aldolase, and lactic dehydrogenase are markedly elevated in the preclinical and early stages of the disease, with levels steadily declining with progression of muscle weakness. The electromyogram shows a typical myopathic pattern, displaying brief duration, low amplitude, and polyphasic muscle action potentials. The muscle biopsy findings are also quite characteristic: the presence of rounded muscle fibers having central nuclei, fibrous tissue proliferation, the presence of basophilic fibers, and the persistence of undifferentiated type 2C muscle fibers. Diagnosis of a carrier state in female siblings can be established by a combination of elevated serum creatine kinase values, electromyogram, and muscle biopsy tests in suspected individuals in approximately 87% of subjects. Prenatal diagnosis of the disease using recombinant DNA techniques around the 15th week of gestation is now possible. Dystrophin, a structural protein normally present in muscles, is almost completely absent in the muscle tissue of patients with Duchenne's dystrophy.

The management is entirely symptomatic. It consists of physical therapy and use of night splints to prevent contractures. Long leg braces may be required when significant weakness of the quadriceps has developed. Use of a wheelchair should be postponed as long as possible, owing to rapid development of kyphoscoliosis once the child becomes wheelchair-bound. Ancillary devices to help the child in activities of daily living, e.g., feeding, may also be needed in the late stages.

Becker's Dystrophy

This X-linked dystrophy differs from Duchenne's dystrophy due to a later age of onset, i.e., around 5 or 6 years, and a slower rate of progression. Survival into mid-adult life is not uncommon. The serum creatine kinase levels are moderately elevated. Myopathic changes are observed on the electromyogram and muscle biopsy. Dystrophin levels in the muscles are between those of Duchenne's dystrophy and normal levels.

Fascio-scapulohumeral Dystrophy

The prototypic form of this illness is character-

ized by development of insidious facial weakness in the first decade, generally causing inability to elevate the corners of the mouth when smiling, or inability to drink from a straw. With time, weakness of the neck flexors and shoulder girdle develops, with the latter leading to significant winging of the scapulae. Weakness of the wrist extensors and hip flexor muscles may also be present. There is relative sparing of flexor muscles in the forearm. The disorder progresses gradually over decades. The clinical picture, combined with moderately elevated serum creatine kinase levels, myopathic changes on the electromyogram, and muscle biopsy help establish the diagnosis.

An infantile variant with almost total paralysis of facial muscles and rapid evolution that results in inability to walk independently by 8-10 years of age has also been described.

Limb Girdle Dystrophy

This is a heterogenous disorder, composed of both autosomal recessive and dominant forms. Most patients have onset of hip girdle weakness in the second or third decades, followed soon thereafter by shoulder girdle weakness. Low backache from weakness of the paraspinal muscles is common. Polymyositis and juvenile spinal muscular atrophy should be considered in the differential diagnosis. Both can be distinguished from limb girdle dystrophy by characteristic muscle biopsy and electromyographic findings.

Glycogen Storage Diseases

A defect in mobilization of muscle glycogen to glucose will result in a deficiency of substrate necessary to generate energy for muscle contraction. A sequence of enzymes is involved in this process, and deficiency of any one can individually result in myopathy with glycogen accumulation. Glycogen storage disease types II, III, IV, and V are the most common of such disorders.

Pompe's or **Type II** glycogen storage disease occurs due to deficiency of the lysosomal enzyme, acid maltase (alpha 1, 4-glucosidase). The infantile variety is characterized by hypotonia and enlargement of the heart, tongue, and liver from glycogen storage. The cardiomyopathy is severe; an enlarged, globular heart may be visualized on the chest x-ray. The diagnosis can be established by muscle biopsy, which discloses glycogen accumulation and deficiency of acid maltase on specific histochemical stains. The disease is progressive and usually fatal by 1-2 years of age. A milder form of Pompe's disease with onset of weakness and contractures in later childhood has also been described.

Type III glycogen storage disease or debrancher enzyme (amylo-1, 6-glucosidase) deficiency causes glycogen storage in the liver as well as skeletal muscle. Hypotonia, muscle fatigue on exertion, and hypoglycemia are commonly seen.

Type IV glycogen storage disease or brancher enzyme deficiency usually causes hypotonia and muscle weakness, along with the more prominent manifestations of failure to thrive and hepatosplenomegaly.

McArdle's or **Type V** glycogen storage disease occurs as a consequence of myophosphorylase deficiency. Muscle cramps, myoglobinuria, and mild to moderate generalized muscle weakness have onset in the first or second decade. The serum creatine kinase may be elevated, particularly during episodes of muscle cramps. As in all other glycogenoses, the ischaemic lactate test is abnormal. The test produces limb ischaemia by inflation of an arm blood pressure cuff in between systolic and diastolic pressures followed by exercise, e.g., squeezing the blood pressure cuff for 60-90 seconds; lactate levels are then drawn from the exercised limb at baseline, 1, 3, 5, 10 and 20 minutes. Under normal circumstances, there should be a 3 to 5-fold increase in lactate, especially at the 3 minute peak. Patients with glycogen storage diseases fail to show this degree of lactate elevation. The diagnosis of McArdle's disease can be confirmed by specific histochemical studies for myophosphorylase on muscle biopsy. A high protein diet may help alleviate the symptoms to some extent.

Myopathy Associated with Carnitine Deficiency

Muscles utilize long chain fatty acids as a source of energy during prolonged exercise and fasting. Before long chain fatty acids can be metabolized by mitochondria, they have to be converted outside the mitochondria into their acyl-CoA esters. Carnitine is a lysine derivative

synthesized in the liver, released into the systemic circulation, and taken up by a variety of organ systems (including brain and skeletal muscle) by active transport. With the help of carnitine acyl-CoA enzymes I and II, carnitine then combines with the acyl-CoA esters to form acyl-carnitine esters and ultimately transports them into the mitochondria, where they undergo beta oxidation to form carbon dioxide, water, and in the liver, ketone bodies also.

Skeletal muscle carnitine deficiency is associated with a lipid storage myopathy. Two major forms have been described: a systemic form in which carnitine concentrations are low in the serum and liver, and a muscular form characterized by normal serum, but low muscle carnitine levels.

Onset of generalized weakness may occur anywhere from infancy to middle age. Intermittent exacerbation of muscle weakness is not uncommon. The systemic form may also be associated with episodic vomiting, hypoglycemia, a Reye syndrome-like picture, and cardiomyopathy.

The serum creatine kinase and aldolase levels may be elevated, thereby mimicking polymyositis. In the systemic form, ketonuria is virtually absent despite prolonged fasting. The electromyogram may demonstrate myopathic features. The hallmark of the myopathy is presence of lipid-laden muscle fibers on biopsy. Carnitine levels of skeletal muscle and serum help confirm the appropriate form of the disorder (systemic vs. muscular).

In both varieties, large doses of oral carnitine coupled with a high carbohydrate, low fat diet ameliorate the symptoms.

Myopathy Associated with Carnitine Acyl-CoA Transferase (CAT) Deficiency

A lipid storage myopathy may also result from deficiency of CAT enzymes I and II consequent to the accompanying failure of transport of long chain fatty acids into the mitochondria. Intermittent muscle cramps, myoglobinuria, and easy fatigability are common. Serum cholesterol and triglycerides may be elevated. The skeletal muscle biopsy shows lipid-laden fibers but normal carnitine concentrations. Specific assays for CAT will demonstrate the enzymatic deficiency.

Congenital "Non-Progressive" Myopathies

This group of disorders is identified by the presence of characteristic morphological abnormalities on muscle biopsy and a relatively static course in most subjects. However, decompensation of respiratory function with infections and occasional fatal outcome are not uncommon. **Nemaline rod disease** is associated with basophilic rod-like structures in the muscle fibers. **Myotubular myopathy** is associated with large central nuclei. In **congenital fiber type disproportion**, type I (oxidative) muscle fibers are smaller in size but more numerous than the type II (glycolytic) fibers. Mild elevation of muscle enzymes may also be seen in congenital fiber type disproportion. All congenital non-progressive myopathies may be accompanied by delayed motor development in infancy, poor sucking and swallowing, congenital hip dislocation, scoliosis, or occasionally, mild intellectual impairment. The group includes autosomal recessive, dominant, and sporadic forms.

Polymyositis and Dermatomyositis

Polymyositis is an inflammatory skeletal myopathy. When associated with characteristic cutaneous lesions, the disorder may be termed dermatomyositis. This definition is, however, a simplication of the distinction between the two disorders. Besides primary dermatomyositis and polymyositis, secondary forms accompanying collagen vascular diseases (e.g., lupus, polyarteritis nodosa, scleroderma, and mixed connective tissue disease) have also been described.

Polymyositis and dermatomyositis are characterized by a vasculopathy with resultant ischemic changes in skeletal muscle fasicles, as well as the presence of lymphocytic infiltration. In adults, dermatomyositis may be a marker of occult malignancy in approximately one third of affected patients. Such an association with malignancy is, however, not found in childhood dermatomyositis.

Subacute, progressive, proximal muscle weakness is present in both disorders. Dysphagia may develop consequent to involvement of the pharyngeal constrictors. Muscle pain and tenderness are elicitable in only a third of the subjects. The dermatomyositis rash may appear before, or along with the skeletal muscle weakness. It is erythematous, blotchy, and sometimes accompanied by edema of the overlying skin. The rash is distributed mainly over the malar region, upper eyelids, and extensor surfaces of joints in the upper extremities. Polymyositis and dermatomyositis tend to run a variable course with spontaneous permanent resolution in some, a progressive remitting and relapsing course in some, and a chronic indolent course in others. Death may occur from involvement of respiratory musculature in a third of the patients.

Both disorders can be suspected on the basis of elevated muscle enzymes (especially CK and LDH); normal levels of such enzymes have been noted on occasion. The EMG demonstrates a myopathic pattern. Muscle biopsy changes are characteristic, with presence of muscle atrophy in the periphery of fasicles, round cell infiltration, and occasional immune complex deposition in blood vessel walls.

Treatment consists of bed rest and immunosuppresive agents. Prednisone, in a dose of 1.5-2.0 mg/kg/day is recommended as the starting dose. The duration of therapy may vary from 6-12 months, depending on the clinical response. There may be a lag of 2-3 weeks between initiation of steroid therapy and improvement in muscle strength. Muscle enzymes should be monitored periodically, especially when the dose is being tapered. A sudden increase in values of the muscle enzymes may indicate relapse, calling for an increase in steroid dosage. Failure of steroid therapy may be an indication for use of other immunosuppressive agents such as methotrexate, cytoxan, or azathioprine.

Trichinosis

Larvae of the dog tapeworm *Trichinella spirallis* can cause a painful generalized myositis. Consumption of undercooked infected meats (especially pork) will result in the adult worms attaching themselves to the small intestine mucosa. Larvae produced by the gravid female worm gain entry into the lymphatic system and thence the systemic circulation. They can lodge in a variety of organs, including muscle; resulting in an acute inflammatory disorder. The replication cycle of *trichinella* comes to a dead end in the human, and ultimately the larvae become inactive, encapsulated, and calcified. Trichinosis is associated with fever, generalized muscle pain, maculopapular rash, periorbital edema, eosinophilia, and moderate elevation of muscle enzymes. A muscle biopsy may demonstrate encysted larvae and an inflammatory exudate. Elevated serum titres on the bentonite flocculation tests are confirmatory. The treatment is entirely supportive. The value of steroids for treatment is uncertain.

Viral Myositis

A transient, painful myositis may occur along with systemic viral infections (especially influenza). There may be symmetric involvement of muscles of the lower extremities, especially the calves, resulting in pain and refusal to walk. Mild to moderate elevation of muscle enzymes may also be present. As the disorder is benign and resolves spontaneously in 1-2 weeks, reports on electromyographic and muscle biopsy features are sparse.

SUGGESTED READING

1. Swift TR and Ignacio OJ. Tick paralysis: electrophysiological studies. Neurology 25:1130, 1975.

2. Rodriquez M, Gomez MR, Howard FM and Taylor WF. Myasthenia gravis in children: long-term follow-up. Ann Neurol 13:504-510, 1983.

3. Ryniewicz B and Badurska B. Follow-up study of myasthenic children after thymectomy. J Neurol 217:133-138, 1977.

4. Vincent A. Immunology of myasthenia gravis: recent developments. Clinics in Immunology and Allergy 1(1): 161-179, 1981.

5. Fenichel GM. Clinical syndromes of myasthenia in infancy and childhood. Arch Neurol 35:97-103, 1978.

6. Drachman DB. Myasthenia gravis. Parts I and II. N Engl J Med 298(3):136-142, 198(4)186-193, 1978.

7. Seybold ME. Myasthenia gravis, a clinical and basic science review. JAMA 250(18):2516-2521, 1983.

8. Moser AE, Singh I, Brown FR, Solish GI, Kelley RI, Benke PJ and Moser HW: The cerebrohepatorenal (Zellweger) syndrome. Increased levels and impaired degradation of very long-chain fatty acids and their use in prenatal diagnosis. N Engl J Med 310:1141-1146, 1984.

9. Sarnat HB. Diagnostic value of the muscle biopsy in the neonatal period. Am J Dis Child 132:782-785, 1978.

10. Kimura J. Principles and pitfalls of nerve conduction studies. Ann Neurol 16(4):415-429, 1984.

11. McKinlay IA and Mitchell I. Transient, acute myositis in childhood. Arch Dis Child 51:135, 1976.

12. Brooke MH. A Clinician's View of Neuromuscular Diseases. Williams and Wilkins, Baltimore, 1978.

13. Dyck PJ, Thomas PK and Lambert EH, eds. Peripheral Neuropathy, Volumes I and II. W.B. Saunders, Philadelphia, 1975.

14. Guillain Barre Syndrome. Proceedings of a conference sponsored by the Kroc Foundation. Ann Neurol, supplement to Vol 9, 1-145, 1981.

15. McKhann GM, Griffin JW. Plasmapharesis and the Guillain-Barre syndrome. Ann Neurol 22:762-763, 1987.

SLEEP DISORDERS IN CHILDREN

Sleep is a cyclical, physiological state of decreased consciousness from which arousal is easily accomplished. Despite that fact that most individuals spend close to a third of their life asleep, little attention had been directed to clinical sleep disorders until very recently. Over the past decade, however, sleep disorders medicine has advanced close to the point of becoming recognized as a formal discipline.

ONTOGENY OF SLEEP

Familiarity with maturational and physiological aspects of sleep is fundamental to understanding sleep disorders in children. Differentiation between wakefulness and sleep becomes apparent by 28-29 weeks conceptional age. By 32 weeks conceptional age, two sleep states are identifiable on the electroencephalogram (EEG): active or rapid eye movement (REM) and quiet or non-REM (NREM) sleep.[1] Characteristics differentiating the two states are outlined in the Table. A premature infant of approximately 32 weeks conceptional age spends about 80% of the total sleep time in REM sleep. By 40 weeks' conceptional age, the time spent in REM sleep has declined to about 50% of total sleep time, and by adolesence, to 20% of total sleep time. REM sleep is associated with higher values of cerebral blood flow as compared to NREM sleep and its abundance in the neonatal period may be a reflection of its underlying role in maturation of the central nervous system.[2]

NREM sleep becomes fully differentiated into four distinct stages by 6 months of age: drowsiness or Stage I, Stage II, Stages III and IV.[3] Isolated vertex sharp wave transients are evident in Stage I. They become more abundant and are associated with spindle activity in stage II sleep. Stage III and IV sleep, together also termed slow wave sleep, are associated with increasing proportions of slow EEG activity in the delta (1 to 4 hertz) range. Most of slow wave sleep is clustered into the first third of night sleep. Sleep cycles consist of a combination of REM and non-REM sleep. They are approximately 55-60 minutes long in the neonatal period. With progressive maturation of the central nervous system, the length of sleep cycles increases to the adult range of 70-90 minutes. In neonates and infants of up to 3 months of age, the transition from wakefulness is initially into REM sleep, with subsequent appearance of NREM sleep. In normal older infants, children, and adults sleep onset is associated with an initial appearance of NREM sleep, to be subsequently followed by REM sleep.

A circadian variation in sleep-wake function develops by 6-12 months of age. Nocturnal growth hormone release selectively in slow wave sleep also evolves by the same age. Normal newborns spend between 18-20 hours a day in sleep, but the need for sleep gradually declines through infancy and early childhood. Daytime naps are still common in children up to the ages of 5-6 years but infrequent thereafter. Around puberty, the physiological increase in the total requirement of sleep reappears.[4] Unfortunately, the lifestyle of most teenagers directly conflicts with their physiological sleep needs. Consequently, it is not unusual to find teenagers remaining relatively sleep-deprived through the weekdays and sleeping-in late on the mornings of holidays and weekends in order to make up for lost sleep. Serotonin, produced mainly by the raphe nuclei of the brainstem is involved in the induction of NREM sleep, whereas norepinephrine (synthesised mainly in the locus coeruleus) plays a role in induction of REM sleep.[5]

POLYSOMNOGRAPHY

This technique of monitoring multiple physiological parameters during sleep is helpful in the study of some sleep disorders. Its greatest value lies in evaluating respiratory disorders associated with sleep (sleep apnea) and in disorders characterized by excessive daytime sleepiness (nar-

colepsy). The procedure[6] consists of simultaneous monitoring of the electroencephalogram (usually four channels—two each from the left and right sides of the scalp), eye movements, chin electromyogram, nasal airflow (using a thermistor), thoracic and abdominal respiratory movements (generally using mercury-filled strain gauges), electrocardiogram, and oxygen saturation. The above parameters are recorded continuously for the entire length of night sleep. Standard criteria for scoring sleep and sleep stages and abnormal events during sleep have been established for both infants[7, 8] and older children.[9]

CLASSIFICATION OF SLEEP DISORDERS

I. **Parasomnias**

    Sleep walking

    Night terrors (pavor nocturnus)

    Sleep talking (somniloquoy)

    Nocturnal enuresis

    Teeth grinding (bruxism)

    Nightmares

II. **Disorders of excessive sleepiness**

    Narcolepsy

    Sleep apnea syndrome

    Psychophysiological disturbances

    Drug intoxication

III. **Disorders of initiating and maintaining sleep**

    Psychophysiological

    Drug withdrawal or intoxication

    Sleep apnea syndrome

    Systemic conditions (e.g., chronic cough and pain)

IV. **Disorders of sleep schedule**

    Delayed sleep phase syndrome

    Jet lag

    Frequently changing shift work

It is beyond the scope of this chapter to review each disorder and only the most common sleep-related problems are discussed. The reader is referred to certain review articles for further details.[10, 11, 16, 17, 22, 29]

NIGHT TERRORS AND SLEEP WALKING (NON-REM DYSSOMNIAS)

Definition

Transient (5-20 minute duration) episodes of altered behavior, autonomic dysfunction, and motor automatisms which occur during non-REM sleep Stages III/IV (deep or slow wave) of which the patient has no recollection upon awakening constitute NREM dyssomnias. These dyssomnias are usually maturational disorders, in most instances resolving spontaneously over time.[10]

Clinical Manifestations

The hallmark of both night "terrors" and sleep walking is the time of occurrence. Both disorders occur exclusively in the domain of slow wave sleep. This type of sleep is normally clustered into the 2nd and 3rd hours after falling asleep. The history should therefore elicit the time of onset of abnormal nocturnal behavior in relation to sleep onset.

Night terrors are common in children between the ages of 2 and 5 years, sleep walking in those 5 to 10 years of age. Persistence of sleep walking beyond 12 years of age may be indicative of an underlying psychiatric disorder.

During night terrors, the child usually wakes up screaming or crying, may be sweating and have a flushed face, and is disoriented and difficult to console. The entire episode lasts 5-10 minutes, following which the child goes right back to sleep and has no recollection whatsoever of the episode the following morning.

Children with somnambulism typically sit up in bed, have a "glassy" facial expression, may walk about clumsily, or talk in an irrelevant manner (somniloquy). The entire episode lasts from 30 seconds to 15-20 minutes, following which the patient resumes normal sleep and has no recollection of the event upon awakening in the morning.

Diagnosis

The typical time of onset and clinical manifestations are by themselves diagnostic.[11] If one is fortunate enough to obtain an electroencephalo-gram during one of the NREM sleep disturbances, characteristic rhythmic 1-2 Hertz generalized delta activity is noted. As patients rarely enter into Stages III and IV of non-REM sleep during daytime naps, the EEG study ideally should be obtained at night.

Differential Diagnosis

Nocturnal partial seizures may on occasion be associated with nocturnal wandering. In contrast to NREM dyssomnias, however, these events have a random, temporal dispersion throughout night-sleep and are generally associated with vertex or parasaggital spike activity on the EEG.

Management

1. Reassurance to parents, indicating that the disorder (sleep walking or night terror) resolves spontaneously in a few months to 1-2 years.
2. If the disorder becomes severe or adversely affects sleep habits of the rest of the family, hypnotic-sedative medications like chloral hydrate (10- 20 mg/kg/dose) can be administered at bedtime in order to suppress slow wave sleep and consequently, the sleep disturbance.

NOCTURNAL ENURESIS

Approximately 10 to 15% of all children between the ages of 4 and 5 years continue to wet the bed.[12] In one study, however, 90% of the children had attained nocturnal dryness by age 7 years, and 97% by 12 years.[13]

Primary nocturnal enuresis (where the child has never been consistently dry since infancy) should be differentiated from secondary enuresis (relapse into bedwetting following a period of normal nocturnal bladder control). The latter is usually consequent to an emotional disturbance and is not a primary sleep disturbance.

Polygraphic studies of sleep had initially indicated that primary nocturnal enuretic events occur mainly in Stage III and IV of sleep, and therefore liable to be clustered within the first third of night sleep. It now appears that such enuretic episodes are uniformly dispersed throughout the night in both REM and NREM sleep.[14] Primary nocturnal enuresis is most likely a maturational disorder of the supranuclear bladder innervation which generally resolves spontaneously over 3-4 years. Although not inherently harmful, it can lead to serious psychological problems. Family life may be altered as undue attention is focussed on the enuretic child through scapegoating, treatment attempts, or the need to maintain a family secret. It may also result in chronic anxiety in the child and lowering of self-esteem.

Treatment

It is important to reassure the family and child of the strong likelihood of spontaneous resolution of the problem in 3-4 years. Pharmacological treatment with Imipramine (25-50 mg at bedtime) is of some value in breaking the cycle of: nocturnal enuresis→reinforcement of anxiety→persistence of enuresis. Treatment should be continued for a period of 3-4 months. Conditioning alarm devices attached to the perineal skin surface which sense moisture and produce an arousal when activated are somewhat more effective (initial cure rate 80%) than Imipramine therapy (initial cure rate 40%).[15] There is a high incidence of relapse, however, with both modalities of treatment. Whenever enuresis persists beyond 12-13 years of age, supportive psychotherapy should be initiated, as emotional problems invariably develop in such children.

NARCOLEPSY

Narcolepsy is a disorder characterized by the tetrad of episodes of irresistible sleepiness, cataplexy, hypnogogic hallucinations, and sleep paralysis. All four manifestations may not necessarily be present in each patient at a given time. Excessive daytime sleepiness and cataplexy are the two most common clinical features.

It is a general misconception that narcolepsy is a disease that affects mainly adults. Yoss and Daly in a review of 400 narcoleptic patients followed at the Mayo Clinic noted that the symptom of excessive daytime sleepiness had appeared in 59% of the subjects by the age of 15 years.[16] The exact prevalence of the disease is unknown. Roth estimated an incidence of

0.03% in Czechoslovakia.[17] Approximately 66,000 narcoleptic patients were believed to be present in the United States in 1974.[17]

Etiology

The etiology of narcolepsy is not yet fully understood. The occasional clustering of patients in families is suggestive of a genetic predisposition. The most interesting recent data in this regard pertain to the strong association of the human leukocyte antigen (HLA) DR2 with narcolepsy. This association has been documented in British, Japanese, and French narcoleptic subjects.[18, 19, 20] The HLA gene is located on the short arm of chromosome 6. The antigen is present in 100% of both familial and nonfamilial narcoleptics. On a neurochemical basis, the abnormality, at least in part, relates to function of the locus coeruleus nucleus, which is responsible for synthesis of the REM sleep-initiating norepinephrine.

Clinical Manifestations

The most invariant clinical feature is the irresistible urge to sleep. The naps may last from 1 to 15 minutes, following which the patient appears momentarily refreshed. The patient may fall asleep while reading, riding in an automobile, and even while talking or walking, thus making him/her susceptible to accidents. Cataplexy is the second most frequent manifestation. It may occur along with the daytime sleepiness or develop within the subsequent 5-10 years. It is characterized by sudden weakness and loss of muscle tone, either generalized or limited to a small muscle group, usually in response to an emotional change such as anger, fright, or laughter. The patient may suddenly feel weak and fall to the floor when experiencing such emotions. Consciousness is fully preserved, and the entire event lasts a few minutes, following which the patient is back to normal. The hypotonia, hyporeflexia, and rapid eye movements that occur along with the cataplexy indicate that it is a reflection of REM sleep intrusion into wakefulness. Hypnogogic hallucinations are vivid visual or auditory experiences at sleep onset. Sleep paralysis is a transient clinical feature which can occur while the patient is falling asleep or waking up from sleep. Narcoleptics frequently also have disturbed nocturnal sleep, with frequent miniature arousals and periodic leg movements. Memory problems may develop in the third or fourth decade.

Diagnosis

Historical data combined with polysomographic and immunological studies are conventionally used to establish the diagnosis. The nocturnal polysomnogram helps exclude other causes of excessive daytime sleepiness such as sleep apnea. Upon awakening from the all-night sleep study, the patient with suspected narcolepsy undergoes a Multiple Sleep Latency Test (MSLT). The test requires that the patient attempt to take a series of 4-5 daytime naps at two hour intervals, with simultaneous monitoring of EEG, eye movements, chin electromyogram, and respiration. The nap is terminated on each occasion within 5-10 minutes of sleep onset. Patients with narcolepsy demonstrate a markedly decreased sleep latency (time from initiation of attempt at napping to sleep onset). The onset of sleep characteristically is marked by appearance of REM rather then the normal NREM sleep. Positive leukocyte studies for the HLA DR2 antigen also aid in establishing the diagnosis.

Differential Diagnosis

Excessive daytime sleepiness following head trauma, viral encephalitis, drug dependency, and the sleep apnea syndrome are disorders which can mimic narcolepsy. Cataplexy may be mistaken for atonic seizures. In most of the above instances, however, the history, electroencephalogram, and polysomnographic findings are distinct from those of narcolepsy.

Treatment

Excessive Daytime Sleepiness. This most disabling feature of narcolepsy requires life-long therapy with central nervous system stimulants. Pemoline sodium (CYLERT), methylphenidate (RITALIN), and dextroamphetamine are the most commonly prescribed agents. It is recommended that the patient be commenced initially on the less potent of the three drugs (pemoline or methylphenidate). If possible, planned daytime naps and observation of regular night sleep

habits may also be beneficial. Children with narcolepsy frequently develop behavioral problems and require supportive psychotherapy.[21]

Cataplexy. Cholinergic pathways in the brainstem seem to mediate cataplexy.[22] Anticholinergic drugs are therefore useful in inhibiting it. Protryptiline (VIVACTIL) in a dosage of 2.5-5mg/ day is the most commonly prescribed agent.

SLEEP APNEA SYNDROMES

Definition

Sleep apnea syndromes are characterized by defective control of breathing during sleep.[23] This abnormality may result from an impairment in the central nervous system control of respiration, a defect in transmission of the neural output to upper airway muscles, anatomical abnormalities in the upper airway, or as a result of weakness of respiratory muscles. Except in very severe cases, the respiratory abnormality is typically undetectable when the patient is awake. Sleep apnea syndrome is defined as the presence of more than 30 apnea episodes during a nocturnal polysomnogram or of more than 5 apneic episodes per hour of sleep, each of a minimum duration of 10 seconds.[23]

Three major kinds of apneic episodes can be distinguished on the polysomnogram:

> **Central apnea**; characterized by simultaneous cessation of nasal airflow, thoracic, and abdominal respiration (Fig. 13-1).

> **Obstructive apnea**; in which cessation of nasal airflow occurs despite persistence of thoracic and abdominal respiratory effort. Such children may have structural abnormalities of the upper airway or manifest airway lumen collapse owing to weakness of upper airway musculature (pharyngeal constrictors).

> **Mixed apnea**; which is a combination of central and obstructive types, with the former always preceding the latter in each episode.

Clinical Features

Two clinical disorders presenting with apnea in children are described:

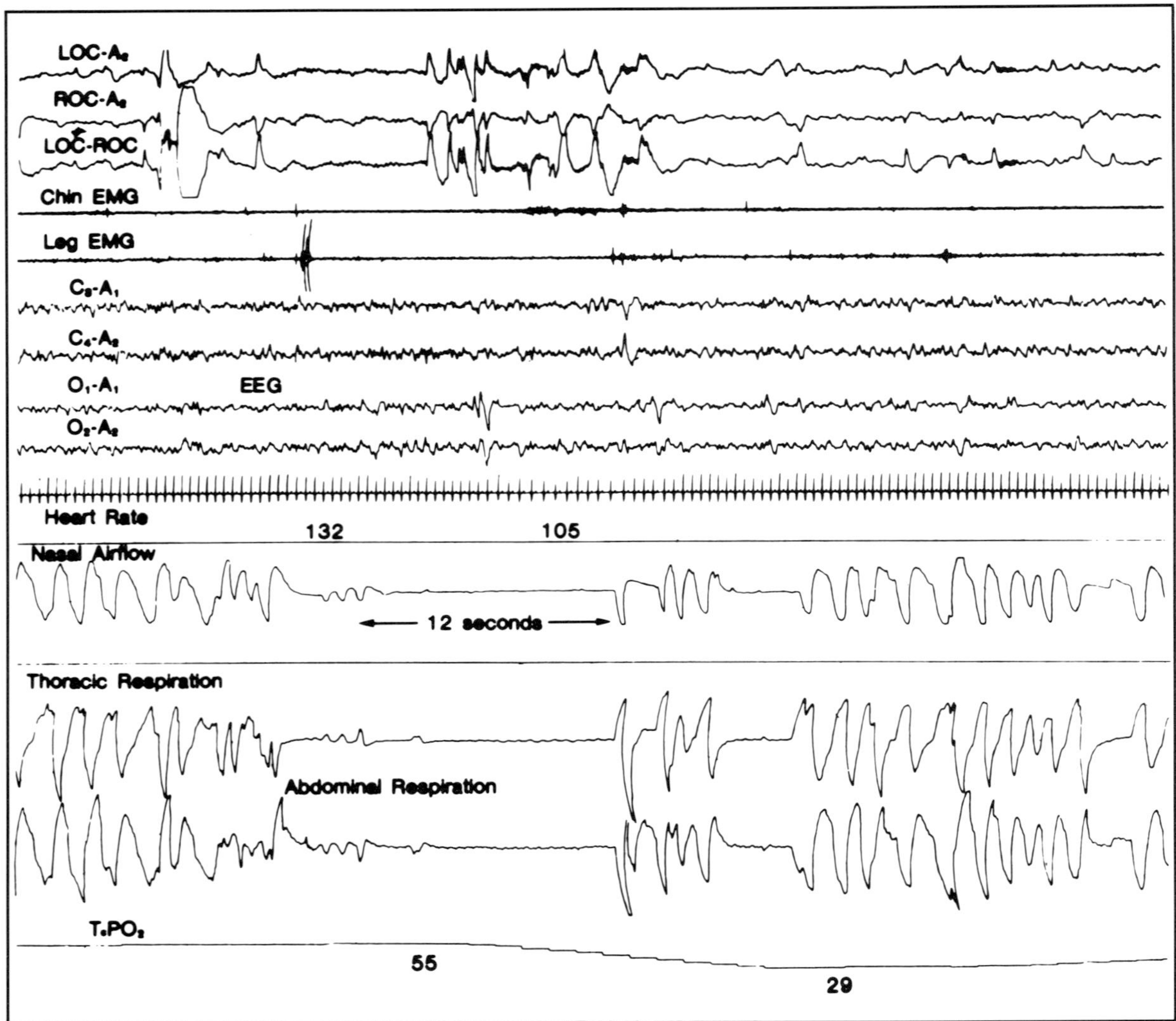

Fig. 13-1. Polysomnogram on a patient with central apnea in sleep, demonstrating hypoxemia and bradycardia. **LOC** = Left outer canthus, **A2** = right ear, **ROC** = right outer canthus (eye movement channel), **EMG** = electromyogram, **C3** = left central region, **C4** = right central region, **01** = left occipital region, **02** = right occipital region, **TcPO$_2$** = transcutaneous pO$_2$.

Central Alveolar Hypoventilation Syndrome. Characterized by central apnea due to defective central nervous system control of respiration during sleep, this condition may be present in infancy[24, 25] (congenital form) or later childhood. Developmental malformations of the brainstem (sometimes only evident at the microscopic level) are common in the congenital variety. Head trauma, bulbar poliomyelitis, metabolic disorders, and neuromuscular diseases are some of the etiological factors. Respiration is generally normal during wakefulness, but periodic breathing, central apnea, and hypoxemia appear during sleep. The central nervous system arousal response to hypoxia and hypercarbia during sleep is very often impaired.[26] The diagnosis of central alveolar hypoventilaion syndrome can be readily confirmed using a polygraphic study of sleep and respiration.

A variety of treatment measures can be attempted, none entirely satisfactory. Theophylline and acetazolamide can be used to enhance chemoreceptivity of brainstem respiratory neurons. A curaiss (shell) respirator applied to the chest wall during sleep and diaphragmatic pacing are other modalities of treatment. The latter may be useful in mild to moderate hypoventilation syndromes. The outcome depends to some extent upon the nature of the underlying illness. Spontaneous resolution can occur in a minority of subjects, especially infants.

Obstructive Apnea. These events may occur at all ages in childhood. In the newborn period they are generally secondary to collapse of the hypotonic upper airway musculature in sleep or congenital malformations (choanal atresia, micrognathia and macroglossia). In older children, tonsillar and adenoidal hypertrophy or the Pickwickian syndrome (obesity and sleep-related respiratory disturbances) are common causes.[27] Nocturnal snoring is also common in older children. Some patients with airway obstruction demonstrate only nocturnal oxygen desaturation, disturbed sleep, and increased respiratory effort, but they may have a minimal number of apneic events per se.

Hypersomnia is frequently observed in older children with obstructive apnea and is a consequence of fragmentation of night sleep due to hypoxia from repeated apneic episodes. This results in suppression of slow wave (Stages III, IV of NREM) and REM sleep, with rebound excessive daytime sleepiness. Another consequence of chronic nocturnal hypoxemia is pulmonary vasoconstriction, chronic cor pulmonale, and failure to thrive.

Children with obstructive sleep apnea may also develop intellectual dysfunction and hyperactivity. The diagnosis of obstructive apnea can be readily established on the nocturnal polysomnogram. Direct visualization of airway collapse during sleep using a fiberoptic camera inserted through the nose is also helpful.

A variety of measures are available for treatment. Weight loss is strongly recommended for any obese individual. Tonsillar and adenoidal hypertrophy can be easily corrected surgically. In infants with airway collapse during sleep, the problem may resolve spontaneously over time or with use of continuous nasal positive pressure breathing during sleep. Uvulo-palato-pharyngoplasty is of benefit in enlarging the oropharyngeal lumen in those obese subjects in whom it is narrow. If the above procedures are not beneficial, one may have to resort to tracheostomy. While tracheostomy produces significant and immediate relief, it makes home management of the patient exceedingly complicated. It should be reserved as a last resort.

HYPERSOMNIA RELATED TO DRUG INTOXICATION

Children with this category of hypersomnia generally have an iatrogenic disorder resulting from prescription of medications such as antihistamines, anticonvulsants, or tranquilizers (e.g., thioridazine). Once the cause of hypersomnia is recognized, the disorder is easily remediable. Hypersomnia in the adolescent from abuse of street drugs is a more difficult management problem. Treatment requires cooperation of the child and family, as well as psychiatric intervention.

DISORDERS OF INITIATING AND MAINTAINING SLEEP

Most children generally fall asleep at night within 15-30 minutes of going to bed and turning off the lights. However, patients with chronic anxiety or depression may have consistent difficulty in initiating sleep. When they do fall asleep, they tend to have frequent nocturnal awakenings and may be unable to sleep past the early morning hours. The carry-over effect into bedtime of stimulant medications administered in the daytime (e.g., pemoline or dextroamphetamine for hyperactivity) is another sleep disturbance which can be resolved by changing the time of drug administration. Hypoxemia as a consequence of the sleep apnea syndrome also reduces the overall quantity and quality of night sleep. Systemic illnesses (bronchial asthma, chronic cough, nasal obstruction, chronic pain) are generally treatable causes of disturbed sleep initiation and maintenance.

A physiological event that is frequently ignored from the standpoint of sleep hygiene is exercise within 2-3 hours of bedtime. It is well known that sleep-wake and body temperature cycles follow a circadian pattern, and that both cycles are biphasic, parallel, and closely synchronized. Wakefulness is generally maximal at a point that the body temperature is at its highest (mid-day) and sleepiness is maximal at a point the body temperature has reached its nadir (early morning). Exercise within 2-3 hours of bedtime raises the core body temperature, thereby inhibiting sleep onset, and therefore should ideally be so timed that it does not interfere with sleep onset.

Table 13-1. Comparison of sleep states

	REM SLEEP	NREM SLEEP
EEG activity	Low voltage, irregular	High voltage; sleep spindles and K complexes present
EMG activity	Intermittent	Continuous
Rapid eye movements	Present	Absent
Respiration	Irregular	Regular
Proportion of sleep	50% (newborn) to 20% (adolescent) of total sleep time	50% (newborn) to 80% (adolescent) of total sleep time
Responsivity of brainstem respiratory neurons to CO2 accumulation	Suppressed	Intact

DELAYED SLEEP PHASE SYNDROME

This is the most common circadian rhythm disorder and accounts for about 10% of all insomnia complaints.[29] It is characterized by a constitutional inability to advance (prepone) sleep onset prior to a given time. The patient is typically a "night person" who is unable to fall asleep prior to 2 or 3 a.m. despite the best of efforts. If allowed to sleep uninterrupted (on holidays for example), the individual will very often sleep untill 11 a.m. or noon, feeling quite refreshed upon awakening. The quantity and quality of sleep are entirely normal. However, on weekdays the patient has to awaken earlier, at a socially acceptable hour, in order to attend school or work. As a consequence, sleep deprivation and excessive daytime sleepiness ensue.

Treatment

The treatment[30] consists of sequentially *advancing* the patient's bed-onset time forwards, around the clock over a period of 2-3 weeks, so that ultimately sleep onset occurs around 9 or 10 p.m.. The patient is then advised to lock in to this bedtime by maintaining regular sleep-wake habits.

EPILEPSY AND SLEEP

The relationship between sleep and epilepsy is well known. Between 0.5 to 24% of epileptics have seizures that occur only during sleep.[31,32,33] Janz, in a study of 2,110 patients with generalized convulsive seizures, reported that 45% had seizures predominantly in sleep.[34] Generalized epileptifom discharges are more liable to occur in Stages I and II of NREM sleep and focal epileptifom discharges in both NREM and REM sleep. Also, sleep deprivation is well known to lower seizure threshold.

Besides convulsive seizures occurring in sleep, two other disorders also deserve mention. One is the syndrome of episodic nocturnal wandering seen in light NREM sleep, associated with temporal or generalized epileptifom discharges.[35] Most such children have a favorable response to anticonvulsants (phenytoin or carbamazepine). The second disorder is characterized by paroxysmal awakenings from sleep coinciding with epileptiform discharges and secondary excessive daytime sleepiness.[36] Most subjects are young to middle-aged adults. Once again, anticonvulsant therapy is beneficial in resolving the hypersomnia.

REFERENCES

1. Dreyfus-Brisac C. Ontogenesis of sleep in human prematures after 32 weeks of conceptional age. Dev Psychobiol 3(2):91-121, 1970.

2. Denenberg V.H. and Thoman E.B. Evidence for a functional role for active (REM) sleep in infancy. Sleep 4(2):185-191, 1981.

3. Coons S. and Guilleminault C. Development of sleep-wake patterns and non-rapid eye movement sleep stages during the first six months of life in normal infants. Pediatrics 69:793-798, 1982.

4. Carskadon M.A., The second decade. In: Guilleminault C, ed. Sleeping and Waking Disorders. Indications and Techniques. Menlo Park, Addison-Wesley, 1982; 99-125.

5. Jouvet M. Biogenic amines and the states of sleep. Science 163:32-41, 1969.

6. Carskadon M.A. Basics for polygraphic monitoring of sleep. In: Guilleminault C, ed. Sleeping and Waking Disorders. Indications and Techniques. Menlo Park, Addison-Wesley, 1982; 1-16.

8. Guilleminault C. and Soquet M. Sleep states and related pathology. In: Korobkin R. and Guilleminault C, eds. Advances in Perinatal Neurology; Vol. 1, New York, Spectrum, 1979; 225-248.

9. Rechtschaffen A. and Kales A, eds. A manual of standardized terminology, techniques and scoring system for sleep stages in human subjects. Los Angeles; UCLA Brain Information Service/Brain Research Institute, 1978.

10. Kales A. and Kales J.D. Sleep disorders. Recent findings in the diagnosis and treatment of disturbed sleep. N Engl J Med 290:487-498, 1974.

11. Anders T.F. and Guillerminault C. The pathophysiology of sleep disorders in pediatrics. Parts I and II. Advances in Pediatrics 22:137-174, 1976.

12. Nesbit REL. Urethrovesical malfunctions and urinary incontinence in female children and adolescents. Pediatr Clin North Am 19:705-716, 1972.

13. Oppel WC, Harper PA and Rider RV. The age of attaining bladder control. Pediatrics 42:614-626, 1968.

14. Fritz GK and Anders TF. Enuresis: the clinical application of an etiologically based classification system. Child Psychiatr and Human Dev 10(2):103-113, 1979.

15. Wagner W, Johnson SB, Walker D, et al. A controlled comparison of two treatments for nocturnal enuresis. J Pediatr 101:302-307, 1982.

16. Yoss RE and Daly DD. Narcolepsy in children. Pediatrics 25:1025-1033, 1960.

17. Zarcone V. Narcolepsy. N Engl J Med 288:1156-1166, 1973.

18. Billiard M, Siegnalet J, Besset, et al. HLA-DR2 and narcolepsy. Sleep 9(1):149-152, 1986.

19. Honda Y, Juji T, Matsuki K, et al. HLA-DR2 and Dw2 in narcolepsy and in other disorders of excessive somnolence without cataplexy. Sleep 9(1):133-142, 1986.

20. Langdon N, Lock C, Welsh K, et al. Immune factors in narcolepsy. Sleep 9(1):143-148, 1986.

21. Kotagal S, Hartse KM, Walsh JK. Characteristics of Narcolepsy in preteenaged children. Pediatrics 85; 1990 (In press)

22. Mitler M and Dement WC. Cataplectic-like behavior in cats after micro-injections of carbachol in pontine reticular formation. Brain Res 68:335-343, 1974.

23. Guilleminault C, Van Den Hoed J and Mitler M. Clinical overview of the sleep apnea syndromes. In: Guilleminault C, ed. Sleep Apnea Syndromes. Alan R Liss, New York, 1978; 1-12.

24. Guilleminault C, McQuitty J, Ariagno RL, et al. Congenital central alveolar hypoventilation syndrome in six infants. Pediatrics 70(5):684-694, 1982.

25. Onal E, Lopata M and O'Connor T. Pathogenesis of apneas in hypersomnia-sleep apnea syndrome. Am Rev Respir Dis 125:167-174, 1982.

26. Farmer WC, Glenn WWL, Gee JBL. Alveolar hypoventilation syndrome. Study of ventilatory control in patients selected for deaphragm pacing. Am J Med 64:39-49, 1978.

27. Guilleminault G, Korobkin R and Winkle R. A review of 50 children with obstructive sleep apnea syndrome. Lung 159:1-13, 1981.

28. Guilleminault C, Ariagno R, Korobkin R et al. Sleep parameters and respiratory variables in "near miss" sudden infant death syndrome infants. Pediatrics 68(3):354-360, 1981.

29. Moore-Ede MC, Czeisler CA and Richardson GS. Circadian time-keeping in health and disease. Parts I and II. N Engl J Med 309(8)469-476 and 309(9):530-535, 1983.

30. Czeisler CA, Richardson GS, Coleman R, et al. Chronotherapy: resetting the circadian clocks of patients with delayed sleep phase insomnia. Sleep 4:1-21, 1981.

31. Gibbard F, Bateson M. Sleep epilepsy: its patterns and prognosis. Br Med J 2:403-405, 1974.

32. Langdon-Down M, Brain W. Time of day in relation to convulsions in epilepsy. Lancet 2:1029-1032, 1929.

33. Patry F. The relation of time of day, sleep and other factors to the incidence of epileptic seizures. Am J. Psychiatr. 87:789-813, 1931.

34. Janz D. The grand mal epilepsies and the sleep-wake cycle. Epilepsia 3:69-109, 1962.

35. Pedley T. and Guilleminault C. Episodic nocturnal wanderings responsive to anticonvulsant drug therapy. Ann Neurol 2:30-35, 1977.

36. Peled R. and Lavie P. Paroxysmal awakenings from sleep associated with excessive daytime somnolence. Neurology 36(1):95-98, 1986.

SUGGESTED READING

1. Guilleminault C. Sleep and Its Disorders in Children. Raven Press, New York, 1987.

CHAPTER XIV

DEVELOPMENTAL ARREST OR REGRESSION

Introduction

Central nervous system neoplasms, hydrocephalus, chronic subdural hematomas, inborn errors of metabolism, toxic encephalopathies, and subacute or slow viral infections can all lead to arrest in the child's development. With progression in the underlying neurologic disorder, there may even be loss of previously acquired milestones. The algorithms presented in this chapter

ALGORITHM A

DEVELOPMENTAL ARREST OR REGRESSION

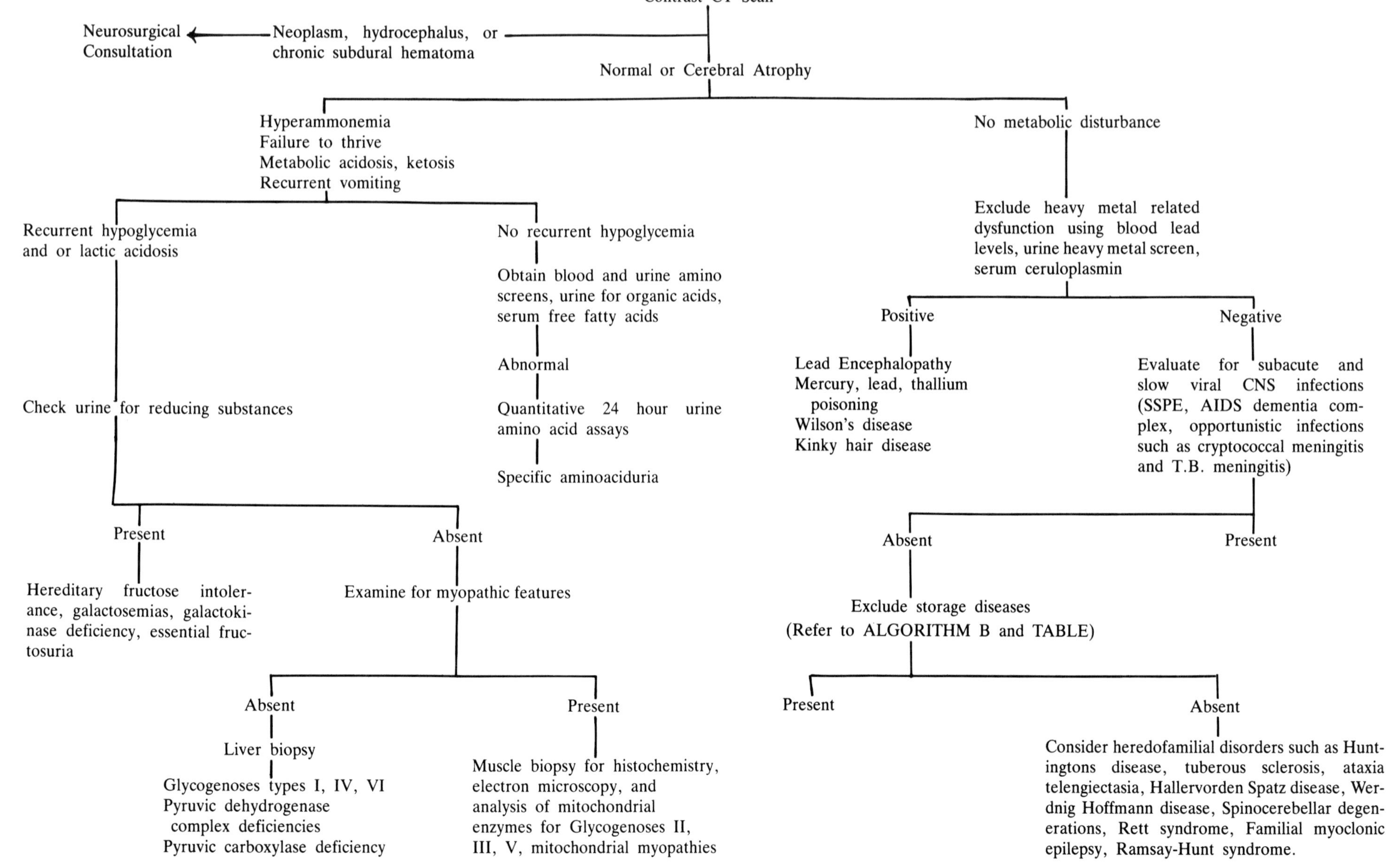

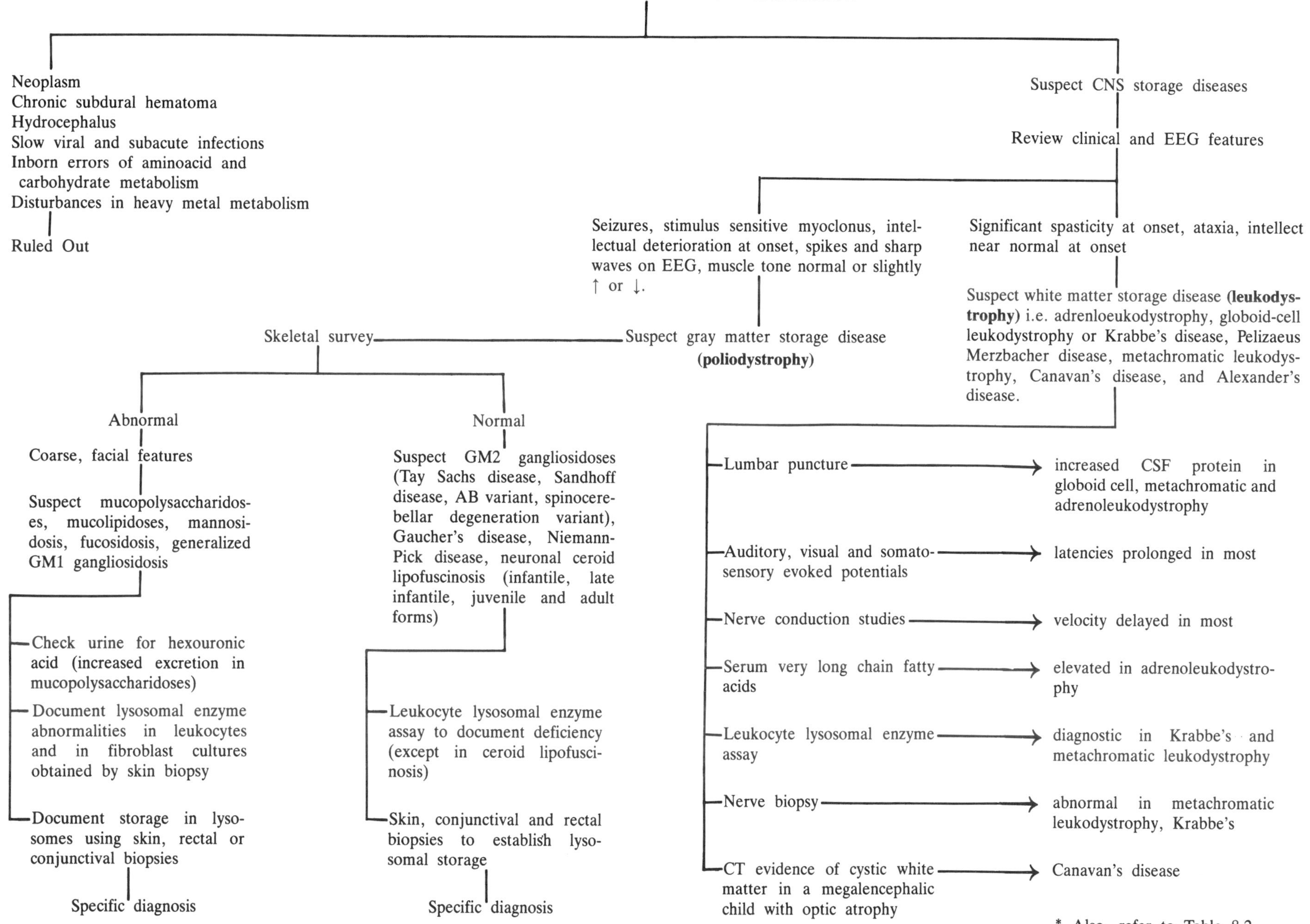

ALGORITHM B

DEVELOPMENTAL ARREST OR REGRESSION*

Neoplasm
Chronic subdural hematoma
Hydrocephalus
Slow viral and subacute infections
Inborn errors of aminoacid and
  carbohydrate metabolism
Disturbances in heavy metal metabolism

Ruled Out

Suspect CNS storage diseases

Review clinical and EEG features

Seizures, stimulus sensitive myoclonus, intellectual deterioration at onset, spikes and sharp waves on EEG, muscle tone normal or slightly ↑ or ↓.

Significant spasticity at onset, ataxia, intellect near normal at onset

Suspect white matter storage disease (leukodystrophy) i.e. adrenloeukodystrophy, globoid-cell leukodystrophy or Krabbe's disease, Pelizaeus Merzbacher disease, metachromatic leukodystrophy, Canavan's disease, and Alexander's disease.

Skeletal survey

Suspect gray matter storage disease (poliodystrophy)

Abnormal

Normal

Coarse, facial features

Suspect mucopolysaccharidoses, mucolipidoses, mannosidosis, fucosidosis, generalized GM1 gangliosidosis

Suspect GM2 gangliosidoses (Tay Sachs disease, Sandhoff disease, AB variant, spinocerebellar degeneration variant), Gaucher's disease, Niemann-Pick disease, neuronal ceroid lipofuscinosis (infantile, late infantile, juvenile and adult forms)

Check urine for hexouronic acid (increased excretion in mucopolysaccharidoses)

Document lysosomal enzyme abnormalities in leukocytes and in fibroblast cultures obtained by skin biopsy

Document storage in lysosomes using skin, rectal or conjunctival biopsies

Specific diagnosis

Leukocyte lysosomal enzyme assay to document deficiency (except in ceroid lipofuscinosis)

Skin, conjunctival and rectal biopsies to establish lysosomal storage

Specific diagnosis

Lumbar puncture

increased CSF protein in globoid cell, metachromatic and adrenoleukodystrophy

Auditory, visual and somato-sensory evoked potentials

latencies prolonged in most

Nerve conduction studies

velocity delayed in most

Serum very long chain fatty acids

elevated in adrenoleukodystrophy

Leukocyte lysosomal enzyme assay

diagnostic in Krabbe's and metachromatic leukodystrophy

Nerve biopsy

abnormal in metachromatic leukodystrophy, Krabbe's

CT evidence of cystic white matter in a megalencephalic child with optic atrophy

Canavan's disease

* Also, refer to Table 8-2

should only be used as a general guide to evaluation. Certain diagnostic steps may be omitted if the clinical features are overwhelmingly suggestive of a specific disorder, e.g., it is not always necessary to obtain a CT scan in a child with metabolic acidosis, vomiting, and failure to thrive who most likely has an inborn error of metabolism.

NEOPLASMS

The majority of brain tumors in children are primary to the central nervous system. Neoplasms tend to be more common in the supratentorial space in infancy but subsequently, 60-70% of neoplasms in childhood occur within the posterior fossa. Choroid plexus papilloma, ependymoma and teratomas are the most common supratentorial neoplasms in infancy. Astrocytoma, medulloblastoma, ependymoma, and brainstem glioma are the most common posterior fossa tumors. Astrocytomas may also arise in the supratentorial space, generally in the region of the diencephalon. Craniopharyngoma is another common supratentorial tumor. It may be located within the sella or the suprasellar space. Brain tumors in children are generally characterized by origin close to the midline, with early impingement on the ventricular system leading to obstructive hydrocephalus. The duration of time between onset of symptoms and clinical presentation is relatively brief—between 2-6 weeks.

Clinical manifestations

These are related partly to increased intracranial pressure, and in part to the location of the tumor. Headache, vomiting, change in personality, dizziness, double vision from extraocular nerve pareses, and unsteadiness of gait from cerebellar system dysfunction are the most common symptoms. Examination may disclose papilledema, macrocephaly, cranial neuropathies, pyramidal signs, gait ataxia, and head tilt (due to incipient tonsillar herniation). Unilateral VI and VII cranial nerve palsy with contralateral hemiparesis or ataxia are common manifestations of a brainstem glioma. Contrast CT or MRI scans are the diagnostic procedures of choice.

Management

Management includes insertion of a ventriculoperitoneal shunt for hydrocephalus, biopsy for determination of tumor type, and resection of as much of the tumor mass as is safely possible. Computer-assisted stereotactic laser techniques, when available, enable removal of deep seated lesions with minimal injury to adjacent normal tissue. Post-operative radiation therapy (5,000 rads) to the craniospinal axis is indicated for astrocytoma, medulloblastoma, and ependymoma.

Prognosis

Complete surgical resection of cerebellar astrocytoma is associated with a 100% five year survival rate; partial resection with approximately a 79% five year survival rate. The five year survival rate for patients with medulloblastoma is 56%, and 25% for ependymoma. Brainstem gliomas have a very poor prognosis owing to inoperability and resistance to radiation therapy, with the overall five year survival being 15-20%.

Follow-up

Patients with craniopharyngomas should have careful pre and postoperative evaluation of neuroendocrine function and visual fields. Children with medulloblastomas, astrocytomas, or ependymomas should undergo serial postoperative CT scans to assess for tumor remnants. Periodic lumbar punctures for tumor cytology, tumor markers (polyamines elevated in medulloblastoma recurrence, alphafetoprotein elevated with germ cell tumor recurrence), and myelography are required to monitor for postoperative tumor seeding and recurrence in the spinal canal in the case of medulloblastomas and ependymomas.

HYDROCEPHALUS (Chapter X)

CHRONIC SUBDURAL HEMATOMA

Headache, increasing head size, apathy, vomiting, and gait disturbance are the most common clinical manifestations, evolving over weeks to months following head trauma. CT scan is the diagnostic procedure of choice, and demonstrates a hypodense extracerebral lesion. With the exception of chronic subdural hematomas in infancy, drainage through a burr-hole is indicated for all, and is generally therapeutic (also see Chapter X).

INBORN ERRORS OF AMINOACID AND CARBOHYDRATE METABOLISM

These inborn errors may present in the neonatal period, infancy, or early childhood. Failure to thrive, recurrent vomiting, ketosis, and persistent metabolic acidosis are present in both categories. Hyperammonemia is suggestive of either primary or secondary dysfunction in the ammonia cycle. Phenylketonuria, maple syrup urine disease, homocystinuria, non-ketotic hyperglycinemia, isovaleric acidemia, and arginosuccinic aciduria are some of the common inborn errors of aminoacid metabolism. Qualitative aminoacid chromatography, combined with determination of blood ammonia, serum lactate, pyruvate, and a urine organic acid assay (e.g., for dicarboxylic acids) are helpful as initial screens. If a particular aminoacid or metabolite is elevated in the serum or urine, it can be specifically identified and the disorder diagnosed using analysis by gas-liquid chromatography or mass spectrometry. Elevated cerebrospinal fluid glycine levels are diagnostic of non-ketotic hyperglycinemia.

Recurrent hypoglycemia is suggestive of inborn errors of carbohydrate metabolism. Glycogen storage diseases (Types I-VII), galactosemia, fructose 1-6 diphosphatase deficiency, and defects in the pyruvic acid dehydrogenase enzyme complex constitute some of the common carbohydrate metabolic disorders. Galactosemia is associated with the presence of reducing substances in the urine, recurrent hypoglycemia, hepatic dysfunction, and cataracts. The absence of galactose-1-phophate uridyl transferase on red cell assay is diagnositc. Hypoglycemia is also common in glycogen storage diseases types I, III, and VI. Glycogenosis Type II (Pompe's disease) is associated with severe generalized hypotonia and cardiomegaly in infancy; types V and VII with recurrent muscle cramps, myoglobinuria, and atrophy. A decision about whether to obtain a skeletal muscle or liver biopsy in suspected glycogenoses depends on the nature of the predominant symptoms (myopathic versus hypoglycemic).

LEIGH'S DISEASE

Also known as subacute necrotizing encephalomyelopathy, Leigh's Disease is associated with progressive spasticity and intellectual and occulomotor dysfunction, with onset in infancy. Lactic acidosis and episodic hyperventilation may also be present. The pathological lesions are similar to those seen in Wernicke's encephalopathy (degeneration of the periaqueductal gray matter, basal ganglia, and spinal cord). Some patients with Leigh's disease have been found to have pyruvate carboxylase/pyruvate dehydrogenase complex deficiencies.

LEAD ENCEPHALOPATHY

This is most commonly seen in children of the preschool age. The acute form is associated with a blood lead level exceeding 80 ugm/ml, stupor from increased intracranial pressure, and convulsions. The subacute form is more prevalent, and is seen with moderate level chronic exposure to lead. Serum lead levels are generally between 30-60 ugm/ml. The child manifests developmental delay, headaches, and behavioral disturbances. The management consists of removing the source of lead (e.g., peeling lead-based paint) from the child's home environment and chelation using Calcium EDTA or penicillamine.

WILSON'S DISEASE

This autosomal recessive disorder is caused by excessive accumulation of copper in the nervous system and liver owing to lack of an alpha globulin (ceruloplasmin) which normally binds over 95% of the circulating copper. It may present either primarily with hepatic dysfunction in the form of jaundice and portal hypertension or as a neurological syndrome characterized by tremor, rigidity, dystonia, salivary drooling, and speech difficulty. By the time neurologic manifestations appear, copper deposition in the Descemet's layer of the cornea is invariably present and visible in the form of the green/yellow/brown Kayser-Fleischer rings. The diagnosis can be established by documentation of low or absent serum ceruloplasmin levels and elevated plasma copper levels. The treatment consists of the removal of excessive amounts of copper using d-penicillamine, and supplementing the diet with pyridoxine to offset the antipyridoxine effect of penicillamine.

KINKY HAIR DISEASE

First described by Menkes and associates, this is an X-linked recessive disorder leading to progressive degeneration of the gray matter commencing in infancy. Patients have low serum copper and ceruloplasmin levels. Copper levels are also reduced in the liver and brain, but elevated in the intestinal mucosa and fibroblasts. Lack of availability of copper for synthesis of various copper containing enzymes in the body (ceruloplasmin, cytochrome oxidase) leads to dysfunction that is most notable in the brain, blood vessels, hair, and bones. Seizures, poor feeding, and hypotonia become apparent in infancy. Microscopic examination of hair reveals a twisted appearance with multiple fractures at regular intervals. Blood vessels become tortuous. X-Rays of long bones may reveal metaphysial spurring. The diagnosis can be established by documenting lack of the physiologic rise in serum ceruloplasmin levels after the first month, as well as low plasma copper levels. Intravenous copper infusions can raise the serum copper levels into the normal range, but it is not clear whether this results in arrest of the neurologic deterioration. An intrauterine diagnosis of Menke's disease can be made on the basis of elevated fibroblast copper levels.

Refer to Chapter IV for subacute sclerosing panencephalitis (SSPE), acquired immune deficiency syndrome, cryptococcal meningitis and tuberculous meningitis.

HUNTINGTON'S DISEASE

This is a progressive, disorder characterized by chorea, dementia, and autosomal dominant transmission. The gene is located on the short arm of chromosome 4. Children with Huntington's disease are most likely to acquire the disorder from the father. Hypokinesia, rigidity, and seizures are characteristic of juvenile Huntington's disease. Although brain catecholamine metabolism is frequently altered, the exact biochemical and genetic predisposing factors remain uncertain. The diagnosis can be established on the basis of the family history, clinical features, and presence of atrophy in the region of the caudate nuclei on the CT scan. The disorder is steadily progressive, leading to death in 6-8 years. No specific treatment is available.

TUBEROUS SCLEROSIS (Chapter XI)

ATAXIA TELANGIECTASIA (Chapter XI)

HALLERVORDEN SPATZ DISEASE

Progressive dementia, seizures, rigidity, athetosis, club feet, and onset prior to ten years characterize this disorder. The underlying defect remains unknown. Axonal degeneration with a predilection for the globus pallidus and substantia nigra is the most common histological feature. It has been postulated that the disorder is associated with a central nervous system perturbation in iron metabolism. The CT scan may reveal low density lesions in the region of the basal ganglia, while the MRI scan shows areas of decreased signal intensity in the same region on the T1 weighted images. No specific treatment is available.

WERDNIG HOFFMANN DISEASE
(Chapter XII)

SPINOCEREBELLAR DEGENERATION

This familial group of disorders causes varying degrees of degeneration in the cerebellum, brainstem, spinal cord, and peripheral nerves. Friedreich's ataxia, hereditary spastic paraparesis, and Charcot Marie Tooth disease are the most common forms.

Friedreich's ataxia is characterized by progressive "dying back" of axons in the peripheral nerves, dorsolateral columns of the spinal cord, and brainstem. It is transmitted as an autosomal recessive trait. Patients are frequently born with high arched feet (pes cavus) and hammer toes. Progressive ataxia from impaired proprioception that commences in the lower extremities, dysarthria, optic atrophy, and deafness become apparent in the second decade. Ocular dysmetria and sudden jerking of the eyes away from and back to the fixation point (square wave jerks) can also be seen. Intellectual function is preserved. Kyphoscoliosis develops in about 80% of the subjects and may lead to progressive restrictive lung disease. Cardiac abnormalities occur in over 90% of patients and are the most common cause of death. They include asymmetric septal hypertrophy, conduction defects, and decreased contractility of the heart. There is also an unusually high incidence of diabetes. Both visual and somatosensory evoked potentials may be abnormal, reflecting dysfunction in the anterior visual pathway and the dorsolateral spinal cord respectively. The CT scan is usually normal. The electrocardiogram, echocardiogram, and evaluation of other family members for minor variants of the disorder (pes cavus, hammer toes, and scoliosis) are also helpful in establishing the diagnosis. Friedreich's ataxia is progressive and usually fatal in 15-20 years after onset of ataxia.

Hereditary spastic paraparesis is a recessive illness, very stereotyped in all afflicted family members, with a slowly evolving ascending myelopathy followed by ataxia and extrapyramidal features in the late stages. Onset of symptoms usually occurs in middle childhood.

Charcot Marie tooth disease; refer to Chapter XII.

RETT SYNDROME

This is a syndrome of autistic behavior, dementia, and purposive hand movements that occurs predominantly in girls. It usually has onset before the age of five years. It is believed to be X-linked, with the condition being incompatible with survival in males. The diagnostic criteria[1,2] for Rett syndrome are:

a. Normal pre and perinatal period; essentially normal psychomotor development through the first 6, often 12 to 18 months of life.

b. Normal head circumference at birth; decceleration of head growth from age 1 to 4 years.

c. Early behavioral, social, and psychomotor regression; evolving communication dysfunction and dementia.

d. Loss of acquired, purposeful hand skills from age 1 to 4 years.

e. Hand wringing, clapping, hand "washing" behaviors.

f. Appearance of gait apraxia and truncal apraxia/ataxia from 1 to 4 years of age.

g. Diagnosis is tentative until 3 to 5 years of age.

The most consistent neuropathological findings are a diffuse reduction in brain size and decreased pigmentation in the substantia nigra. Abnormalities in central nervous system biogenic amines have been postulated, but no consistent defect has been detected. The electroencephalogram frequently shows non-specific findings in the form of diffuse slowing, multifocal, or generalized spikes and sharp waves. The diagnosis is to some extent, one of exclusion. The management is essentially symptomatic.

FAMILIAL MYOCLONUS EPILEPSY OF UNVERRICHT

This autosomal recessive disorder is characterized by onset between the ages of 5 to 15 years of myoclonic and generalized tonic-clonic seizures (some of which may be stimulus-sensitive), progressive dementia, and cerebellar ataxia. Degeneration of the dentate nucleus in the cerebellum, substantia nigra, hippocampus, and reticular formation is present. Characteristic concentric amyloid inclusions (Lafora bodies) are seen within the cytoplasm of neurons and muscle fibers. The EEG demonstrates repetitive, generalized spike and wave discharges. The etiology and treatment remain unknown and the disorder is invariably fatal by the age of 20-30 years.

RAMSAY HUNT SYNDROME

Also known as dentatorubral atrophy, this disorder is associated with myoclonic epilepsy and progressive ataxia, with onset in the second or third decade and little or no intellectual deterioration. The disorder may be a form of mitochondrial encephalomyopathy.

CENTRAL NERVOUS SYSTEM STORAGE DISEASES

Deficiency, qualitative abnormality, or lack of activator proteins for lysosomal and peroxisomal enzymes can lead to storage diseases. Most storage diseases are secondary to deficiencies of specific lysosomal enzymes that normally degrade glycoproteins, glycolipids, or mucopolysaccharides. When these substances cannot be properly degraded, they accumulate within lysosomes of neuronal and glial cells. This leads to alteration in normal cellular protein synthesis and, ultimately, a progressive impairment of synaptic, axonal, neuronal, and glial membrane function. When the stored substance is ill-defined, but likely to include mucopolysaccharides and glycolipids, the disorder is termed a mucolipidosis.

Peroxisomal enzymes are responsible mainly for degradation of very long chain (C_{24-26}) fatty acids. Severe peroxisomal disorders such as Zellweger syndrome are associated with complete absence of peroxisomes, whereas others (childhood adrenoleukodystrophy) are associated with the presence of peroxisomes, but only the deficiency of oxidative activity for very long chain fatty acids, this leading to elevated serum levels of the fatty acids.

Adrenoleukodystrophy is an X-linked disorder of peroxisomal function. It is characterized by the presence of a normal number of peroxisomes in cells, but impaired oxidation of very long chain (C_{24} to C_{26}) fatty acids.

The patients display normal growth and development until 2-3 years of age, at which point hyperactivity, incoordination, impaired auditory discrimination, and spasticity become apparent. Dementia and blindness may evolve with time. There is symmetric demyelination of the hemispheric white matter that is maximal in the parieto-occipital regions. Adrenal insufficiency is mainly subclinical, but frequently the child may have a bronzed appearance and hyperpigmentation over the palmar creases, abdomen, and scrotum.

The CT scan usually shows areas of symmetric hypodensity over the parieto-occipital regions. Serum very long chain fatty acid levels are elevated.

Adrenomyeloneuropathy is an allied peroxisomal disorder that has its onset in the second or third decade in the form of spastic paraparesis or sensory deficits. Some may have Addison's disease without neurologic involvement. Once again, the elevated serum very long chain fatty acid levels are diagnostic.

Neonatal adrenoleukodystrophy is characterized by a reduced number of peroxisomes and deficiency of multiple perioxisomal enzymes. It is transmitted in an autosomal recessive manner. The patients have mildly dysmorphic facial features, hypotonia, hepatomegaly, and sensorineural hearing loss. Serum phytanic acid levels, very long fatty acids, and pipecolic acid are all increased.

The diagnosis of most **lysosomal enzyme disorders** can be established by documenting low leukocyte or serum levels of the specific lysosomal enzyme. Electron microscopic examination of skin and conjunctival biopsy specimens is useful in the diagnosis of gangliosidoses and mucopolysaccharidoses (membranous-cytoplasmic and "zebra" bodies seen) (Fig.14-1). Cultured fibroblasts provide an unlimited supply of cells and are useful when analysis of a number of enzymes is required. With a few exceptions (Hunter's syndrome, X-linked), the majority of lysosomal enzyme disorders are transmitted in an autosomal recessive manner. Heterozygotes have levels of lysosomal enzymes that are intermediate to those of affected homozygotes and normal individuals. Antenatal diagnosis of most lysosomal disorders is now possible using enzymatic assays on cultured amniotic cells. Antenatal diagnosis of peroxisomal disorders is also possible by analysis of very long chain fatty acid levels in cultured amniotic cells.

Neuronal ceroid lipofuscinosis. Ceroid is a waxy lipopigment present normally in the brain, but in the various forms of neuronal ceroid lipofuscinosis (NCL) an autofluorescent material termed dolichol accumulates in the nervous system, muscle, eccrine glands, and pancreas. It is a long chain polyisoprenoid, which is an important component of cell membranes. The exact biochemical disturbance is unknown.

Infantile NCL (Santavouri type) is characterized by onset of intellectual deterioration, ataxia, and myoclonic and tonic-clonic seizures between the ages of 9-18 months. The age of onset is therefore later than that of the classical Tay Sachs disease, which develops between the ages of 3-6 months. Macular degeneration is present, but macular cherry red spots are generally not visible. The electroretinogram is extinguished owing to storage of dolichols in the retinal rods and cones. This is also distinct from the findings in Tay Sachs disease, in which the electroretinogram is preserved owing to sparing of the retinal rods and cones and storage predominantly in the retinal ganglionic cell layer. Granular inclusion bodies may be seen on

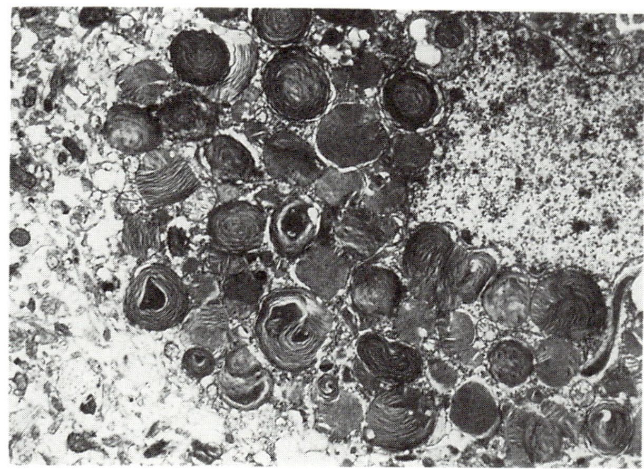

Fig. 14-1. Electron micrograph of a conjunctival biopsy specimen from a patient with GM$_2$ gangliosidosis, demonstrating circumscibed, membranous cytoplasmic bodies.

Fig. 14-2. Macular cherry red spot in a patient with GM$_2$ gangliosidosis.

electron microscopic examination of lymphocytes of patients with the infantile form of NCL.

The **late infantile** (Batten-Bielschowshy) form of NCL is characterized by onset between the ages of 2 to 4 years, progressive intellectual deterioration, ataxia, intractable seizures, and blindness. The electroencephalogram may show high amplitude waves in the occipital regions, with photic stimulation at low frequencies (1 to 3 hertz). The electroretinogram is extinguished

early. Dolichols may be recovered from the urinary sediment. Electron microscopic examination of skin and conjunctival biopsy specimens discloses storage material in the form of "curvilinear bodies" and "finger-print bodies".

In the **juvenile** (Spielmeyer-Vogt) form of NCL, onset of symptoms generally occurs between the ages of 6 to 14 years in the form of visual loss and intellectual deterioration. Seizures and ataxia are not seen. The electroretinographic, skin and

Table 14-1. Clinical distinctions between gray matter and white matter storage diseases

	GRAY MATTER STORAGE DISEASES	**WHITE MATTER STORAGE DISEASES**
Intellectual dysfunction	Early	Intermediate to late
Seizures	Early	Intermediate to late
Muscle tone	Initially decreased, increased in late stages	Initially increased, decreased in intermediate stages
Macular degeneration	Present in some (ceroid lipofuscinosis, gangliosidoses) See Fig. 14-2.	Absent
Optic atrophy	Intermediate or late	Early
CSF protein	Usually normal; may be elevated in some mucopoly-saccharidoses	Usually elevated
EEG	Generalized spikes and sharp waves	Generalized slowing
Nerve conduction velocity	Normal	Impaired in intermediate and late stages of ALD, MLD, Krabbe's disease.

conjunctival biopsy findings are similar to those in the late infantile form.

When a child is suspected of having a central nervous system storage disorder, the diagnostic possibilities can generally be further narrowed down and unnecessary investigations avoided by clinically distinguishing gray matter storage diseases or poliodystrophies (GM_2 gangliosidoses, GM_1 gangliosidosis, mucopolysaccharidoses, mucolipidoses, neuronal ceroid lipofuscinosis) from white matter storage diseases or leukodystrophies (adrenoleukodystrophy, metachromatic leukodystrophy, globoid cell leukodystrophy) as indicated in Table 14-1.

Table 14-2. Central Nervous System Storage Disorders

DISORDERS	CLINICAL FEATURES	ENZYMATIC DISORDERS	USEFUL ASSAY SPECIMEN
Mucopolysaccharidosis (MPS) Type I H (Hurler's syndrome)	Cloudy cornea, coarse features, mental retardation, hepatosplenomegaly, dwarfism, death by age 10 years, autosomal recessive, dystosis multiplex	α-L idouronidase	Fibroblasts
MPS Type I S (Scheie syndrome)	Stiff joints, cloudy cornea, normal intelligence, aortic valvular disease, near normal life span, dysostosis multiplex, autosomal recessive	α-L idouronidase	Fibroblasts
MPS Type II (Hunter's disease)	Dysostosis multiplex, no corneal clouding, gradual intellectual deterioration, sensorineural deafness, myocardial and valvular disease, X-linked recessive	Idouronate sulfatase	Fibroblasts
MPS Type III (Sanfilipo disease)	Minor skeletal abnormalities, severe mental retardation and behavioral abnormalities, marked hirsutism, autosomal recessive	Heparan sulfatase	Fibroblasts
MPS Type IV (Morquio's syndrome)	Platyspondyly, genu valgum, normal intellect, short neck, autosomal recessive	Galactosamine 6-sulfate sulfatase	Fibroblasts
MPS Type VI (Maroteaux-Lamy syndrome)	Dysostosis multiplex, corneal clouding, growth retardation, near normal intellect	Arylsulfatase B	Serum, fibroblasts
MPS Type VII (Sly syndrome)	Dysostosis multiplex, somatic and mental retardation, hepatosplenomegaly, hirsutism, autosomal recessive	β-glucuronidase	Fibroblasts
Mucolipidosis I (MLI or Sialidosis)	Onset infancy to adulthood, Cherry-red macular lesions, variable skeletal changes, mental retardation, autosomal recessive	Neuraminidase	Fibroblasts
Mucolipidosis II (ML II or I cell disease)	Dysostosis multiplex, Hurler syndrome-like appearance, onset in infancy, thoracic deformity, hepatosplenomegaly	Lack of "recognition marker" that enables acid hydrolases to enter lysosomes; lysosomal enzyme levels are elevated in serum, deficient in fibroblasts	Fibroblasts — presence of inclusions and deficient in: β-glucuronidase β-galactosidase α-L idouronidase
Fucosidosis	Dysostosis multiplex, coarse facial features, cardiomegaly, frequent infections, progressive psychomotor retardation	α-fucosidase	Leukocytes, fibroblasts
Mannosidosis	Dysostosis multiplex, coarse facial features, hepatosplenomegaly, hearing loss, psychomotor retardation	α-mannosidase	Leukocytes, fibroblasts

Table 14-2. Central Nervous System Storage Disorders (cont.)

DISORDERS	CLINICAL FEATURES	ENZYMATIC DISORDERS	USEFUL ASSAY SPECIMEN
GM_2 gangliosidosis, Tay Sachs variant	Normal facial features, progressive intellectual deterioration in infancy, epileptic and non-epileptic myoclonus, macular "cherry red" lesions, blindness, death by age 2-3 years	Severe deficiency of β-N-acetyl hexosaminidase A	Serum, leukocytes, fibroblasts
GM_2 gangliosidosis, Sandhoff variant	Identical to Tay Sachs variant	Severe deficiency of both hexosaminidase A and B	Serum, leukocytes, fibroblasts
GM_2 gangliosidosis, Juvenile variant	Onset between 2-5 years, gradually progressive ataxia, spasticity, dysarthria, stimulus sensitive, non-epileptic myoclonus, blindness only in late stages, death by age 15 years	Partial deficiency of hexosaminidase	Serum, leukocytes, fibroblasts
GM_2 gangliosidosis AB variant	Identical to Tay Sachs variant	Deficiency of protein that activates hexosaminidase A-related hydrolysis, normal levels of hex A and B	Fibroblasts
GM_1 gangliosidoses	a. Infantile generalized form has dystosis multiplex, hepatosplenomegaly, seizures, blindness, apathy, coarse features, death by age 2 years. b. Juvenile form has slower progression, with onset around 1 year, ataxia, mental deterioration, spasticity, normal facies, mild skeletal changes and seizures. c. Adult form has onset in adolescence, progressive ataxia, minimal intellectual impairment, no seizures, recessive.	β-galactosidase	Leukocytes, fibroblasts
Fabry's disease	Painful extremities, angiokeratoma on trunk, polyneuropathy, X-linked	α-galactosidase A	Plasma leukocytes, fibroblasts
Niemann Pick disease	Type A has progressive intellectual deterioration, seizures, hepatosplenomegaly, and foamy histiocytes in bone marrow. Type B causes hepatosplenomegaly but spares the CNS. Type C similar to Type A, but with onset between 2-4 years. Type D similar to Type C, but seen in Nova Scotia.	Sphingomyelinase absent in Types A,B; normal in Type C, but activator protein absent	Fibroblasts
Gaucher's disease	a. Infantile form has rapid intellectual deterioration, seizures, blindness, spenomegaly, elevated serum acid phosphatase, anemia and presence of Gaucher's cells on bone marrow examination. b. Juvenile form has slowly evolving ataxia, spasticity, intellectual deterioration, hepatosplenomegaly and presence of Gaucher's cells on bone marrow examination.	β-glucosidase	Leukocytes, fibroblasts
Neuronal ceroid lipofuscinoses	a. Infantile (Santavouri) form has onset prior to age 2 years of marked visual loss, absent electroretinogram (ERG), myoclonic seizures, severe developmental delay. Granular or amorphous lymphocytic inclusions on electron microscopy (EM).	Unknown	Lymphocyte, skin and conjunctival examination under EM for characteristic inclusion bodies

Table 14-2. Central Nervous System Storage Disorders (cont.)

DISORDERS	CLINICAL FEATURES	ENZYMATIC DISORDERS	USEFUL ASSAY SPECIMEN
Neuronal ceroid lipofuscinoses (cont.)	b. Late infantile (Jansky-Bielchowsky) form has onset between 2-4 years of ataxia, intellectual deterioration, myoclonic seizures, abnormal ERG, presence of curvilinear and finger print bodies on EM. c. Juvenile (Speilmeyer-Vogt) form has onset between 4-puberty, visual loss, occasional seizures, mild ataxia, abnormal ERG, fingerprint bodies on EM of lymphocytes.		
Krabbe's disease (globoid cell leukodystrophy)	A number of variants; progressive spastic quadriparesis, psychomotor retardation, dysphagia, elevated CSF protein, globoid cells in the CNS, polyneuropathy in the late stages from myelin degeneration, optic atrophy	Galactosyl ceramide, β-galactosidase	Fibroblasts, leukocytes
Metachromatic leukodystrophy (sulfatide lipidosis)	A number of variants; progressive spastic paresis commencing in early childhood to adulthood, polyneuropathy, elevated CSF protein, optic atrophy, psychomotor retardation	Arylsulfatase A	Serum leukocytes, urine fibroblasts
Pelizaeus Merzbacher disease	X-linked, onset prior to age 3 months of arrhythmic and roving eye movements, optic atrophy, spasticity, severe developmental delay, normal CSF examination	Uncertain	Brain biopsy or post mortem examination
Canavan's disease	Onset between age 2-4 months of delayed development, optic atrophy, seizures, spasticity, megalencephaly, cystic appearance of white matter on CT scan	Uncertain	Brain biopsy or post mortem examination
Alexander's disease	Onset in the first year of progressive intellectual impairment, spasticity, megalencephaly, seizures, diffuse white matter hypodensity (especially frontal) on CT, eosinophilic deposits along pial surface of brain.	Uncertain	Brain biopsy or post mortem examination of brain
Adrenoleukodystrophy, childhood form	Perioxisomal disorder, X-linked, onset between 4-8 years of progressive spasticity, ataxia, optic atrophy, increased pigmentation of the skin, white white matter hypodensity on CT (usually parieto-occipital), elevated CSF protein, diminished adrenocortical reserve on ACTH stimulation test	Defective oxidation of very long chain fatty acids (C_{24-26})	Serum ($\uparrow$ levels of VLFA), fibroblast ($\downarrow$ turnover of VLFA)
Adrenoleukodystrophy, neonatal form	Perosixomal disorder, autosomal recessive, progressive hypotonia and seizures in the neonatal period, spasticity in later stages, fatal by age 1-2 years		
Zellweger syndrome	Peroxisomal disorder, autosomal recessive, high forehead, wide open anterior fontanelle, poor sucking and swallowing since birth, hepatomegaly, renal cortical cysts, skeletal malformations, severe hypotonia and apathy, fatal by age 6 months	Severe defect in oxidation of very long chain fatty acids (C_{24-26})	$\uparrow$ serum VLFA levels, $\downarrow$ fibroblast turnover of VLFA

REFERENCES

1. Burd L, Gascon G. Rett syndrome: review and discussion of current diagnostic criteria. J Child Neurol 3:263-268, 1988.

2. Hagberg B, Goutieres F, Hanefeld F, et al. Rett syndrome: criteria for inclusion and exclusion. Brain Dev 7:372-373, 1985.

SUGGESTED READING

1. Bloom HJG. Intracranial tumors: response and resistance to therapeutic endeavors, 1970-1980. Int J Radiation Oncology Biol Phys 8:1083-1113, 1982.

2. Walker RW and Allen JC. Pediatric brain tumors. Pediatric Annals 12:383-394, 1983.

3. Kun LE, D'Souza B and Tefft M. The value of surveillance testing in childhood brain tumors. Cancer 56:1818-1823, 1985.

4. Kelly PJ, Kall BA, Goerss S and Cascino TL. Results of computer-assisted stereotactic laser resection of deep-seated intracranial lesions. Mayo Clin Proc 61:20-27, 1986.

5. Werlin SH, Grand RJ, Perman JA, Watkins JB. Diagnostic dilemmas of Wilson's disease: diagnosis and treatment. Pediatrics 62:47-57, 1978.

6. Danks DM, Campbell PE, Stevens BJ, Mayne V, Cartwright E. Menkes' kinky hair syndrome: an inherited defect in copper absorption with widespread effects. Pediatrics 50:188-201, 1972.

7. Dayan AD, Oegenden BG and Crome L. Necrotizing encephalo-myelopathy of Leigh: neuropathological findings in 8 cases. Arch Dis Child 45:39-48, 1970.

8. Heredodegenerative diseases. In: Menkes JH, ed. Textbook of Child Neurology. Lea and Febiger, Philadelphia, 3rd edition, 1985; 123-168.

9. Dyken P and Krawiecki N. Neurodegenerative diseases of infancy and childhood. Ann Neurol 13:351-364, 1983.

10. Burton BK. Inborn errors of metabolism: the clinical diagnosis in early infancy. Pediatrics 79(3):359-369, 1987.

11. O'Brien JF. The lysosomal storage diseases. Mayo Clin Proc 57:192-197, 1982.

12. Neufeld EF, Fratantoni JC. Inborn errors of mucopolysaccharide metabolism. Science 169:141-146, 1970.

13. Sandhoff K and Christomanou H. Biochemistry and genetics of gangliosidoses. Hum Genet 50:107-143, 1979.

14. Naidu S, Moser AE, Moser HW. Phenotypic and genotypic variability of generalized perioxisomal disorders. Pediatr Neurol 4:5-12, 1988.

CHAPTER XV

DEVELOPMENTAL DISABILITIES

Mental Retardation

Cerebral Palsy

Normal Language Development

Causes of Delayed Speech and Language Development

Evaluation and Management of Delayed Language Development

Algorithm

MENTAL RETARDATION

DEFINITION

The World Health Organization defines mental retardation as incomplete or insufficient development of mental capacities. An individual performing two standard deviations below the expected mean for age on standardized psychometric tests also meets the criteria. However, a low intelligence quotient (IQ) is not always a reliable measure of the level of intellectual function. The incidence of mental retardation in the United States is approximately 3%. The disorder has profound socio-economic implications for the patient, the family, and the community.

COMMON CAUSES

Table 15-1 lists the common causes of mental retardation and groups them into eight categories.

Table 15-1. Common causes of mental retardation

Prenatal Factors
- a. Chromosomal anomalies such as Trisomies 13, 18, 21, X-linked mental retardation, and partial deletion syndromes.
- b. Maternal exposure to toxins such as radiation and alcohol.
- c. Congenital intrauterine infections such as toxoplasmosis, cytomegalovirus, rubella, herpes simplex, and syphilis.
- d. Miscellaneous: placental insufficiency, severe dietary inadequacies, maternal metabolic disorders, intrauterine cerebrovascular accidents, and genetic factors leading to dysmorphic syndromes.
- e. Congenital malformations like hydranencephaly, holoprosencephaly, porencephaly, lissencephaly (agyria).

Perinatal Factors
Birth trauma
Bacterial meningitis
Viral encephalitis
Severe hypoxic-ischemic encephalopathy

Inborn Errors of Metabolism
- a. Disorders of carbohydrate metabolism such as galactosemia.
- b. Disorders of aminoacid metabolism such as phenylketonuria.
- c. Disorders of lipid metabolism such as Tay Sachs disease.
- d. Disorders of purine metabolism such as Lesch Nyhan syndrome.
- e. Disorders of endocrine and mineral metabolism such as hypothyroidism, and pseudohypoparathyroidism.

Head Trauma (Cerebral contusion or laceration)

Bacterial or **Viral Meningoencephalitis in Infancy or Early Childhood**

Phakomatoses
Tuberous sclerosis
Neurofibromatosis
Incontinentia pigmenti
Hypomelanosis of Ito
Sturge-Weber syndrome
Multiple lentigines syndrome
Sjogren Laarson syndrome
Linear sebaceous nevus of Jadassohn

Toxic Encephaopathies
Lead intoxication
Chronic renal or hepatic disease

CLASSIFICATION

Mental retardation is divided into three classes:

Mild. IQ between 50-70, educable up to the 5th or 6th grade at school and trainable for a simple occupation and in self-care skills. Eighty percent of retarded individuals fall into this category.

Moderate. IQ between 25-50, trainable generally only for self-care skills.

Severe. IQ below 25, requires custodial care. As has been indicated earlier, the application of IQ scores to classify a child as retarded, and the degree of retardation, is not always accurate in gauging the level of intellectual functioning. Poor speech development, systemic illnesses, and cultural factors may lead to underestimation of mental capabilities. Psychometric studies should therefore be repeated every 2-3 years. A functional assessment of the patient with regard to his lifestyle and daily activities at home is also helpful in assessing the degree of retardation.

CLINICAL FEATURES

Some abnormal physical features that commonly accompany syndromes with mental retardation are listed in Table 15-2, along with the underlying disorders.

Particular attention should be paid to determining hearing and visual loss, seizures, and nutritional disorders. A developmental and functional assessment should also be undertaken in order to assess the ability of the individual to function independently within the home, community, and school.

DIFFERENTIAL DIAGNOSIS

Environmental deprivation. Children who have failed to receive adequate parental stimulation are frequently delayed in their language skills and social behavior. A rapid improvement is noted when they are placed in a nurturing environment.

Cerebral Palsy. This term indicates a static central nervous system insult acquired prenatally or in early infancy and childhood. Musculo-skeletal defects are most common. While two thirds of patients with cerebral palsy are clearly mentally retarded, others may be near normal intellectu-

ally, e.g., the athetoid form, characterized by predominantly subcortical brain dysfunction.

Autism. (see page 142).

TREATABLE CAUSES

There are a number of treatable causes of mental retardation:

1. Hypothyroidism

2. Some inborn errors of metabolism (phenylketonuria, B12-responsive methylmalonic acidemia, biotin responsive propionic acidemia).

3. Severe protein-calorie malnutrition

4. Lead and other toxic encephalopathies

5. Untreated hydrocephalus

DIAGNOSTIC SCREENING

Diagnostic screening is available for a number of disorders which are likely to cause mental retardation.

1. Phenylketonuria (in the neonatal period).

2. Hypothyroidism (in the neonatal period).

3. Pregnancy in women over 35 years (at risk to have offspring with Down's syndrome, amniocentesis available).

4. School-age girls unexposed to or unimmunized against rubella (at risk for having offspring with the congenital rubella syndrome).

5. X-linked mental retardation (patient or carrier-state detection using amniocentesis)

COMMON NEUROPATHOLOGICAL CORRELATES

Gross examination

Micrencephaly, hydranencephaly, holoprosencephaly, porencephaly, lissencephaly, agenesis of the corpus callosum, intracranial calcification, cortical atrophy, or cerebellar hypoplasia can be detected on gross examination of the brain.

Table 15-2. Clinical features of mental retardation

Head

1. Microcephaly at birth: chromosomal anomalies, intrauterine infection, exposure to teratogens.
2. Macrocephaly: hydrocephalus, mucopolysaccharidoses, mucolipidoses, neurofibromatosis, X-linked mental retardation.
3. Brachycephaly: Down's syndrome.
4. Frontal bossing: hydrocephalus.

Hair

1. Low hairline: Arnold-Chiari malformations.
2. Alopecia: Cockayne syndrome, incontinentia pigmenti, Menke's disease, progeria.
3. Kinkiness: Menke's disease.
4. Coarseness: mucopolysaccharidosis, Sjogren-Laarson syndrome.
5. Abnormal pigmentation: albinism, Waardenburg syndrome, ataxia telangicetasia.
6. Hirsutism: de Lange syndrome, Trisomy 18, Hurler, Hunter San Filipo syndromes.

Face

1. Micrognathia: some partial deletion syndromes, Turner's and Zellweger syndrome, Trisomy 8 or 18, Meckel and de Lange syndromes
2. Cleft palate: Trisomies 13, 18, Treacher-Collins syndrome, de Lange and cri-du chat syndrome, fetal alcohol syndrome.
3. Short philtrum: fetal alcohol and oro-facio-digital syndromes.
4. Long philtrum: Weaver and William's syndromes.

Abdomen

1. Protuberance: cretinism, mucopolysaccharidosis, Duchenne's muscular dystrophy.
2. Umbilical hernia: Beckwith-Wiedemann, mucopolysaccharidosis, hypothyroidism, Trisomies 13 and 18.
3. Hepatosplenomegaly: achondrogenesis, Zellweger and Chediak-Higashi syndromes, mucopolysaccharidoses.

Skin

1. Cafe-au-lait spots: neurofibromatosis.
2. Ash-leaf-shaped hypopigmented spots: tuberous sclerosis.
3. Adenoma sebaceum: tuberous sclerosis.
4. Shagreen patches: tuberous sclerosis.
5. Facial hemangiomta: Sturge Weber syndrome, linear sebaceous nevus syndrome, ataxia-telengiectasia.
6. Icthyosis: Sjogren-Laarson and Rudd syndromes.
7. Whorled, hyperpigmented lesions: incontinentia pigmenti.
8. Whorled, hypopigmented lesions: Hypomelanosis of.
9. Ito Albinism: oculocutaneous albinism, Chediak Higashi syndrome.

Eyes

1. **Palpebral fissure slant: Apert, Coffin-Lowry, cri-du chat, Down's, Pfeiffer, Rubinstein-Taybi, Soto's syndromes.**
2. Epicanthal folds: Down's, Noonan's, Turner's, Zellweger's syndromes, X-linked mental retardation, William's syndrome.
3. Hypotelorism: Holoprosencephaly with or without Trisomy 13.
4. Hypertelorism: Apert's, fetal hydantoin, Soto's, Pfeiffer's and 4p-, 13q-syndromes.
5. Cataracts: congenital rubella, Lowe syndrome, galactosemia.
6. Chorioretinitis: congenital rubella, Lowe syndrome, galactosemia.
7. Optic nerve hypoplasia: septo-optic dysplasia.
8. Optic nerve atrophy: longstanding hydrocephalus, leukodystrophies.
9. Macular degeneration: gangliosidosis, ceroid lipofuscinosis.
10. Vacuolar retinopathy: Aicardi syndrome.
11. Iris hamartomata: neurofibromatosis.
12. Microphthalmia: Hallerman-Streiff, oculo-dento-digital, rubella, Trisomy 13 syndromes.
13. Corneal clouding: congenital syphilis, Hurler's, Maroteaux-Lamy and rubella syndromes.

Neck

Webbed neck: Noonan's and Turner's syndromes.

External genitalia

1. Enlarged: X-linked mental retardation.
2. Small: Prader-Willi, Down's, Turner's, Laurence-Moon-Biedl, Fanconi syndromes.
3. Ambiguous: Kleinfelter's syndrome.

Back

1. Gibbus: mucopolysacharidoses.
2. Kyphoscoliosis: basal cell nevus, Coffin-Lowry syndromes.

Hands

1. Nail hypoplasia: fetal hydantoin syndrome, William's syndrome.
2. Bilateral simian creases: Down's syndrome.
3. Subungual fibromata: tuberous sclerosis.
4. Broad thumbs: Rubinstein-Taybi syndrome.

Histology

Histological findings in mental retardation include:

a. Paucity of neurons in the cerebral cortex.

b. Lack of the normal cellular laminar arrangement in the cerebral cortex.

c. Neuronal heterotopias

d. Dendrites relatively devoid of spines; those present are more liable to be elongated and slender rather than short and thick as seen normally.

DIAGNOSTIC STUDIES

The following diagnostic studies are useful:

1. CT head scan (above mentioned gross lesions can be detected).

2. EEG (may help detect seizures, identify seizure type, assess degree of cortical maturation).

3. Blood and urine amino acid screens, urine organic acid studies, serum thyroxine and thyroid stimulating hormone levels.

4. Chromosomal studies (to detect trisomy or partial deletion syndromes, X-linked mental retardation).

5. Psychometric testing (to determine exact level of mental function and intellectual strengths/deficits, as well as formulate an appropriate educational program).

6. Audiogram or brainstem auditory evoked responses to exclude sensorineural deafness.

MANAGEMENT

Care of medical and physical handicaps (anticonvulsants for seizures, physical therapy for spasticity and contractures, occupational therapy to teach self-care skills).

Monitoring the nutritional status of the moderately and severely mentally retarded if feeding difficulties are present.

Mainstreaming. Placement of a mildly retarded child in a regular classroom for the first 1-2 years of school education is desirable. This environment is liable to be more stimulating and enhance learning. Potential ostracization by normal children because of the visible physical and mental handicaps is a potential drawback.

Special education programs. When mainstreaming is not possible, placement of mildly or moderately retarded children in appropriate special classrooms that emphasize developing self-confidence, communication ability, and self-care skills is recommended.

Provision of emotional support. The mildly mentally retarded adolescent may become overanxious, hyperactive, or depressed. A firm, consistent, but loving environment is necessary.

"Normalization." Vocational guidance may facilitate finding work for the mildly retarded in a sheltered workshop and thereby develop a feeling of self-confidence. With some supervision, the mildly retarded may also be able to live independently in group homes.

"Institutionalization." It is desirable that the retarded individuals be maintained in the mainstream of society. However, when families are no longer able to care for them (especially the severely impaired), placement in a residential institution may become necessary.

CEREBRAL PALSY

DEFINITION

Cerebral palsy is a static encephalopathy secondary to an insult to the immature nervous system, with resultant motor, intellectual, and neuromuscular handicaps. The term encompasses a group of disorders with diverse etiopathology. The central nervous system insult is usually acquired prenatally, perinatally, in infancy, or early childhood. The estimated incidence in the United States is between 1.5 to 5 per 1000 live births.

CAUSES

Table 15-3 lists three categories of causes for cerebral palsy.

No apparent cause can be identified in about 20-30% of instances. In a study of 189 children with cerebral palsy, maternal mental retardation, birth

Table 15-3 Causes of cerebral palsy

Prenatal insults
Intrauterine infections (toxoplasmosis, cytomegalovirus, rubella, syphilis, herpes simplex)
Chromosomal disorders
Exposure to toxins (radiation, alcohol)
Maternal metabolic diseases (diabetes mellitus, toxemia of pregnancy)

Perinatal insults
Severe hypoxic encephalopathy
Intracranial hemorrhage
Metabolic encephalopathies, e.g., hypoglycemia
Bilirubin encephalopathy (kernicterus)
Bacterial meningitis

Illnesses during infancy
Head trauma
Bacterial meningitis
Viral encephalitis
Sequel of toxic and metabolic encephalopathies

weight below 2001 grams, breech presentation and fetal malformations were found to be the leading risk factors.[9] Perinatal asphyxia by itself was responsible for only 9% of cerebral palsy in this study.

With regard to the association between Apgar scores and cerebral palsy, the 5 minute Apgar score of 0-3 was associated with an 8% death rate in the first year and a 1% risk of cerebral palsy in survivors. On the other hand, a 20 minute Apgar score of less than 3 was associated with a 59% death rate in the first year and a 57% incidence of cerebral palsy in survivors.

CLASSIFICATION

Based upon clinical features, the various types of cerebral palsy can be identified (Table 15-4).

Spastic diplegia is most frequently observed in premature infants who suffer periventricular leukomalacia. Spastic tetraparesis occurs as a consequence of diffuse, bihemispheric insults such as anoxic encephalopathy. Spastic hemiparesis usually occurs from a focal insult such as porencephaly. Athetosis is frequently associated with basal ganglia lesions due to perinatal hypoxia or hyperbilirubinemia. Developmental malformations, especially cerebellar hypoplasia, are common in children with atonic cerebral palsy. Ataxic

cerebral palsy is probably a non-entity, being composed of children with metabolic or heredofamilial disorders affecting the cerebellar system.

CLINICAL FEATURES

Developmental delay. This usually becomes most apparent by the latter half of the first year and is universal. Very often attention is drawn to the child because of difficulty in assuming a sitting position or a lag in motor development relative to intellectual development.

Abnormal motor performance. In children with hemiplegic cerebral palsy, hand preference (normally not developed until age 2-2 1/2 years) may become apparent during infancy. Toe walking develops in those with contractures of the Achilles tendon secondary to spasticity. Some infants with hemiplegia or diplegia do not crawl, but may resort to propelling themselves forward on their knees and elbows. Walking is frequently delayed. Most children with cerebral palsy who are able to develop independent walking skills do so by the age of five or six years . Pseudobulbar palsy, frequently present along with spastic quadriparesis, leads to swallowing difficulties and recurrent aspiration pneumonitis.

Abnormal muscle tone. Most children with cerebral palsy manifest an initial period of hypotonia. Evolution to hypertonia commences around 2-3 months of age. The hypertonia may interfere with the child's ability to assume a sitting position. The increase in tone is exacerbated when

Table 15-4

TYPE	APPROXIMATE PERCENTAGE[8]
Spastic	61.4
Hemiparesis	
Paraparesis (diplegia)	
Quadriparesis	
Athetoid	12.7
Ataxic	4.7
Rigid	8.0
Atonic	0.8
Tremor	0.2
Mixed	12.2

the child is held in the upright or semi-upright positions. Asymmetrically increased muscle tone in the extraocular muscles may lead to strabismus, which is present in approximately 80% of children with cerebral palsy. If uncorrected, the strabismus may interfere with the development of stereoscopic vision.

Abnormal movements and postures. Patients with pyramidal tract lesions frequently keep their hands fisted. Scissoring of the lower extremities from hypertonicity may be elicited by holding the child upright. There may be adduction at the hips from hypertonia. Longstanding increase in muscle tone combined with limited mobility at various joints may lead to contracture formation. Children with extrapyramidal manifestations may develop a stooped, dystonic posture or athetosis (slow, twisting movements along the long axis of a distal extremity). Opisthotonus suggests failure of the cerebral cortex to inhibit the vestibulospinal and reticulospinal projections originating within the brainstem.

Abnormal reflexes. Tendon reflexes may be exaggerated in segments of the body affected by pyramidal lesions. Undue persistence of developmental reflexes (e.g., persistent Moro in a 7 month old) may suggest delay in development of cortical inhibitory projections. Children with impaired neck and trunk righting reflexes are unable to maintain a sitting position. The "parachute" response which normally appears by 8 to 9 months of age may be absent in the child with a brainstem or cerebellar dysfunction. Persistence of primitive reflexes like the tonic neck, Moro, and obligate extensor posturing upon vertical suspension beyond the age of 24 months indicate an unfavorable prognosis for walking.

Intellectual dysfunction This is the most serious associated disability. Approximately one third of all children with cerebral palsy are intellectually normal, a third are mildly mentally retarded, and another third function in or below the range of moderate retardation. Patients with quadriparetic and atonic forms show the greatest degree of intellectual impairment, and those with the hemiparetic and choreoathetoid forms the least. Nearly one half in the hemiparetic category have normal intellectual function. Abnormal muscle tone, posture, and coordination may lead to underestimation of the intellectual potential due to underachievement on the performance items of psychometric tests.

Seizures. The overall incidence of seizures is about 50%. They may be generalized tonic-clonic, minor motor, partial complex or partial simple in type. Though anticonvulsants are helpful in decreasing the frequency of the majority of seizure types, minor motor and partial seizures may be especially difficult to control.

Sensory disturbances. Patients with hemiparesis may demonstrate hemianopsia, impaired two point discrimination, stereognosis over the affected side of the body, as well as higher level perceptual disturbances.

Disordered growth. Failure to thrive is common in patients with moderate to severe cerebral palsy, especially those with spastic quadriparesis. The exact cause for growth failure is uncertain. Patients with parietal lobe lesions (especially right hemispheric, e.g., porencephaly) manifest retardation of growth over the contralateral extremities. This is partly secondary to loss of the normal trophic influence of upper motor neurons on skeletal maturation.

Orthopedic complications. Contractures at the ankles and knees that prevent effective ambulation may necessitate tendon lengthening procedures. Surgical correction of hip flexor and adductor contractures may prevent progressive coxa vara and femoral anteversion, which can lead to hip dislocation if uncorrected. Scoliosis from asymmetric contraction of the paraspinal muscles may require a brace or, infrequently, surgical correction.

MANAGEMENT

The management of a child with cerebral palsy requires a team approach that includes the family, patient, physical and occupational therapists, and the physician.

Feeding difficulties. Proper positioning of the patient, with slight flexion at the hips and neck may reduce gagging and choking with liquids. If the pseudobulbar state is severe, placement of a gastrostomy tube may be necessary to maintain adequate nutrition. Swallowing may be facilitated by using semisolid food and teaching the caretaker to depress the child's upper lip and elevate the lower lip by using the index finger and second finger.

Physical and occupational therapy. The goal of physical therapy is mainly prevention of disuse atrophy and contractures. A variety of programs have been designed to enhance sensorimotor coordination and motor development. The value of these programs is at this point debatable. After the child has reached 2-3 years of age, involvement of an occupational therapist may help the child master activities involved in daily living. This can in turn foster self respect and boost self-image. Therapists are also an additional source of emotional support for the family.

Bracing of the lower extremities when contractures are developing may prevent their progression and assist in achieving independent walking. Bracing of the spine can minimize scoliosis and also inhibit unwanted trunk movements in cerebral palsy complicated by dystonic postures.

Associated disabilities. Treatment of seizures with anticonvulsants and spasticity with diazepam/ dantrolene sodium/ baclofen can be tried. The antispasticity agents are effective only in a limited number of patients. Drowsiness is a major limiting factor in the use of these drugs. Athetosis may be minimized by a trial of trihexyphenidyl(AR-TANE).

Education. If the child is of near-normal intellect and modifications in the school environment can be made for accommodating the child, e.g., use of a wheelchair, placement in a regular classroom should be encouraged. However, if intellectual and physical disabilities preclude functioning in a normal classroom, placement in a special school program among children with similar disabilities should be sought. Vocational guidance and training are necessary in adolescents with mild cerebral palsy in order to facilitate a smooth transition into adulthood.

Emotional disturbances. These are common in most mild to moderately impaired children with cerebral palsy. They arise as a direct consequence of the physical handicaps and may require supportive psychotherapy.

Surgical procedures. Tendon lengthening may be required in case contractures impair the quality of gait, and extraocular muscle resection in case of strabismus.

PROGNOSIS

Ambulatory mild to moderately impaired patients with cerebral palsy have a near normal life span, but only approximately one third are gainfully employed as adults. Approximately 50% of children with severe cerebral palsy (spastic quadriparesis) die by age 10 years and the rest by age 20-25 years, usually as a result of intercurrent infections or seizures during sleep.

NORMAL LANGUAGE DEVELOPMENT

Language acquisition is a dynamic process which commences in early infancy, coinciding with the development of the ability to attend to and discriminate speech sounds. The reproduction of verbal labels for visualized objects commences by 7-8 months of age and progresses rapidly thereafter. The ability to communicate in phrases evolves by 18-24 months, and in simple declarative sentences between 24-36 months. As abstract intellectual function develops, verbs, adjectives, and prepositions are introduced steadily into speech. Symbol and shape recognition (as used in solving puzzles) precedes the ability to match graphemes (written language symbols) with phonemes (spoken speech). This in turn corresponds with the development of reading skills. Language development is based upon multiple factors — genetic traits, environmental stimulation, and the presence or absence of brain dysfunction. The left hemisphere is dominant for language in almost all right-handed persons and a majority of left-handed individuals. The posterior two thirds of the superior temporal gyrus and the angular gyrus (Wernicke's area) are essential for language decoding, whereas the inferior frontal gyrus and adjacent areas of the frontal cortex are essential for speech encoding. While the semantic and phonemic aspects of language are controlled in most individuals by the left hemisphere, the right hemisphere plays a role in controlling the emotive and prosodic elements of speech, e.g., appreciation of melody.

Clinical language function assessment requires testing the comprehension of spoken and written language, naming ability, auditory memory, repetition, speech fluency, and language competence. A structured interview with the child and parents provides information about his speech repertoire.

Formal standardized instruments which can also be used to assess language function include the Weschler Preschool and Primary Scale of Intelligence (WPPSI), the Picture Peabody Vocabulary and Stanford-Binet tests, as well as the Illinois Test of Psycholinguistic Abilities.

CAUSES OF DELAYED LANGUAGE DEVELOPMENT

Deafness

Hearing loss may be conductive or sensorineural, and difficult to detect in the office setting in an infant or toddler. Speech output is sparse or defective in its enunciation. Deaf children who do not have associated central nervous system lesions are able to communicate using gestures. The degree of speech impediment depends upon the age of onset, severity, and duration of hearing loss. Central nervous system infections such as cytomegalovirus and bacterial meningitis and inherited disorders are the most common etiologies for deafness.

Articulation Defects

Pseudobulbar states accompanying cerebral palsy are frequently associated with defective articulation. These children have defective coordination of tongue, lip, and soft palatal movements. Their speech is frequently high pitched at the onset, then fades off gradually into a whisper. Oromotor apraxia is another cause of defective articulation and is characterized by normal lip, tongue, and palatal movements on command, but inability to spontaneously emit speech sounds requiring identical peripheral oromotor activity. They have defective encoding of the speech program at the cortical level. Cleft palate is a common congenital lesion associated with defective articulation, frequently conferring a hypernasal quality to the speech. Children with neuromuscular disease may also manifest hypernasal speech as a consequence of the soft palatal weakness interfering with closure of the nasopharynx during talking.

Mental Retardation

Patients with mental retardation have impaired comprehension of spoken and written language, impaired speech, as well as difficulty in use of gestures. This pervasive, global impairment of language function is accompanied by delayed problem solving ability as well as impaired adaptive and social behavior.

Developmental Language Disorders

A child is considered as having a developmental language disorder (DLD) if language/speech delay is unassociated with peripheral hearing loss, mental retardation, dysarthria, or anatomical abnormalities of the vocal passage. While there are no gross anatomical correlates, faulty synaptogenesis is present at the ultrastructural level to a variable degree in most cases. The delay in language development is often erroneously ascribed to their being "shy," "lazy," or too little need to verbalize because parents and older siblings readily anticipate and provide for the child's needs. Most children with developmental language disorders become frustrated by their inability to communicate effectively and may develop secondary behavioral problems. About two thirds demonstrate gradual improvement during the preschool years. There are a number of different types of developmental language disorders:

Auditory verbal agnosia. This developmental language disorder is characterized by inability to decode speech, with resultant faulty encoding of speech. The child is frequently mute or has speech that is marked by paucity and misarticulations. The ability to communicate with gestures, interest in surroundings, and meaningful play remains intact. Behavioral disorders may develop as a consequence of the communication disorder. A subgroup consisting of children of less than age 5-6 years who develop focal temporal or generalized paroxysmal discharges, which may or may not be associated with seizures, has been identified.[13] There is no clear relationship, however, between severity of the language disorder or laterality of the seizure focus with the degree of improvement in speech following anticonvulsant therapy.

Autism. This syndrome is characterized by onset generally prior to age 30 months of a pervasive lack of responsiveness to others, severe and global impairment of language, bizarre responses to the environment (resistance to change, attachment to inanimate objects, lack of eye contact), as well as absence of hallucinations, delusions, and loose associations that characterize schizophrenia. Speech may develop normally in some autistic children till age 12-14 months and then regress, whereas in others it may be slow to develop right from early infancy. There is a preponderance of boys over girls by a ratio of 5:1. X-linked mental retardation can also manifest as an autistic syndrome in males and in heterozygous females. Rett syndrom may underlie autism in girls (See Chapter XIV). Approximately 75% of autistic children function in the mentally retarded range. Between 7-28% develop seizures by age 18 years. Failure to develop communication skills or use age-appropriate toys by age 5 years is associated with a poor longterm prognosis for the ultimate development of communicative skills.

Semantic pragmatic syndrome. These children have defective comprehension of discourse and use of language, commonly manifested in the form of anomia in spontaneous speech. In order to compensate for the difficulty in retrieving verbal labels for objects and pictures, they may use speech in profusion, but with a loose, tangential quality to it ("cocktail party chatter"). The syndrome is most commonly seen in children with hydrocephalus.

Mixed phonologic-syntactic syndrome. This is the most common form of developmental language disorder, characterized by relatively normal language comprehension but the presence of significant difficulty in speech that is often nonfluent, sparse, and supplemented by the use of gestures or head nods. As language comprehension is near normal, the child may become easily frustrated because of his expressive difficulties. Oromotor apraxia is present in some of these children.

Phonologic programming deficit syndrome. These children have an extreme form of expressive impediment, almost amounting to mutism. The expressive disability is therefore much more severe than in the phonologic-syntactic syndrome. Language comprehension remains strikingly normal.

Environmental deprivation

Speech comprehension and expression may be impaired in extreme forms of environmental deprivation. Aberrant social and adaptive behavior are frequently present also. Assuming that there is no associated organic brain dysfunction, such children demonstrate a rapid and almost complete recovery of language function upon being placed in a nurturing and stimulating environment.

EVALUATION AND MANAGEMENT OF DELAYED LANGUAGE DEVELOPMENT

Early diagnosis and initiation of appropriate therapy are necessary in all instances (preferably between the ages of 30-36 months). A multidisciplinary team comprised of the physician, psychologist, speech pathologist, and occupational therapist is necessary.

The child should be assessed for hearing loss. Since conventional hearing tests in preschool age children frequently provide unreliable results, the audiologist may need to use Evoked Response Audiometry (Brainstem Auditory Evoked Potentials). The severity of the hearing loss, if present, should be determined and whether or not the child can be helped by speech amplification devices (conductive deafness).

Psychometric, speech, and language evaluation by a psychologist and speech pathologist help determine the strengths and weaknesses in both the verbal and nonverbal areas of intellectual function. An appropriate individualized educational program can then be formulated based upon the above findings.

EEG and CT scan are necessary in those children with focal neurological deficits or a history suggestive of seizures.

Intensive speech therapy, either through an individualized program or in a group setting, is necessary for almost all children with developmental language disorders. Hearing impaired children and certain children with developmental language disorders (auditory verbal agnosia) benefit from being taught "total communication"— a combination of sign language, lip reading, and speech training.

Children with severe expressive language impairment (those with cerebral palsy complicated by oromotor apraxia/ pseudobulbar states) may be able to enhance their communication ability using communication boards composed of pictures or words. Automated, microcomputer-aided speech

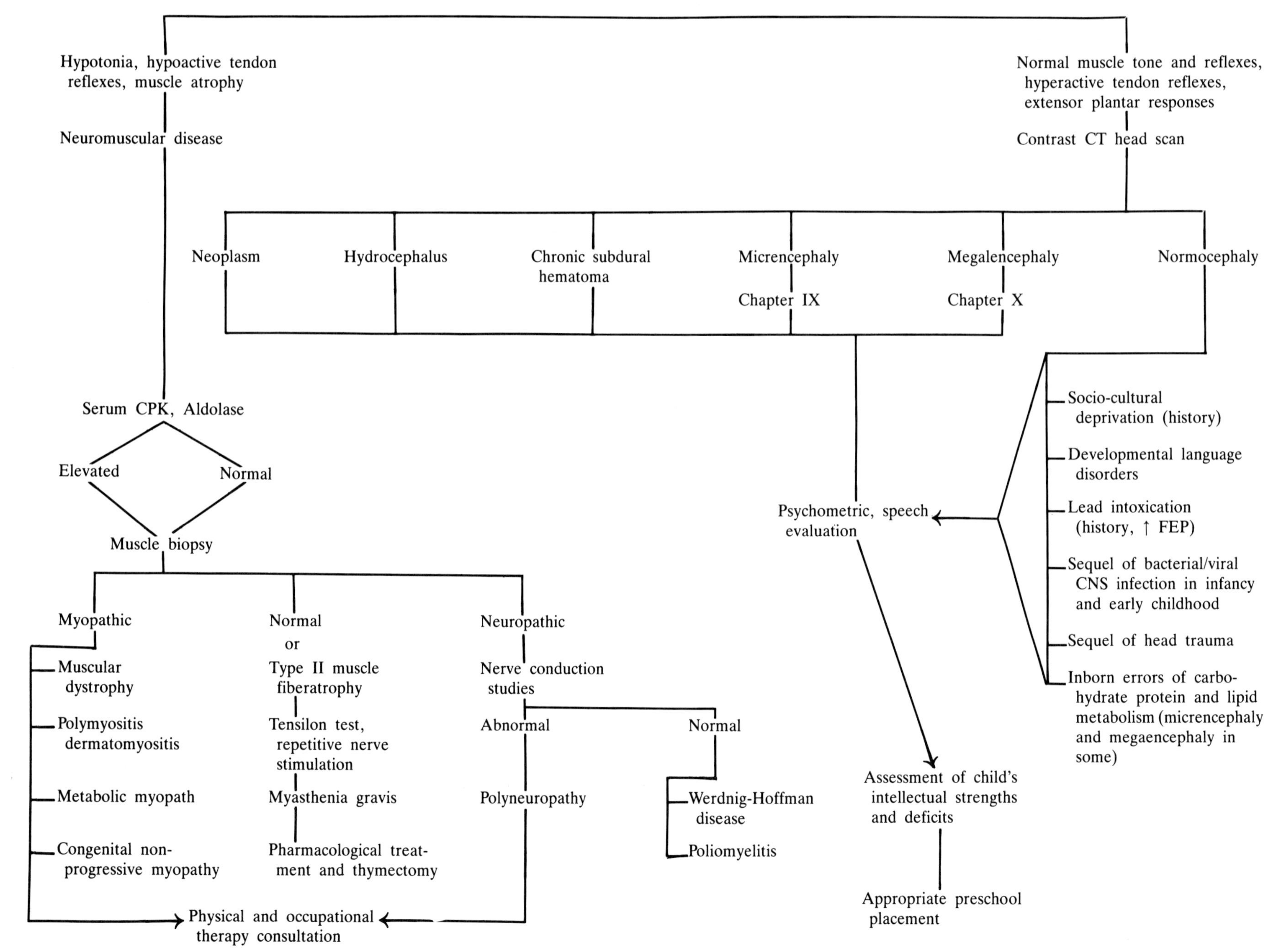

DELAYED DEVELOPMENT
Hypotonia, hypoactive tendon reflexes, muscle atrophy
Normal muscle tone and reflexes, hyperactive tendon reflexes, extensor plantar responses
Neuromuscular disease
Contrast CT head scan
Neoplasm
Hydrocephalus
Chronic subdural hematoma
Micrencephaly
Chapter IX
Megalencephaly
Chapter X
Normocephaly
Serum CPK, Aldolase
Elevated
Normal
Muscle biopsy
Socio-cultural deprivation (history)
Developmental language disorders
Lead intoxication (history, ↑ FEP)
Sequel of bacterial/viral CNS infection in infancy and early childhood
Sequel of head trauma
Inborn errors of carbohydrate protein and lipid metabolism (micrencephaly and megaencephaly in some)
Psychometric, speech evaluation
Myopathic
Normal or Type II muscle fiberatrophy
Neuropathic
Muscular dystrophy
Tensilon test, repetitive nerve stimulation
Nerve conduction studies
Polymyositis dermatomyositis
Abnormal
Normal
Metabolic myopath
Myasthenia gravis
Assessment of child's intellectual strengths and deficits
Congenital non-progressive myopathy
Pharmacological treatment and thymectomy
Polyneuropathy
Werdnig-Hoffman disease
Poliomyelitis
Physical and occupational therapy consultation
Appropriate preschool placement

synthesizers are also now available and may be useful in a limited number of such patients.

Behavioral modification using conditioning techniques is necessary in autistic children in order to minimize self-stimulatory behavior and enhance interaction with family members and peers.

Psychopharmacological agents are sometimes required in order to enhance concentration during speech therapy and minimize hyperactivity or self mutilatory behavior. Drugs commonly used include: thioridazine (MELLARYL) 10-60 mg/day, haloperidol (HALDOL) 0.25-2 mg/day, pemoline (CYLERT) 18.75-125 mg/day, and methylphenidate (RITALIN) in doses of 5-40 mg/day.

While some children with developmental language disorders are able to function normally in regular school programs with supplemental speech therapy, the majority continue to need placement in a special schools.

SUGGESTED READING

1. Jones KL, ed. Smith's Recognizable Patterns of Human Malformation. WB Saunders, Philadelphia, 4th edition, 1988.

2. Smith DW and Simons FER. Rational diagnostic evaluation of the child with mental deficiency. Am J Dis Child 129:1285-1290, 1975.

3. Nelson RP and Crocker AC. The medical care of mentally retarded persons in public residential facilities. N Engl J Med 299:1039-1044, 1978.

4. Lapierre YD and Reesal R. Pharmacologic management of aggressivity and self-mutilation in the mentally retarded. Psychiatr Clin North Am 9(4):745-755, 1986.

5. Turner G, Robinson H, Laing S and Purvis-Smith S. Preventive screening for the fragile X syndrome. N Engl J Med 315(10):607-609, 1986.

6. Nelson KB and Deutschberger J. Head size at one year as a predictor of four-year IQ. Dev Med Child Neurol 12:487-495, 1970.

7. Ferry PC. Infant stimulation programs. A neurologic shell game? Arch Neurol 43:281-282, 1986.

8. O'Reilly DE. Care of the cerebral palsied: outcome of the past and needs for the future. Dev Med Child Neurol 17:141-149, 1975.

9. Nelson KB and Ellenberg JH. Antecedents of cerebral palsy. Multivariate analysis of risk. N Engl J Med 315:81-86, 1986.

10. Molnar GE and Taft LT. Cerebral palsy and spinal cord injuries. In Current Problems In Pediatrics. Ped Rehab 7(3):3-40, 1977.

11. Disorders of oral and written language. In: Rapin I, ed. Children with Brain Dysfunction, Raven Press, New York, 1982; 131-156.

12. Damasio AR. Autism (editorial). Arch Neurol 41:481, 1984.

13. Mantovani JF and Landau WM. Acquired aphasia with convulsive disorder: course and prognosis. Neurology 30:524-529, 1980.

14. Ludlow CL. Children's language disorders: recent research advances. Ann Neurol 7:497-507, 1980.

15. Chudley AE and Hagerman RJ. Fragile X syndrome. J Pediatr 110:821-831, 1987.

CHAPTER XVI

ATAXIA OF ACUTE ONSET

Posterior Fossa Tumor

Posterior Fossa Abscess

Posterior Fossa Hemorrhage

Cerebral Concussion

Post-meningitic Ataxia

Neuromuscular Disorders

Basilar Migraine

Acute Labyrinthitis

Drug Intoxications

Heat Stroke

Acute Cerebellar Ataxia

Seizure Disorders

Cerebral Vasculitis

Metabolic Diseases

Algorithm

INTRODUCTION

Children with acute ataxia frequently present with a history of excessive falling or inability to maintain standing or sitting positions. The lesion may involve the cerebellum, brainstem, labyrinths, spinal cord, peripheral nerves, and occasionally, the frontal cortex. Accompanying clinical manifestations such as papilledema, somnolence, and weakness are helpful in establishing etiology and determining the management, which varies with the underlying disorder. Table 16-1 shows the various etiologies of ataxia.

Ataxia with Meningeal Irritation or Increased Intracranial Pressure

POSTERIOR FOSSA TUMORS

Although these tumors generally result in ataxia that evolves over weeks, a sudden increase in size due to hemorrhage within the tumor may lead to an acute presentation owing to development of acute hydrocephalus or compression of adjacent cerebellar or brainstem structures. The ataxia induced by medulloblastoma, ependymoma, and astrocytoma is usually accompanied by acute hydrocephalus and bilateral papilledema. Patients with brainstem gliomas, on the other hand, have ataxia associated with ipsilateral cranial neuropathies and contralateral long tract signs such as hemiparesis or extensor plantar response, but signs of increased intracranial pressure are generally lacking. MRI or contrast CT scan are the diagnostic procedures of choice when a posterior fossa tumor is suspected.

POSTERIOR FOSSA ABSCESS

This abscess is most often localized to the cerebellopontine angle and originates from a septic

Table 16-1. Etiologies of acute ataxia

I. Ataxia accompanied by signs of meningeal irritation or increased intracranial pressure.
  Posterior fossa neoplasm
  Posterior fossa abscess
  Cerebral concussion
  Posterior fossa hemorrhage
  Viral meningoencephalitis and bacterial meningitis
  Lead encephalopathy

II. Ataxia associated with weakness
  Tick paralysis
  Guillain-Barre syndrome
  Acute transverse myelitis

III. Ataxia with vomiting, nausea or headache but no signs of increased intracranial pressure.
  Migraine
  Labyrinthitis

IV. Ataxia with somnolence, but no signs of increased intracranial pressure, nausea, vomiting, or headache.
  Toxic encephalopathies from ingestion of:
    Phenobarbital
    Phenytoin
    Diazepam
    Alcohol
    Other hypnotic-sedatives.

V. Miscellaneous
  Heat stroke
  Acute cerebellar ataxia
  Seizure disorders
  Cerebral vasculitis
  Hartnup's and maple syrup urine disease
  Opsoclonus-myoclonus syndrome

process in the petrous or mastoid bones. Infected posterior fossa dermoid cysts are generally located in the dorsal midline cerebellum. Fever, signs of meningeal irritation, and increased intracranial pressure may accompany the abscess. Lumbar puncture is contraindicated. MRI and contrast CT scans are the diagnostic procedures of choice.

POSTERIOR FOSSA HEMORRHAGE

Posterior fossa hemorrhage is generally secondary to a ruptured arterio-venous malformation, vasculopathy (Moya-Moya syndrome), or a bleeding disorder such as hemophilia. If large, the mass lesion may cause increased intracranial pressure and require urgent surgical intervention (ventriculostomy followed by decompression of the posterior fossa). CT scan is the diagnostic procedure of choice.

CEREBRAL CONCUSSION

Cerebral concussion may be accompanied by ataxia in the acute stage due to the attendant brainstem, cerebellar, or labyrinthine dysfunction. The history and presence of low density, non-enhancing lesions in the posterior fossa on CT scan is helpful in establishing the diagnosis. There is complete recovery over a period of weeks in most instances.

BACTERIAL MENINGITIS

Ataxia following bacterial meningitis is seen in the recovery phase, and may correlate clinically with areas of cerebellar inflammation on CT or MRI scans. It almost always completely resolves spontaneously within a few months.

VIRAL MENINGOENCEPHALITIS

Viral meningoencephalitis may also be accompanied by ataxia at the onset resulting from involvement of the brainstem or cerebellum. The disorder is generally transient. The cerebrospinal fluid shows a characteristic lymphocytic pleocytosis, elevated protein, and normal glucose concentrations.

Ataxia Related to Neuromuscular Disorders

Guillain Barre Syndrome (refer to Chapters XII and XIX)

Tick Paralysis (refer to Chapters XII and XIX)

Acute Transverse Myelitis (refer to Chapter XIX.)

Ataxia with Vomiting, Nausea, Headache But No Signs of Increased Intracranial Pressure

BASILAR MIGRAINE

Basilar migraine can occur in children of any age and is associated with acute, episodic dizziness, nausea, vomiting, double vision, visual field defects, ataxia, and headache. It is accompanied by hypoperfusion in the region of distribution of the vertebro-basilar vessels. The neurologic deficit may last from hours to three or four days, and resolves completely in most instances. A family history of migraine is helpful in establishing the diagnosis, which is based mainly upon the historical data, clinical findings, and presence of a normal contrast CT scan. The frequency and intensity of the episodes gradually diminishes with age. Continuous prophylaxis with phenytoin is recommended in those with frequent recurrences.

ACUTE LABYRINTHITIS

This condition is generally of viral origin. It is accompanied by severe vertigo, nausea, vomiting, and ataxia. The vertigo is characteristically made worse by movement of the head. Nystagmus, either unilateral or bilateral, is present alongwith it. The caloric response may be absent. Gradual resolution over a 3-4 week period is the rule.

Ataxia with Somnolence But No Nausea, Vomiting, Headache, or Signs of Increased Intracranial Pressure

DRUG INTOXICATIONS

Drug intoxications may be accidental (in toddlers), resulting from an inadvertent overdose (e.g., anticonvulsants in a child being treated for seizures), or a consequence of psychiatric disturbances in the adolescent. The ataxia has abrupt onset and is unassociated with fever or signs of meningeal irritation. If alcohol has been ingested, its smell may be apparent in the breath. Bilateral horizontal and vertical nystagmus may be present in intoxication with barbiturates, phenytoin, or diazepam. Signs of intoxication become apparent with phenobarbital and phenytoin when levels exceed 30 and 20 ug/ml respectively. Ataxia from lead encephalopathy generally occurs with blood levels of above 60 ug/ml and may be accompanied by signs of increased intracranial pressure. Hallucinogens such as phencyclidine and phenothiazine may also occasionally induce ataxia. A change in mental status accompanies all patients with toxic encephalopathies and may vary from agitation to lethargy, delerium, and coma. The diagnosis of a toxic encephalopathy should be suspected whenever acute onset of altered mental status and ataxia is unaccompanied by trauma or inflammatory disease. Urine and serum drug screens help confirm the diagnosis. Blood alcohol levels should be obtained when a smell of alcohol is present on the breath. The serum free erythrocytic protoporphyrin and lead levels are elevated and metaphysial opacification ("lead lines") apparent in patients with lead encephalopathy.

MISCELLANEOUS

HEAT STROKE

This condition is caused by exposure to intense heat and sunlight and is accompanied by a derangement in the heat dissipating mechanisms of the body, with resultant hyperpyrexia, dry skin, confusion, coma, convulsions, and shock. Degeneration of the Purkinje cells in the cerebellar cortex is the most remarkable feature upon autopsy. Survivors are frequently left with ataxia, which resolves spontaneously over weeks to months.

ACUTE CEREBELLAR ATAXIA

This is usually observed in children under the ages of 6-8 years. It frequently develops within 2-3 weeks of an acute viral illness. Association with varicella, influenza, enterovirus, and Epstein Barr virus has been noted. The child generally develops severe gait and truncal ataxia, resulting in falls or inability to sit independently. Nystagmus or other forms of abnormal eye movement are found in half the instances. There are no signs of increased intracranial pressure. The mental status remains normal. Hypotonia, pendular tendon reflexes, and scanning speech may be present. Systemic signs of acute illness (fever, malaise) are characteristically absent. A CT scan should be obtained in order to exclude a mass lesion, but is invariably normal. The cerebrospinal fluid discloses pleocytosis and mild protein elevation in about 25% of the patients. The disorder most likely represents immunological cerebellar dysfunction that has been triggered by the viral illness. Occult neuroblastoma may accompany ataxia in some of the patients. Complete remission within 3-4 months is seen in approximately 70% of the patients, but 30% remain with some degree of residual incoordination.

SEIZURE DISORDERS

Patients with seizure disorders may develop ataxia secondary to the underlying neurological

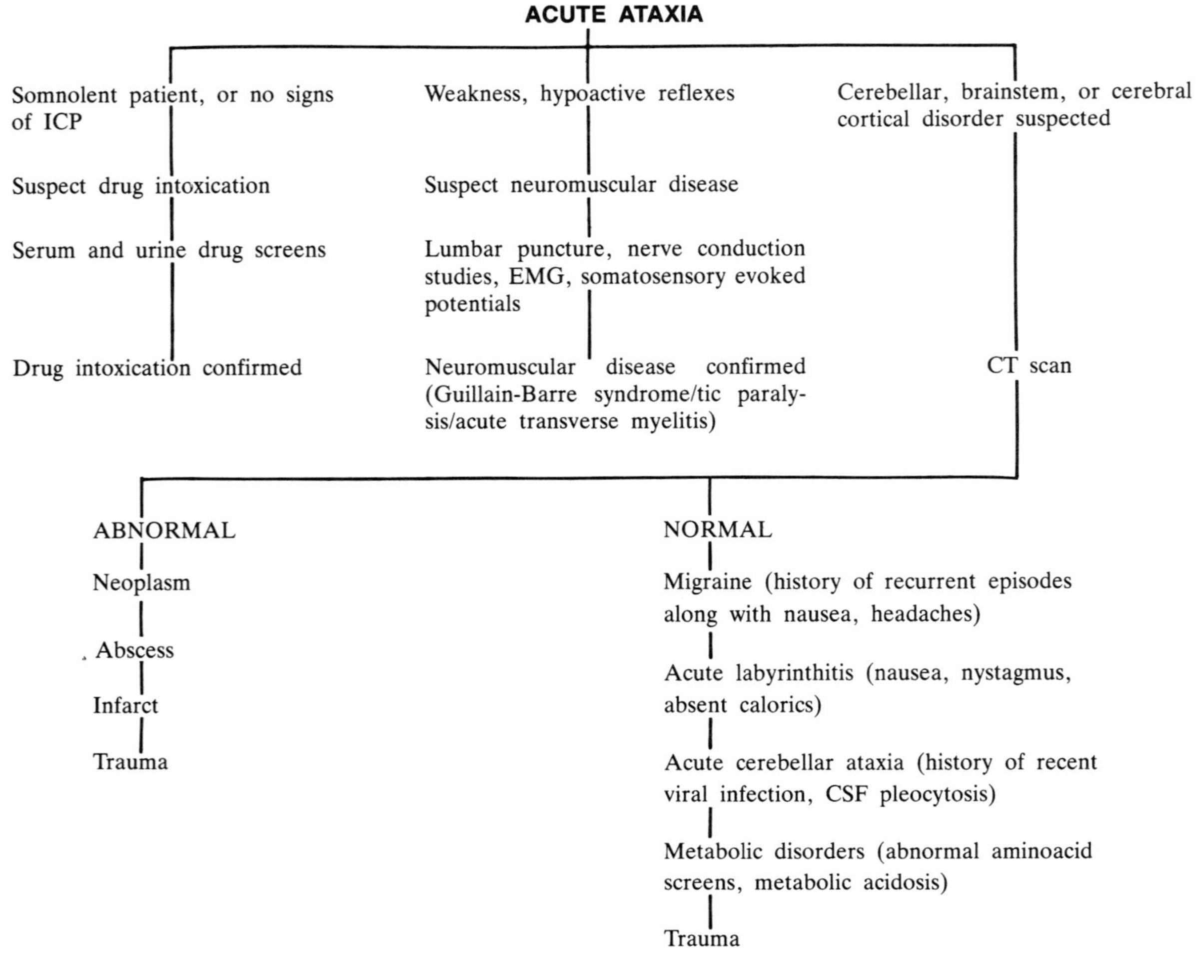

disorder, anticonvulsant intoxication, or, infrequently, as a direct consequence of cortical dysfunction from poor seizure control, with resultant alteration in function of the crossed fronto-pontocerebellar pathways.

CEREBRAL VASCULITIS

This condition most frequently accompanies systemic lupus erythematosus or polyarteritis nodosa. Alterations in mental status and systemic manifestations are invariably present. The erythrocytic sedimentation rate is elevated. Serum antinuclear antibodies, circulating immune complexes, and systemic evidence of disease are also present in this condition.

METABOLIC DISEASES

Hartnup's disease is a disorder of transport of neutral aminoacids which is accompanied by intermittent ataxia, episodes of psychotic behavior, a photosensitive dermatitis, and renal aminoaciduria. Occasionally patients with maple syrup urine disease also manifest intermittent ataxia coinciding with intermittent increased urinary excretion of valine, leucine, and isoleucine. Plasma levels of these branched chain ketoacids may be elevated during the acute episode of ataxia. The urine ferric chloride test may show a blue discoloration. Pyruvic dehydrogenase complex abnormalities may also present with intermittent ataxia, hypoglycemia, and lactic and pyruvic acidosis.

OPSOCLONUS-MYOCLONUS SYNDROME

This is characterized by bursts of chaotic, arrythmic, irregular eye movements termed opsoclonus. The syndrome of opsoclonus-myoclonus consists of acute or subacute onset of a combination of the eye movement disturbance along with non-epileptic myoclonus and dysmetria involving the distal extremities. The disorder has a diverse etiology. It may represent a non-metastatic manifestation of an occult neuroblastoma. In other instances, it may follow exposure to toxins or viral infections. An autoimmune mechanism is operant in the majority of patients. Examination of the cerebrospinal fluid may disclose mild pleocytosis and elevated gamma globulin levels. Investigations to exclude an occult neuroblastoma are recommended in most patients and consist of chest and abdominal X-Rays, bone marrow examination, and 24-hour urinary collections for catecholamines and vanilmandelic acid. Most patients have a self-limited disorder that resolves in 2-3 months. Corticosteroid therapy for 6-8 weeks may be beneficial in those who do not improve spontaneously.

SUGGESTED READING

1. Autoimmune and postinfectious diseases. In: Menkes JH. Textbook of Child Neurology, 3rd edition, Lea and Febiger, Philadelphia, 1985; 462-463.

2. Walker RW and Allen JC. Pediatric brain tumors. Pediatric Annals 12:383-394, 1983.

3. Healy GB. Hearing loss and vertigo secondary to head trauma in children. N Engl J Med 306:1029, 1982.

4. Perlstein P and Attala R. Neurologic sequlae of plumbism in children. Clin Pediatr 5:292-298, 1966.

CHAPTER XVII
NEONATAL NEUROLOGY

Neonatal Seizures

Perinatal Hypoxic Encephalopathy

Periventricular-Intraventricular Hemorrhage

Intracerebellar Hemorrhage

Perinatal Bilirubin Encephalopathy

Arthrogryposis Multiplex Congenita

Cephalhematoma

Subgaleal Hemorrhage

Primary Subarachnoid Hemorrhage

Subdural Hemorrhage

Brachial Plexus Injuries

Spinal Cord Injuries

Cerebral Infarction

NEONATAL SEIZURES

Introduction

Seizures are by far the most common manifestation of neurological disease in the newborn. They are an important reason for neurological consultation in the Nursery. Based on a review of 54,000 pregnancies between 1959 and 1966, the incidence of neonatal seizures in the Collaborative Perinatal Project was found to be 0.5%.[1] Neonatal seizures differ from those in older infants in nosology, etiology, clinical manifestations, and outcome. The diagnosis is frequently difficult. There is also reason to believe that prolonged seizure states in the neonate may lead to adverse long term consequences.

Classification

The International Classification of Seizures is not applicable at this age. One widely accepted classification[2] is shown in Table 17-1.

Table 17-1. Classification of neonatal seizures

Tonic Seizures
Episodes of stiffening of the trunk and extremities resembling opisthotonus.

Multifocal Clonic Seizures
Rhythmic clonic movements of different parts of the body in various seizures.

Focal Clonic Seizures
Repetitive clonic movements of the same segment of the body in serial seizures.

Subtle Seizures
Episodes of stereotyped bicycling, sucking, and swallowing movements.

Myoclonic Seizures
Isolated or repetitive brief jerks of the body.

If one were to assess neonates for seizures solely relying on clinical observations, it is likely that the seizures would go unrecognized in some neonates.[3] On the other hand, they may be over-diagnosed in other neonates due to the interpretation of non-epileptic rhythmic activity originating at subcortical levels as seizures. Applying video-EEG telemetry studies, Mizrahi and Kellaway[4] have recently developed an alternate classification (Table 17-2).

From the practical standpoint, Volpe's classification[2] is recommended to the clinician. The Mizrahi and Kellaway classification[4] may ultimately lead to a better understanding of the pathophysiology of seizure phenomena in neonates.

Table 17-2. Alternate classification of seizures

I. Seizures with a Close Association with EEG Seizure Discharges
- **Focal Clonic**
  - Unifocal
  - Multifocal
    - Alternating
    - Migrating
    - Hemiconvulsive
    - Axial
- **Myoclonic**
  - Generalized
  - Focal
- **Focal Tonic**
  - Asymmetric truncal
  - Eye deviation
- **Apnea**

II. Seizures with Inconsistent or no Relationship to EEG Seizure or Discharges
- **Motor Automatisms**
  - Oral-buccal-lingual
  - Ocular signs
  - Progressive movements
    - Pedaling
    - Stepping
    - Rotary arm movements
  - Complex, purposeless movements
- **Generalized tonic**
  - Extensor
  - Flexor
  - Mixed extensor/flexor
- **Myoclonic**
  - Generalized
  - Focal
  - Fragmentary

III. Infantile Spasms

IV. EEG Seizures without Clinical Seizures.

Pathophysiology

The neonatal brain is incapable of generating sustained high frequency electrical discharges. A combination of tonic and clonic events in the same seizure is therefore rare at this age. Premature infants have even less capability of generating well synchronized seizure activity. Owing to the relative paucity of synapses and myelination, seizures in the newborn are often fragmentary, poorly sustained, and sometimes focal even in the presence of a diffuse cerebral insult. It is unclear whether stereotyped seizure-like movements without an EEG paroxysmal correlate (e.g., subtle or generalized tonic seizures)[4] constitute seizure activity originating at subcortical levels or whether they are non-epileptic—representing a subcortical release phenomenon due to cerebral cortical dysfunction.

Using in vivo phosphorus 31 nuclear magnetic spectroscopy, Younkin et al.[5] documented a decrease in brain phosphocreatine by approximately 33% during seizures in four neonates. Simultaneously, oxidative metabolism increased by approximately 45%. Immediate administration of phenobarbital in one of the four led to a prompt increase in brain phosphocreatine. Perlman and Volpe measured blood flow velocity during seizures in the anterior cerebral arteries using Doppler in 12 premature infants.[6] A marked increase in blood flow velocity during the seizures was documented in all infants. This was accompanied by a marked increase in systemic blood pressure and intracranial pressure. They felt that the increase in cerebral blood flow may be maladaptive in the newborn, who has vulnerable capillary beds such as the periventricular germinal matrix.

In a study of immature (4 day old) rats, a single two hour episode of status epilepticus induced by flurothyl irreversibly curtailed brain weight and brain DNA.[7] Rats subjected to status epilepticus also subsequently showed delayed behavioral milestones and reduced seizure thresholds. It is conceivable that even in the human neonate, serial seizures may permanently impair myelination, synaptogenesis, and cerebellar growth.

Etiology

Hypoxic ischemic encephalopathy, cerebral infarction, and intracranial hemorrhage (subdu-

Table 17-3. Common etiologies of neonatal seizures

Metabolic Derangements

Hypoxic-ischemic encephalopathy
Hypocalcemia
Hypomagnesemia
Hypoglycemia
Hyponatremia

Inborn error of metabolism
Phenylketonuria
Methylmalonic acidemia, maple syrup urine disease
Galactosemia
Ammonia cycle disorders
Non-ketotic hyperglycinemia
Zellweger syndrome and neonatal adrenoleukodystrophy
Pyridoxine deficiency and dependancy states

Intracranial Hemorrhage

Primary subarachmoid
Subdural hemorrhage following birth trauma
Intraventricular hemorrhage (especially Grades III and IV)

Infections

Congenital intrauterine (syphilis, acquired immune deficiency syndrome, toxoplasmosis, cytomegalovirus herpes simplex, rubella)

Bacterial meningitis
Viral meningoencephalitis (e.g., herpes simplex)

Cerebral Malformations

Trisomies (e.g., trisomy 18)
Partial deletion syndromes
Holoprosencephaly
Porencephaly
Hydranencephaly
Lissencephaly, without Miller-Dieker syndrome
Septo-optic dysplasia
Aicardi syndrome

Drug Induced

Withdrawal (heavy maternal use of hypnotics, opiates)
Toxic (topical anesthetics administered to mother for pudendal block)

Vascular

Cerebral infarction
Vein of Galen malformation (rare)

Miscellaneous

Benign familial neonatal seizures
Incontinentia pigmenti
Tuberous sclerosis
Sturge Weber syndrome

---

ral, subaracnoid, or intraventricular) are the most prevalent etiologic factors. Some of the common etiologies are listed in Table 17-3.

Seizures related to hypoxic encephalopathy, trauma, pyridoxine dependency, and hypoglycemia typically develop in the first 48 hours after birth.[8] Multiple metabolic derangements may frequently coexist, or occur in conjunction with a structural disease.[8] **Hypocalcemia** is defined as the presence of a serum calcium of less than 8 mg/dl in a term infant and less than 7.5 mg/dl in a preterm infant. Early hypocalcemia (within 72 hours of birth) is seen in infants with hypoxia, infants of diabetic and hyperparathyroid mothers, osteopetrosis, the Di George syndrome, and with intrauterine growth retardation. Late onset hypocalcemia (between 4 to 7 days after birth) is usually seen with excessive phospate load in the diet, e.g., with use of cow's milk. **Hypoglycemia** is defined as a blood glucose value of less than 20 mg/dl in a preterm infant and less than 30 mg/dl in a term infant. It is commonly encountered in infants of diabetic mothers, intrauterine growth

retardation, methylmalonic acidemia, maple syrup urine disease, galactosemia, and septo-optic dysplasia.

Clinical Assessment

Family members may not be physically present in the Nursery and frequently need to be contacted over the phone to obtain additional history. A thorough history should address maternal age, gravida, para, gestational age when pregnancy was diagnosed, illnesses during pregnancy, drug use, exposure to toxins, labor, Apgar scores, need for resuscitation at birth, complications after birth, and presence of a family history of seizures or mental retardation. A discussion with the nursing staff is always important because it frequently provides valuable information about seizure type and the seriousness of the encephalopathy (e.g., presence or absence of irritability and feeding difficulties).

A neonate with seizures who is small for gestational age may have chromosomal anomalies, congenital intrauterine infections, or intrauterine exposure to a toxin. Dysmorphic facial features such as hypotelorism, hypertelorism, small palpebral fissures, or low set ears are frequently a clue to cerebral dysgenesis. Neurocutaneous syndromes that can be diagnosed in the Nursery include the Sturge Weber syndrome, incontinentia pigmenti, and tuberous sclerosis. Patients with congenital cytomegalovirus infections may manifest petechial skin hemorrhages and hepatosplenomegaly.

The neurological examination should include assessment of: reactivity and habituation to external stimuli, abnormalities in the resting posture, fundoscopy (for cataracts, chorioretinitis, lacunar retinopathy, and optic disc hypoplasia), eye movements, tendon and developmental reflexes, head size, fullness of the anterior fontanel, and the spine. Seizures may be undiagnosed or underestimated in critically ill neonates who are on respirators and require skeletal muscle paralysis for management of the respiratory illness. A high index of suspicion and serial electroencephalographic monitoring is necessary for diagnosis of seizures in these infants.

Investigations

1. Check serum calcium, magnesium, electrolytes, and blood glucose in all cases.

2. Unless the etiology is very obvious, obtain a lumbar puncture in all neonates to exclude bacterial meningitis, viral encephalitis, and subarachnoid hemorrhage.

3. Suspect an inborn error of metabolism if the patient has unexplained lethargy, metabolic acidosis, reducing substances in the urine or ketonuria. Obtain blood ammonia, urine amino and organic acid screens.

4. Obtain a neurosonogram to exclude structural central nervous system lesions such as hemorrhage, infarction, porencephaly, or hydranencephaly.

5. Magnetic resonance/computed tomographic scan and chromosomal analysis are called for if the child has dysmorphic features suggesting central nervous system malformation.

6. The electroencephalogram (EEG) helps to confirm the diagnosis in patients with suspected seizures, establish a prognosis, and guide the length of anticonvulsant therapy. Serial studies are recommended. EEG patterns recorded during seizures include rhythmic delta, theta and alpha-like activity, and repetitive sharp wave discharges that may be uni or multifocal. Interictal abnormalities of the background are probably of greater significance than ictal patterns in establishing a prognosis.[9] Rowe et al. prospectively evaluated 74 term and preterm infants with neonatal seizures up to an average age of 33 months.[10] All infants had EEG studies in the neonatal period within 72 hours of the seizures. Normal EEG studies were associated with normal outcome in 22/26 (94.6%) of subjects. Severely abnormal EEGs (low voltage/electrocerebral inactivity/burst suppression) were associated with moderate to severe neurologic sequalae in 36/37 (97.3%) of the population.

7. Chromosomal analysis is performed in patients with dysmorphic features. Urine cytomegalovirus cultures and serum titres for toxoplasmosis, rubella, cytomegalovirus, herpes, and syphilis are done in patients with suspected congenital intrauterine infection.

Differential Diagnosis

Jittteriness. Exaggerated segmental reflexes in hypoxia, hypocalcemia, hypomagnesemia, and drug withdrawal states may induce rhythmic to and fro movement of the jaw or limbs. Jittery movements can be easily distinguished from seizures owing to the fact that they are abolished by relaxing the affected group of muscles, and are not associated head segment automatisms, and because the EEG does not show simultaneous paroxysmal discharges.

Benign Neonatal Sleep Myoclonus. These repetitive jerks of the body are present during all sleep states, but greatest during quiet sleep. The neurologic examination and subsequent development are normal. Transient neurotransmitter imbalance and genetic factors may play a causative role.[11]

Treatment

1. Correct hypoglycemia if present. Use 10% dextrose in 0.25% normal saline intravenously at a rate of 2 ml/kg, followed by 8 ml/kg over 24 hours.

2. Correct hypocalcemia if present. Use calcium gluconate 200 mg/kg slow IV with monitoring of the heart rate for bradycardia.

3. Correct hypomagnesemia if present. Use magnesium sulfate 0.25 mg/kg IM of 50% solution. When the patient has a combination of hypocalcemia and hypomagnesemia, both deficits need simultaneous correction in order to effect a clinical improvement.

4. Correct hyponatremia if present. Use 3% normal saline IV 12 ml/kg, with correction of 50% of the deficit immediately and the remainder over the ensuing 24 hours.

5. Exclude pyridoxine dependancy by administering 100 mg of pyridoxine IV, preferably with simultaneously monitoring of the EEG. Paroxysmal discharges should subside within 20-25 minutes of infusion.

6. If the metabolic derangements listed above are absent or have been corrected, but the seizures persist, then use Phenobarbital 20 mg/kg slow IV; this may be repeated as a 10-20 mg/kg bolus if necessary. If seizures persist, use phenytoin (DILANTIN) 20 mg/kg slow IV at a rate not exceeding 30 mg/minute, monitoring for bradycardia and hypotension.

   OR

   Lorazepam 0.05 mg/kg/dose IV[12]; this may be repeated X 2 or 3 every 15-20 minutes if necessary.

Gal et al. noted that seizures could be controlled in 85% of 60 neonates when phenobarbital was used in doses of up to 40 mg/kg.[13] Maintenance doses of 2-4 mg/kg/day are sufficient to maintain therapeutic levels. Owing to a gradual decline in the plasma half life over the first four weeks,[14] serial monitoring of serum phenobarbital levels is necessary in order to maintain a therapeutic phenobarbital level. Also, owing to poor oral absorption, serum phenytoin levels may drop precipitously when the patient is switched from intravenous to oral phenytoin. Concerns have been raised about the adverse effects of phenobarbital on the developing nervous system.[15,16] Anticonvulsant therapy for neonatal seizures should therefore be discontinued as soon as it becomes safe to do so. In a study by Brod et al.,[17] normal initial electroencephalograms in the Nursery were found to be a reliable indicator of successful discontinuation of anticonvulsant therapy in 18 of 22 term neonates. In preterm infants, subsequent normal EEG studies were a reliable indicator of successful weaning in 9 of 10 infants.

Prognosis

The Perinatal Collaborative Project prospectively enrolled 54,000 pregnant women between 1959 and 1966.[1] The offspring included 277 with neonatal seizures, most of whom were followed up to the age of seven years. The mortality rate was 34.8%. Of the 181 survivors, 70% were normal. Thirteen percent had a combination of cerebral palsy, epilepsy, and mental retardation. Twenty percent had epilepsy. A low Apgar score after 5 minutes of age, need for resuscitation, low birth weight, and early onset of seizures correlated with adverse outcome. However, the data were not correlated with seizure etiology and reflect management prior to an era of major advances in neonatal intensive care.[14] It is possible that seizure etiology itself, e.g., hypoxic encephalopathy, has a greater bearing on the outcome than seizures per se.[9] When specific etiologies were also examined, Berman et al. found that 53% of neonates with hypoxic encephalopathy and/or intracranial hemorrhage had moderate to severe sequlae on follow up for 12 to 60 months.[18]

PERINATAL HYPOXIC ENCEPHALOPATHY

Perinatal hypoxia accounts for between 30-70% of all neonatal seizures and constitutes an important, frequently preventable disorder.

Pathophysiology

Hypoxic hypoxia is characterized mainly by exclusion of oxygen from the system, with relative preservation of blood pressure and cerebral perfusion, e.g., following meconium aspiration. Ischemic hypoxia on the other hand, is associated with hypotensive states and diminished tissue perfusion such as that following antepartum hemorrhage. It leads to impaired clearance of metabolites from the brain, which can further adversely impact cellular function. Hypoxic hypoxia tends to impair the function of cortical and subcortical structures without regard to vascular territories, whereas ischemic hypoxia is liable to maximally affect areas lying within watershed (boundary) zones. Watershed zones are those that lie between the territorial distribution of two major arterial systems, thus receiving only the very terminal branches from either system and therefore being most vulnerable to the effects of diminished tissue perfusion in hypotensive states. In term infants, involvement is generally seen in the cortical watershed zones, whereas preterm infants demonstrate a predisposition for infarction in watershed zones of the periventricular white matter.

Hypoxia leads to depletion of high energy phosphates (ATP, creatine phosphate). This in turn leads to an inability to maintain the integrity of the cell membrane, which causes cellular swelling and calcium entry into the cytoplasm. Consequently, there is inactivation of endoplasmic reticular and mitochondrial function. Edema as a consequence of cell swelling may further compromise cerebral perfusion. The accumulation of aspartate and glutamate in the extracellular spaces in the hippocampus and neocortex also leads to further opening up of the calcium channels and calcium entry into the neurons.

Hippocampal regions of the cerebral cortex, the cerebellar cortex, superior colliculi, and the thalamus are most vulnerable to hypoxic insults in term infants. Periventricular leukomalacia and intraventricular hemorrhage are most often observed in preterm infants.

Clinical Manifestations

A five minute Apgar score of less than 6, metabolic acidosis, and hypotension are generally suggestive of significant asphyxia in term infants. However, in preterm infants the five minute Apgar score may not always provide a reliable estimate of the severity of asphyxia, and extended 10, 15 and 20 minute scores may be more relevant.

Ninety percent of all asphyxial insults have an in utero onset, frequently secondary to prolapsed umbilical cord, placenta previa, abruptio placenta, and intrauterine growth retardation. In only approximately 10% of instances does asphyxia have a distinct, post-natal onset, e.g., with congenital heart disease or recurrent apneic spells.

The mildly asphyxiated infant (Stage I) may manifest a hyperalert appearance, tremouslesness, poor feeding, exaggerated tendon reflexes, tachycardia, and pupillary dilatation. The EEG is invariably normal during this stage, and seizures are infrequent.

The moderately asphyxiated neonate (Stage II) is usually lethargic, hypotonic, and may have seizures and paroxysmal changes on the EEG.

The severely asphyxiated neonate (Stage III) is generally comatose, hypotonic, and has impaired brainstem occulomotor reflexes. The anterior fontanelle may be full and bulging due to the presence of cerebral edema. The EEG demonstrates low voltage, periodic, or multifocal paroxysmal changes.

In both moderate and severely asphyxiated infants, the seizure frequency may increase concurrent with the improvement in sensorium that is usually seen by the second or third day of life.

After the first week, most asphyxiated infants show gradual improvement in muscle tone (frequently evolving from hypotonic to hypertonic states), and retain impaired sucking and swallowing functions and alterations in sleep-wake cycling (e.g., inability to sustain sleep for more than 1-2 hours at a time).

General Principles in Management

Ensure adequate oxygenation and cerebral perfusion; pressor agents may be needed if hypotension develops as a consequence of myocardial hypoxic injury, or respiratory support if respiratory insufficiency develops from pulmonary/brain stem dysfunction.

Exclude any coexisting metabolic, infectious, or structural central nervous system insults and treat when indicated. Hypoglycemia, hypocalcemia, and hypomagnesemia are the most common disturbances that accompany asphyxia.

Control seizures by correcting any metabolic derangements or with the use of anticonvulsants.

Treat cerebral edema in severely hypoxic infants with coma and bulging anterior fontanelle with the use of mannitol 0.25gm/kg IV (one dose only) or dexamethasone 0.2 mg/kg/day in four divided doses for 2-3 days.

Monitor for fluid overload and restrict fluids to 2/3 of maintenance volume until cerebral edema has resolved.

Prognosis

In a study of 38,405 consecutive deliveries, the impact of asphyxia on mortality was seen to increase with increasing gestational age.[8] Mortality was seen to increase twofold above normal in asphyxiated infants of 27-28 weeks gestation and more than a hundredfold in infants of over 36 weeks gestation. Between 20-40% of preterm infants who survive perinatal asphyxia are left with moderate to severe neurologic sequele. The low birth weight infant who is small for gestational age is more liable to be neurologically impaired than an "appropriate" for gestational age infant.

Between 10-20% of asphyxiated term infants with hypoxic ischemic encephalopathy die within the first decade, and another 20-45% have moderate to severe neurologic sequlae.

The extended Apgar scores at 10, 15 and 20 minutes are of greater value than the five minute score in estimating mortality and morbidity. Mortality is about 18% in term infants with 10 minute Apgar scores of 0-3, but climbs to 59% when the score remains depressed in this range at 20 minutes after birth. The incidence of cerebral palsy is 5% in infants with a score of 0-3 at 10 minutes after birth, 9% in those with a 0-3 Apgar score at 15 minutes, and 57% with such a low score at 20 minutes.

Cerebral edema, status epilepticus, stupor or lethargy persisting beyond the first week, CT evidence of hypodense lesions involving both the gray and white matter; as well as periodic, low-voltage, or multifocal patterns on the EEG are all indicative of a poor outcome, with a strong likelihood of permanent sequlae. Patients with mild or moderate encephalopathy (Stage I or Stage II) generally have a normal outcome.

PERIVENTRICULAR INTRAVENTRICULAR HEMORRHAGE

Increasing survival of premature infants in modern neonatal intensive care units has been associated with an increase in the recognition of periventricular hemorrhage-intraventricular hemorrhage (PH-IVH). The incidence in infants under 1500 grams undergoing routine CT scan or ultrasound examinations is between 32 and 44%. Infrequently, the disorder may also be seen in full term infants.

The hemorrhage has venous or capillary origin from the periventricular germinal matrix, usually at the level of the head of the caudate nucleus (Fig. 17-1). With enlargement in size, it may rupture into the ventricular system or the parenchyma. Post-hemorrhagic hydrocephalus may result from obstruction of the flow of CSF (Fig. 17-2). Lateralized deficits become evident in infancy and childhood in survivors with large parenchymal extensions. Involvement of the periventricular region may compromise the ultimate migration and maturation of precursors of glial cells located in the periventricular germinal matrix, thus affecting myelination of the brain and leading to spasticity and hyperreflexia.

Pathophysiology

Preterm infants, especially those of less than 32 weeks gestation, are especially vulnerable to PH-IVH for a variety of reasons:

a. There is increased vascularity in the periventricular region relative to that in the cerebral cortex.

b. Hypoxic injury to fragile periventricular vessels renders them liable to rupture.

c. There may be increased cerebral venous pressure due to heart failure and use of pressure ventilators.

d. There is loss of autoregulation in the cerebral vasculature with hypoxia, as a consequence of which the vascular system becomes pressure-passive and liable to be affected by any systemic fluctuations in blood pressure.

e. Lack of stromal tissue support to vessels in the periventricular germinal matrix in premature infants.

f. High fibrinolytic activity in vessels of the periventricular region, interfering with clot formation once the hemorrhage has occurred. PH-IVH may be seen infrequently in term infants, in which case it usually originates from the choroid plexus or arteriovenous malformations involving the vein of Galen.

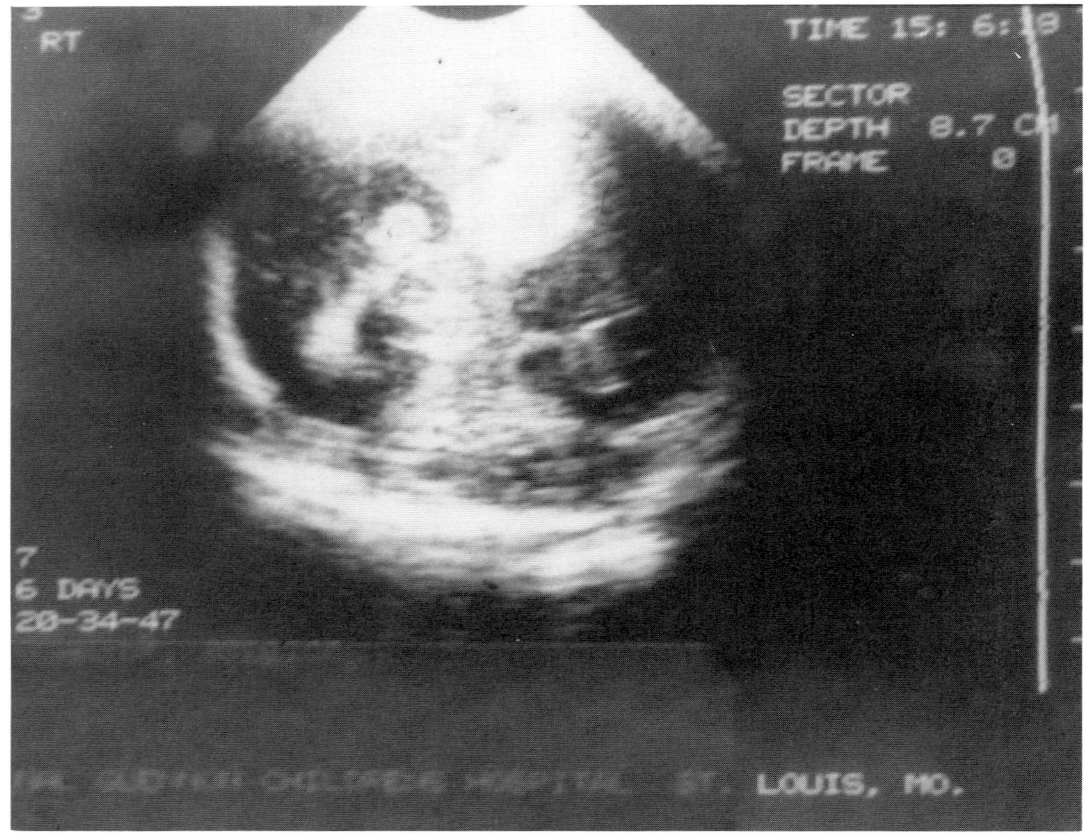

Fig. 17-1. Coronal section of a neonatal neurosonogram, demonstrating echodense lesions in the right lateral ventricle and in the region of the left caudate nucleus. The right lateral ventricle is also mildly enlarged.

Clinical Features

Most PH-IVH has onset 12-72 hours after birth. The following clinical presentations may be observed:

Catastrophic deterioration. The preterm infant with respiratory distress abruptly develops seizures, opisthotonus, a tense and bulging anterior fontanelle, and occulomotor and pupillary abnormalities. This coincides with extension into the ventricle of a large volume of blood with resultant acute hydrocephalus and rise in intracranial pressure.

Saltatory deterioration. Lethargy, seizures, and apneic spells evolve gradually over 3-4 days. It is associated with mild to moderate intraventricular bleeding.

Asymptomatic. There may be no clinical manifestations when the hemorrhage is small and restricted to the periventricular region. Such asymptomatic lesions may be detected only in the course of routine serial ultrasound or CT examinations.

Post-hemorrhagic hydrocephalus. Monitoring using serial cranial ultrasound studies is recommended through the first 6-8 weeks after birth.

Craniomegaly in posthemorrhagic hydrocephalus. This may lag behind ventricular enlargement by 7-10 days owing to the soft consistency of the deep white matter.

Prognosis

The outcome depends to a large extent upon whether or not the hemorrhage has ruptured into the ventricular system, on the amount of blood within the ventricles, and the presence or absence of parenchymal extension. With small

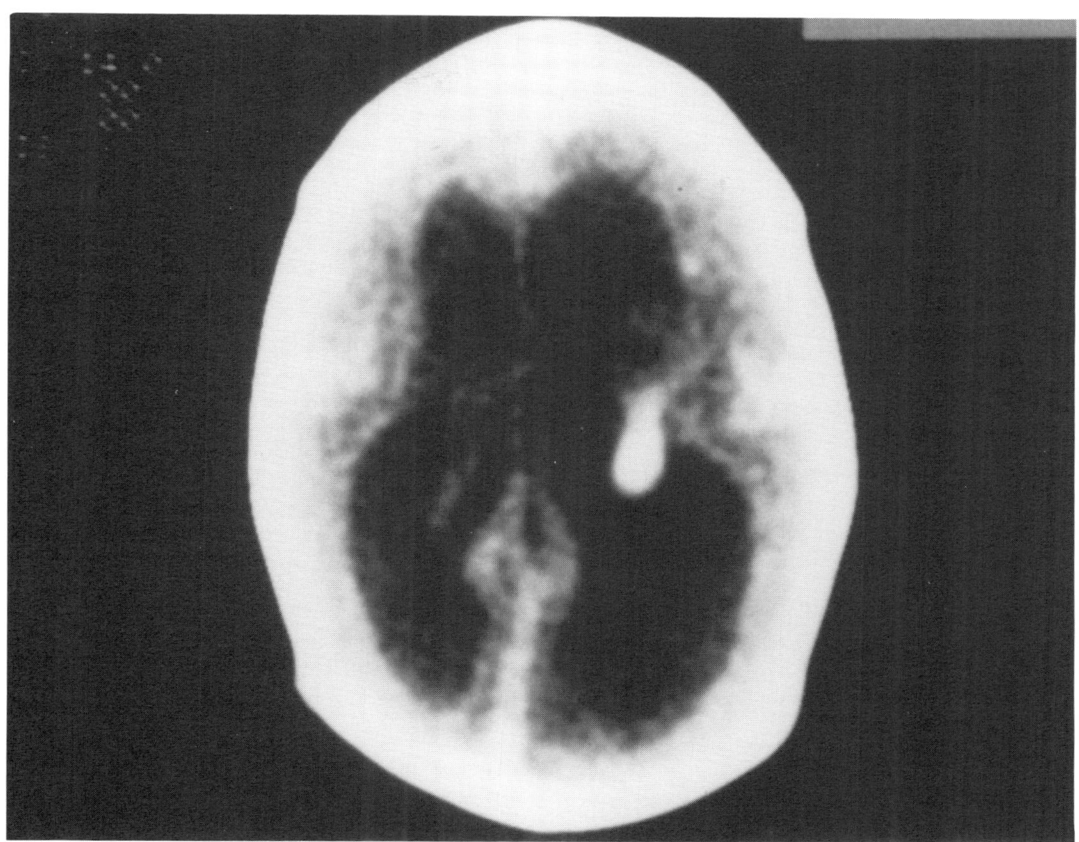

Fig. 17-2. Non-contrast CT scan in a neonate recovering from intraventricular hemorrhage, demonstrating hydrocephalus with symmetric lateral ventricular enlargement.

lesions restricted to the periventricular region, survival is the rule and no sequele are likely.

With moderate hemorrhagic lesions that have extended into the ventricles, the mortality rate is approximately 10% and the incidence of post-hemorrhagic hydrocephalus approximately 20%.

With severe lesions (generally seen with a catastrophic clinical picture from large intraventricular and intraparenchymal extensions), mortality varies between 50-60%. Between 65-100% of survivors have neurological sequele; these sequele are most frequently seizures, spastic tetraparesis, severe hypotonia, and visual field deficits.

Management of Post-hemorrhagic Hydrocephalus

If the patient has signs of acutely increased intracranial pressure, neurosurgical consultation should be immediately sought to obtain a ventricular tap to decrease the intracranial pressure. An indwelling intraventricular cannula helps drain the blood gradually over a period of days. Such patients generally require insertion of a ventriculoperitoneal shunt once the ventricular fluid protein has dropped below 150-200 mg/dl.

If there are no signs of acute intracranial hypertension, the infant should be monitored with serial ultrasound studies obtained every 3-4 days. A small percentage of patients in this group have transient hydrocephalus which arrests spontaneously, and therefore do not require any further intervention.

If there is sub-acute progressive ventricular enlargement, medical treatment to reduce the rate of formation of CSF may be tried (acetazolamide or furosemide for a period of 7-10 days, with close monitoring of fluid-electrolyte, acid/base balance, and ventricular size). There is no proof that medical therapy is superior to surgical therapy. However, a trial may be warranted in those with mild to moderate, slowly evolving hydrocephalus.

If the infant has progressive ventricular enlargement, with or without medical therapy, insertion of a ventriculoperitoneal shunt is indicated. The procedure is not free of complications, however, a number of infants require revision of the shunt over time due to occlusion.

INTRACEREBELLAR HEMORRHAGE

Between 15-25% of premature infants of less than 32 weeks gestation develop perinatal intracerebellar hemorrhage. The hemorrhage may be due to venous infarction of the cerebellar parenchyma, rupture of fragile capillaries in the cerebellar periventricular germinal matrix, or a caudal extension of banal intraventricular hemorrhage. Molding of the occipital bone during birth, with resultant traction on the posterior fossa dura and hypoxic ischemic injury to cerebellar vessels, may play a role in the pathogenesis.

When the hemorrhage is large and compressing posterior fossa structures, acute hydrocephalus with resultant apnea, skew deviation of the eyes, coma, opisthotonus, and loss of pupillary reflexes are seen. When small (less than 0.5-1.0 cm), the hemorrhage does not cause compression of the ventricular system, remains clinically silent, and may be noted incidentally upon CT or autopsy examinations.

Surgical evacuation is called for only when the patient is developing acute hydrocephalus as a result of compression of the fourth ventricle. If this is not apparent, only supportive care is necessary.

PERINATAL
BILIRUBIN ENCEPHALOPATHY

While brain dysfunction secondary to hyperbilirubinemia in term infants with uncomplicated hemolytic disease is now infrequent, it is still a concern in preterm infants, and in those term infants whose clinical course is complicated by systemic metabolic derangements like sepsis, hypoglycemia, or acidosis.

Pathogenesis

Term and preterm infants are exposed to a high systemic bilirubin load compared to older infants. This is due to the high mean neonatal corpuscular RBC volumes, decreased RBC life span, hemolytic disease of the newborn, prolonged enterohepatic circulation of bilirubin, and decreased elimination of bilirubin from the liver. Systemic factors such as acidosis, hypoglycemia, cold stress, and presence of certain drugs (salicylates, sulfonamides, furosemide) may displace bilirubin from the bilirubin-albumin complex, thereby increasing concentrations of free or acid bilirubin, which in turn can penetrate the blood-brain barrier.

The blood-brain barrier in the neonate is immature, and this facilitates entry of unbound bilirubin into the central nervous system. However, the degree of immaturity of the blood-brain barrier in the neonate has probably been overestimated. Presence of concurrent hypoxic encephalopathy or cerebral hemorrhage may enhance penetration of bilirubin into the central nervous system.

The exact mechanism of brain injury from high levels of acid bilirubin remains uncertain. The end result, however, is disruption of neuronal membrane and mitochondrial function.

Yellow staining of affected areas of the brain upon post-mortem in hyperbilirubinemia is termed kernicterus. The globus pallidus, corpus striatum, subthalamic nuclei, cerebellum, cochlear nuclei, and the periaqueductal gray matter are most vulnerable to kernicterus. With the exception of involvement of Ammon's horn of the hippocampus, the cerebral cortex is generally spared.

The exact level of total bilirubin at which the central nervous system dysfunction occurs is variable. While levels over 20 mg/dl have been traditionally considered dangerous in uncomplicated hyperbilirubinemia of term infants, the presence of acidosis, hypoxia, or intracranial hemorrhage necessitate a downward revision in the level of serum bilirubin to be regarded as noxious. In preterm infants, levels above 8-10 mg/dl require careful monitoring, especially if the aforementioned systemic complications are present.

Clinical Features

1. In the acute stage (usually 3-5 days after birth), lethargy and feeding difficulties are seen.

2. Hypertonia, mainly in the truncal musculature, becomes apparent 7-14 days after birth in the form of opisthotonus. Seizures are relatively infrequent, occurring only in approximately 15% of subjects.

3. The hypertonia increases progressively during infancy, along with nerve deafness and delayed motor and intellectual development. Upward gaze may be restricted owing to involvement of the periaqueductal gray matter. Intelligence is usually normal in nearly 75% of patients.

4. Dyskinesia, the most remarkable physical finding in affected older survivors, becomes apparent by 1-2 years of age in the form of athetosis, dysarthria, and hypertonia.

Management

Efforts to decrease prematurity and the incidence of hemolytic disease of the newborn, e.g., by administration of anti Rh antibodies to mothers soon after delivery, should indirectly help decrease the overall incidence of bilirubin encephalopathy.

Careful monitoring of the serum bilirubin in all high risk infants is necessary. Exchange transfusions should be carried out when the total bilirubin concentration (in mg/dl) reaches 1% of the body weight (in grams). Elevated, but lower, levels should be managed with phototherapy.

Prevention of risk factors like acidosis, cold stress, and hypoglycemia and avoiding drugs which displace bilirubin from the bilirubin-albumin complex are important.

ARTHROGRYPOSIS MULTIPLEX CONGENITA

Arthrogryposis multiplex congenita is a condition of multiple joint deformities at birth from contractures of heterogeneous etiology. Approximately 25% of patients have contracture formation from connective tissue dysfunction following restriction of fetal movements because of oligohydramnios or uterine malformations (orthopedic arthrogryposis). The remainder have the neuromuscular form, due to myopathies, diseases of the anterior horn cells, or ventral nerve roots. A history of diminished fetal movement is frequently present in all cases.

Myopathic disorders associated with arthrogryposis include myotonic dystrophy and congenital non-progressive myopathies. Spinal muscular atrophy and hypotrophy of the ventral (motor) nerve roots constitute some neurogenic causes. Spinal muscular atrophy is characterized by intrauterine degeneration of anterior horn cells, preserved sensation, autosomal recessive (rarely dominant) transmission, and presence of grouped muscle fiber atrophy on the skeletal muscle biopsy. Spinal muscular atrophy in infants with arthrogryposis differs from that in the classical Werdnig Hoffmann disease owing to the presence of a relatively non-progressive course in the former.

Contractures in most patients with arthrogryposis occur around the hips, knees, elbows, wrists, and interphalangeal joints. While most manifest a flexion deformity, an occasional patient may develop contractures in extension. Muscular weakness and hypoplasia are present in the neuromuscular forms. Contractures around the temporomandibular joint may confer a rounded appearance to the face. Club feet and cerebral malformations accompany about 10% of patients.

A skeletal muscle biopsy is generally normal in orthopedic arthrogryposis, but abnormal in the neuromuscular forms. Based upon the histological findings, a distinction can also be made between the neurogenic and myopathic subtypes of neuromuscular arthrogryposis. An electromyogram may also enable distinction of myopathic from neurogenic dysfunction.

Physical therapy to enhance the range of movement and prevent further contractures should be prescribed in all patients. Orthopedic arthrogryposis may resolve gradually over months. Patients with neuromuscular disorders may decompensate during infancy and early childhood in the presence of respiratory illnesses.

CEPHALHEMATOMA

A complication of birth trauma, this subperiosteal hemorrhage is almost always localized over the parietal region. Primiparity and application of forceps are important predisposing factors. The hematoma appears as a soft swelling under the scalp, restricted to the parietal region by suture margins. A linear skull fracture may underlie approximately 25% of cases. The cephalhematoma does not by itself cause any clinical manifestations, and resolves spontaneously over 6-8 weeks. In rare instances, it may undergo calcification. No intervention is necessary. Efforts at needle aspiration should especially be avoided as they are liable to expose this sterile collection of blood to infection.

SUBGALEAL HEMORRHAGE

Hemorrhage underneath the galea (epicranial aponeurosis) produces a soft, boggy scalp swelling. Blood loss into the subgaleal space can be substantial enough (200-250 ml) to cause anemia. The hemorrhage tends to resolve spontaneously over 3-4 weeks; when large, however, aspiration with a wide-bore needle may become necessary.

PRIMARY SUBARACHNOID HEMORRHAGE

Hemorrhage restricted to the subarachnoid space (not an extension of subdural, intraparenchymal, and intraventricular hemorrhage) is seen in both term and preterm infants.

Pathogenesis

The delicate skull of the preterm infant may be unable to protect the arachnoid matter from shearing external forces during the process of birth, and this can lead to subarachnoid hemorrhage.

Large for gestational age full term infants with cephalopelvic disproportion may also develop primary subarachnoid hemorrhage from birth trauma. In both term and preterm infants, the hemorrhage is of venous origin, frequently located in the interhemispheric fissure or over the convexity of the cerebral hemispheres.

Clinical Features

The hemorrhage may remain clinically asymptomatic, being noted only as an incidental finding on computed tomography or a neurosonogram.

Irritability and seizures may be seen in full term neonates who otherwise appear well.

Infrequently, coma with progressive deterioration in hemispheric and brainstem function may be present. Most such infants, however, have also concurrently suffered severe asphyxia or parenchymal injury.

Diagnosis

A non-contrast CT scan of the head or a neurosonogram will demonstrate the hemorrhage in the first 3-4 days of life, and also help exclude other intracranial lesions.

Lumbar puncture discloses xanthochromic cerebrospinal fluid with high red blood cell counts and protein concentration.

Prognosis

Ninety percent of patients have an excellent outcome, with normal development and spontaneous resolution of seizures. The remainder may develop communicating hydrocephalus. Serial neurological evaluations during infancy are therefore necessary.

SUBDURAL HEMORRHAGE

With the exception of an occasional patient with hemophilia or Vitamin K deficiency, most subdural hemorrhage in the neonate is a consequence of birth trauma.

Pathophysiology

The hemorrhage is almost always venous, originating from sinuses located in the falx cerebri or the tentorium cerebelli. Malpresentations (breech, face), narrow birth canal, prematurity, large fetus, and application of vacuum or forceps for extraction of the head are common predisposing factors.

Tears in the tentorium may lead to hemorrhage from the vein of Galen or straight sinus into the posterior fossa, with resultant compression of the brainstem. Tears of the falx may lead to rupture of the inferior saggital sinus and bleeding in the interhemispheric fissure. Occipital osteodiastasis is a traumatic separation of the cartilaginous joint between the squamous and lateral portions of the occipital bone. The occipital sinuses are frequently torn, causing severe compression of posterior fossa structures from hemorrhage. Tears in venous channels over the surface of the brain are likely to result in hemorrhage localized over the convexity, with resultant lateralized neurologic deficits. It is not unusual for the torque force that causes dural tears to also cause tears and contusion in the adjacent cerebral tissue. Morbidity and mortality are generally related to this parenchymal injury.

Clinical Features

1. Evidence of brainstem dysfunction due to posterior fossa hemorrhage (coma, skew deviation of the eyes, pupillary abnormalities, apnea and opisthotonic posturing) may be seen as a consequence of tentorial tears or occipital osteodiastasis.

2. Hemorrhage localized over the surface of one cerebral hemisphere may present with irritability, focal seizures, or hemiparesis.

3. Infrequently, convexity hemorrhages remain clinically silent in the neonatal period but enlarge gradually in size during infancy to form a chronic subdural hematoma. This generally presents with excessive cranial enlargement, vomiting, and a bulging anterior fontanelle.

Diagnosis

Non-contrast CT examination is the diagnostic procedure of choice. When this is unavailable, tapping the subdural space through the open anterior fontanelle may yield blood. Skull X-rays may demonstrate fractures or occipital osteodiastasis.

Management

Surgical evacuation of the clot from the posterior fossa is indicated when there is evidence of compression of posterior fossa structures. A subdural hematoma located over the convexity of the brain causing mass effect can be removed either by aspiration through a wide-bore subdural needle directed through the anterior fontanelle, or using open drainage. Mannitol and dexamethasone to control cerebral edema, anticonvulsants for seizures and respiratory support should be used when necessary.

BRACHIAL PLEXUS INJURIES

Traction injury to the brachial plexus during delivery can manifest as a C5-C6 nerve root lesion (Erb's paralysis), involvement of all brachial plexus nerve roots, or infrequently, with involvement of C8-T1 nerve roots (Klumpke's paralysis). Difficulty in delivery of the shoulders and head due to the presence of a large baby, narrow birth canal, and malpresentation (breech, face, or occipitoposterior) underlie most brachial plexus injuries. Additionally, hypoxia from umbilical cord compression during a prolonged second stage of labor may render the fetus hypotonic, and therefore more vulnerable to traction injury.

In the majority of instances, there is a partial breach in the continuity of the nerve roots. Complete avulsion is less likely to occur, but when present, is associated with little or no recovery of function.

Clavicular and humeral fractures or dislocation of the shoulder joint may be present along with severe brachial plexus injuries.

Clinical Manifestations

Erb's palsy is the most common clinical syndrome. This C5-C6 lesion affects the function of the deltoid, serratus anterior, supraspinatus, infraspinatus, biceps, and brachioradialis muscles. As a consequence, the affected arm is flaccid, immobile, kept adducted, and internally rotated. There is extension and pronation at the elbow, flexion at the wrist ("policeman taking a tip" position). When severe, the C4 root may also be avulsed, thus paralysing the ipsilateral diaphragm and leading to respiratory insufficiency. Sensory deficit is usually minimal and generally characterized by anesthesia over the upper one third, lateral aspect of the shoulder.

Pure Klumpke's (C8-T1) paralysis is relatively infrequent. It usually comprises the residue of recovery from a complete brachial plexus injury. The intrinsic hand muscles are paralyzed, with impaired flexion of the wrist and fingers. The grasp reflex may be absent. Interruption of the cervical sympathetic nerves may cause an ipsilateral Horner's syndrome (miosis, ptosis, enophthalmos, anhidrosis).

Investigations

1. Fluroscopy of the diaphragm in affected infants with respiratory distress to exclude diaphragmatic paralysis.

2. X-Rays of the clavicle, arm, and cervical spine to exclude any fracture/ dislocation.

3. Somatosensory evoked potentials help differentiate nerve root from peripheral brachial plexus lesions. The response normally evoked at the Erb's point (in the supraclavicular space) following median nerve stimulation is lost with proximal nerve root lesions, but remains intact with distal lesions.

4. Myelography is not recommended in the neonatal period, but when performed at a later stage in infancy in subjects with little or no improvement, it helps to identify complete nerve root avulsion.

5. Electromyographic studies after the first month may help to determine the presence of complete denervation, which usually carries a poor outlook for recovery.

Management

1. Supporting respiration temporarily in infants with hypoventilation as a consequence of diaphragmatic paralysis.

2. Range of motion exercises and use of splints to prevent contractures. The parents should also be taught to support the hypotonic shoulder and extremity in order to prevent subluxation while handling.

3. Tendon transplantation in subjects with partial lesions in order to improve hand functions like pronation and grasping.

SPINAL CORD INJURIES

While the overall incidence of trauma has decreased with improvements in obstetrical care, the still encountered occasional patient with spinal cord injury continues to have a high mortality and morbidity.

Pathogenesis

Seventy-five percent of patients with neonatal spinal cord injuries are breech presentations. Presence of a footling breech and hyperextension of the neck (beyond 90 degrees) are important predisposing factors. Further extension of the neck during delivery causes partial or complete transection of the cord. The level of the lesion is generally lower cervical to upper thoracic (most frequently C8-T1).

The remaining 25% of patients are vertex presentations in which an effort has been made to manually rotate the head in the birth canal. The torsion force in such instances interrupts spinal cord function at a higher cervical level (C2-C7).

When spinal cord injury is extensive, it may be accompanied by hemorrhage into the posterior fossa or tonsillar herniation.

Clinical Manifestations

1. Flaccid quadriplegia at birth, with preservation of chewing, sucking, and swallowing movements. When there is sparing of C6 function in lower cervical injuries, the hand may be kept in a "pistol" posture with extension in the first and second metacarpophalangeal joints, flexion at the third, fourth, and fifth joints.

2. Irreversible apnea is the rule in lesions above C4; hypoventilation may accompany lower level lesions. The patient may not survive in either instance unless respiration is supported artificially.

3. Presence of a sensory level sensitive to pinprick on the upper chest.

4. Autonomic dysfunction; there may be lack of sweating below the involved cervical segment. A neurogenic bladder is invariably present— initially being atonic and subsequently developing retention with overflow.

5. Hypoxic encephalopathy due to lack of respiratory effort at birth may complicate the clinical picture. One should be wary of labelling neurologic deficit in a hypotonic neonate as exclusively the consequence of hypoxia if motor, sensory, and autonomic levels are present over the upper trunk or neck.

6. Recovery of some degree of motor function and improvement in muscle tone in the neonatal period may indicate an incomplete lesion. Presence of intact somatosen-

sory evoked potentials may also point to an incomplete lesion.

Management

Respiration needs to be supported while the diagnosis, level, and extent of lesion (complete or incomplete transection) are being determined.

Care of the bowel, bladder function, and skin is important as in all patients with spinal cord injuries. Patients with lesions above C7 segment survive for a maximum of 2-3 years.

C8-T1 level spinal cord lesions are compatible with survival, but associated with a tendency to develop respiratory and genito-urinary infections.

NEONATAL CEREBRAL INFARCTION

Infarction denotes focal death of tissue secondary to inadequate blood supply. Barmada et al., in an autopsy survey in 1979, documented a prevalence rate of 5.4% for cerebral infarcts in arterial distribution.[16] Increasing survival rates for critically ill infants over the past decade have led to increasing survival of neonates with cerebral infarction and its greater recognition in the Nursery. Presently, cerebral infarction is considered the second most common cause of neonatal seizures, second only to diffuse hypoxic-ischemic encephalopathy. Periventricular leukomalacia is excluded from this discussion.

Risk Factors

1. Hypoxic-ischemic encephalopathy may at times lead to focal infarction in term infants, especially in the parasaggital watershed zones.

2. Persistent pulmonary hypertension may be associated with abnormal development of the musculature of blood vessels and depletion of circulating fibrinolysins.

3. Disseminated intravascular coagulation on the basis of sepsis and indwelling (umbilical) catheters have been associated with thromboembolic complications involving multiple organs.

4. Polycythemia, seen in infants of diabetic mothers and following feto-fetal transfusions, may cause sludging of blood flow and lead to predominantly venous infarcts.

5. Inherited deficiencies of antithrombin III and protein C, embolism, birth trauma to the carotid vessels, congenital malformations of the cerebral vessels, bacterial meningitis, maternal cocaine abuse, and extracorporeal membrane oxygenation are other risk factors for neonatal stroke.

Pathology

The infarcts may develop prenatally, intrapartum postnatally. They may be due to arterial or venous occlusion. Arterial infarcts are most often seen in the distribution of the middle cerebral artery. Preterm infants generally develop small, multiple infarcts, whereas full term infants are more liable to demonstrate single, large infarcts. Microscopically, the infarcts demonstrate degenerating neurons, foamy macrophages, and proliferation of astrocytes.

Clinical Features

Seizures in the neonatal period are by far the most common feature, developing in over 80% of all subjects, most often 6-12 hours after birth. Consistently unifocal seizures in the absence of any metabolic derangement, or those that persist unifocally despite the correction of accompanying metabolic derangements are especially pathognomonic. A high index of suspicion for cerebral infarcts should be maintained in infants who have been pharmacologically paralyzed for treatment of severe respiratory disorders. Only frequent EEG studies and neurosonograms may be able to detect cerebral infarction in these infants.

Abnormal motor function may also be seen, most often in the form of diffuse hypotonia. Lateralized neurological deficits are rare, becoming apparent only when the infant is 2-3 months old. Depressed sensorium, abnormal eye movements (gaze paresis) and autonomic instability are other manifestations.

Investigations

Neurosonograms may show a focal area of echo density, but do not help in making the distinction between intracerebral hemorrhage and infarction. The CT scan may show a wedge-shaped area of decreased density. Administration of contrast during the CT study is useful in demonstrating a filling defect in the venous sinuses in infarcts due to sinus thrombosis. The MRI scan is capable of detecting infarcts earlier than the CT scan in term infants. However, in the preterm infant, the MRI scan is unable to differentiate the normal watery white matter from the increased white matter water content that accompanies infarction. Therefore, in the premature infant suspected of having infarction, ultrasound still remains the diagnostic modality of choice.

Management

This consists of controlling seizures and maintaining adequate cerebral perfusion by maintaining the blood pressure, oxygenation saturation, pCO_2 and blood viscosity in the normal range.

Outcome

Data on long term outcome are presently unavailable. Patients whose infarcts accompanied asphyxia have a 60 to 70% incidence of moderate to severe sequelae. On the other hand, patients with "idiopathic" infarction or infarction secondary to polycythemia may have a better prognosis.

REFERENCES

1. Holden KR, Mellits DE, Freeman JM. Neonatal seizures. I. Correlation of prenatal and perinatal events with outcomes. Pediatrics 70:165-176, 1982.

2. Volpe J. Neonatal seizures. Clin Perinatol 4:43-63, 1977.

3. Clancy RR, Legido A, Lewis D. Occult neonatal seizures. Epilepsia 29:256-261, 1988.

4. Mizrahi EM, Kellaway P. Characterization and classification of neonatal seizures. Neurology 1837-1844, 1987.

5. Younkin DP, Delivoria-Papadopoulos M, Donlon E, et al. Cerebral metabolic effects of neonatal seizures measured with in vivo 31P NMR spectroscopy. 20:513-519, 1986.

6. Perlman JM, Volpe JJ. Seizures in the preterm infant: effects on cerebral blood flow velocity, intracranial pressure, and arterial blood pressure. J Pediatr 102:288-293, 1983.

7. Wasterlain CG. Effects of neonatal status epilepticus on rat brain development. Neurology 26:975-986, 1976.

8. Painter MJ, Bergman I, Crumrine P. Neonatal seizures. Pediatr Clin North Am 33:91-109, 1986.

9. Camfield PR, Camfield CS. Neonatal seizures: a commentary on selected aspects. J Child Neurol 2:244-251, 1987.

10. Rowe JC, Holmes GL, Hafford J, et al. Prognostic value of the electroencephalogram in term and preterm infants following neonatal seizures. EEG and Clin Neurophysiol 60:183-196, 1985.

11. Resnick TJ, Moshe SL, Perotta L, et al. Benign neonatal sleep myoclonus. Arch Neurol 43:266-268, 1986.

12. Deshmukh A, Wittert W, Schnitzler E, et al. Lorazepam in the treatment of refractory neonatal seizures. Amer J Dis Child 140:1042-1044, 1982.

13. Gal P, Toback J, Boer HR, et al. Efficacy of phenobarbital monotherapy in treatment of neonatal seizures. Neurology 32:1401-1404, 1982.

14. Painter MJ, Pippenger C, MacDonald H, et al. Phenobarbital and diphenylhydantoin levels in neonates with seizures. J Pediatr 92:315-319, 1978.

15. Diaz J, Schain RJ. Phenobarbital: effects of long term administration on behaviour and brain of artificially reared rats. Science 90-91, 1978.

16. Bergey GK, Swaiman KF, Schrier BK, et al. Adverse effects of phenobarbital on morphological and biochemical of fetal mouse spinal cord neurons in cultures. Ann Neurol 9:584-589, 1981.

17. Brod SA, Ment LR, Ehrenkranz RA, et al. Predictors of success for drug discontinuation following neonatal seizures. Pediatr Neurol 4:13-17, 1988.

18. Bergman I, Painter MJ, Hirsch RP, et al. Outcome of neonates with convulsions treated in an intensive care unit. Ann Neurol 14:642-647, 1983.

SUGGESTED READING

1. Ahmann PA, Lazarra A, Dykes FD, Brann AW and Schwartz JF. Intraventricular hemorrhage in the high-risk preterm infant: incidence and outcome. Ann Neurol 7:118-124, 1980.

2. Fenichel GM, ed. Arthrogyryposis. In: Neonatal Neurology. 2nd edition, Churchill Livingstone, New York, 1985.

3. Bergman, I, Painter MJ, Hirsch RJ, Crumrine PK and David R. Outcome in neonates with convulsions treated in an intensive care unit. Ann Neurol 14:642-647, 1983.

4. Broderson R. Bilirubin transport in the newborn infant, reviewed with relation to kernicterus. J Pediatr 96(3):349-356, 1980.

5. Chaplin ER, Goldstein GW, Myerberg DZ, Hunt JV and Tooley WH. Posthemorrhagic hydrocephalus in the preterm infant. Pediatrics 65:901-909, 1980.

6. Donat JF, Okazaki H, Kleinberg F. Cerebellar hemorrhages in newborn infants. Amer J Dis Child 133:441, 1979.

7. Koch BM and Eng GM. Neonatal spinal cord injury. Arch Phys Med Rehabil 60:378-381, 1979.

8. Rose AL and Lombroso CT. Neonatal seizure states: a study of clinical, pathological and electroencephalographic features in 137 full-term babies with a long-term follow up. Pediatrics 45:404-425, 1970.

9. McDonald HM, Mulligan JM, Allen AC and Taylor PM. Neonatal asphyxia. I. Relationship of obstetric and neonatal complications to neonatal mortality in 38, 405 consecutive deliveries. J Pediatr 96:898-902, 1980.

10. Sarnat HB and Sarnat MS. Neonatal encephalopathy following fetal distress. A clinical and electroencephalographic study. Arch Neurol 33:696-705, 1976.

11. Serfontein GL, Rom S, Stein S. Posterior fossa subdural hemorrhage in the newborn. Pediatrics 65:40-43, 1980.

12. Shinnar S, Molteni RA, Gammon K, D'Souza BJ, Altman J and Freeman JM. Intraventricular hemorrhage in the premature infant. A changing outlook. N Engl J Med 306(24):1464-1468, 1982.

13. Volpe JJ. Neonatal seizures. Clin Perinatol 4:43-63, 1977.

14. Volpe JJ. Neonatal intraventricular hemorrhage. N Engl J Med 304(15):886-890, 1981.

15. Mizrahi EM, Kellaway P. Characterization and classification of neonatal seizures. Neurology 37:1837-1844, 1987.

16. Barmada MA, Moosy J, Shuman RM. Cerebral infarcts with arterial occlusion in neonates. Ann Neurol 6:495-502, 1979.

17. Clancy R, Malin S, Laraque D, et al. Focal motor seizures heralding stroke in full term infants. Arch Dis Child, 1985.

CHAPTER XVIII

HEAD INJURIES

Dynamics and Pathophysiology

Mild Closed Head Injury

Severe Closed Head Injury

Battered Child Syndrome

Algorithm

Approximately one in ten children suffers a blow to the head severe enough to impair consciousness. Boys are two to three times more liable to suffer head injuries than girls. Ninety percent of the injuries are closed, i.e., there is no accompanying breach in continuity of the dura mater. Traumatic lesions in the neonate are considered in Chapter XVII.

DYNAMICS AND PATHOPHYSIOLOGY

The **gelatinous consistency** of the incompletely myelinated subcortical white matter in infants and young children renders it more mobile relative to the cerebral cortex, and thereby vulnerable to white matter tears, even following seemingly minor trauma.

The physical forces causing head trauma can induce either **acceleration** (being struck by a blunt object) or **decceleration** (fall) within the cranial cavity. Skull fractures may occur when the force exceeds a certain magnitude. However, absence of a fracture does not exclude serious parenchymal injury. Accelerating forces are liable to cause contre coup injuries (e.g., frontal and temporal lobe tears after being struck over the occipital region). Decelerating injuries on the other hand, are likely to cause the greatest damage around the area of impact. Distortion of the brainstem may also occur with decelerating injuries.

Cerebral concussion denotes a transient state of loss of consciousness, usually of instantaneous onset, which is completely reversible within 24 hours. It is accompanied by a temporary disturbance in axoplasmic transport. While most patients have no structural changes, axonal tears may be present on some occasions.

Cerebral contusion and laceration are more severe forms of head trauma. Orbital surfaces of the frontal lobes, and medial and anterior aspects of the temporal lobes are most susceptible. Gross or microscopic hemorrhages signify the presence of tissue laceration. In both contusion and laceration, alterations in permeability of the injured cerebral microvasculature coupled with a transient initial increase in cerebral blood flow lead to the development of edema, which is most prominent in the deep white matter. The brain edema can lead to herniation, which further compromises cerebral perfusion and tissue integrity.

Acute epidural and subdural hemorrhage may accompany parenchymal injury. Epidural hemorrhage is usually seen in older children, results from rupture of the middle meningeal artery, and may or may not be accompanied by a linear fracture across the temporal bone or by a brief, lucid hiatus in consciousness before the patient becomes symptomatic. Mass effect from the hematoma leads to displacement of the underlying brain. It is invariably fatal unless surgically drained. Acute subdural hemorrhage is of venous origin, can also increase intracranial pressure, and is frequently associated with cerebral contusion.

Some amount of **subarachnoid hemorrhage** is generally present in most patients with severe head trauma. When extensive, the hemorrhage may precipitate reflex alterations in cortical blood flow and seizures.

MILD CLOSED HEAD INJURY

The majority of closed head injuries in children fall under this category, also termed cerebral concussion.

Clinical Features

1. Unconsciousness, lethargy, crying, confusion, vomiting, or unsteadiness in gait develop immediately after or within 6-8 hours of head trauma. Transient blindness or memory loss may also be present. With the exception of nystagmus or extensor plantar responses, neurological signs are not seen.

2. Skull fractures may or may not be present.

3. There is complete resolution of the symptom complex within 24 hours of trauma. However, an occasional patient may develop the post-concussive syndrome, characterized by dizziness, headache, or memory deficits that persist for 4-6 months.

Management

If the family is capable of monitoring the child's respiration and level of consciousness (altered in those who develop increased intracranial pressure) for 24-36 hours, and there is ready access to an Emergency Room, hospitalization is not necessary. The presence of a skull fracture by itself does not warrant admission, unless it is depressed, complicated, or located over the middle meningeal artery vascular markings. The family should be advised to rush the patient back to the hospital should respiratory status or sensorium deteriorate, or if seizures develop.

If the family is likely to have difficulty in monitoring the child at home, admission to the hospital for observation for 24-36 hours is recommended.

SEVERE CLOSED HEAD INJURY

Patients with a history of trauma who are unconscious upon presentation to the hospital, or who have depressed/compound skull fractures and visceral injuries should be assumed as having severe head trauma (contusion or laceration) until proven otherwise.

Clinical Features

1. The patient may be **stuporous** or **comatose**. Those in coma may make stereotyped responses to noxious stimuli such as decerebration, or be totally unresponsive.

2. The **respiratory pattern** is frequently abnormal, being characterized by a shallow and irregular rhythm, central neurogenic hyperventilation, or the Cheyne Stokes pattern. Hypoxia and hypercarbia can result from shallow respiration and may be further exacerbated by sucking wounds in the chest.

3. So long as the course is not complicated by brain herniation, the **pupils** are equal, mildly constricted to mildly dilated, and reactive to light. With onset of uncal herniation, a unilaterally dilated, poorly reactive pupil is seen. Central herniation leads to symmetrically pinpoint pupils. Progressive rostrocaudal deterioration in function may accompany some, but not all, patients with herniation syndromes.

4. **Papilledema** from increased intracranial pressure may not be apparent within the initial 3-4 hours of trauma, but the fundus should be monitored every 4-6 hours for evaluation of such a change. Presence of subhyaloid hemorrhage is seen with subarachnoid hemorrhage.

5. Signs of **brainstem dysfunction** commonly seen include tonic downward deviation of the eyes (from pressure on the pretectal region of the midbrain due to hydrocephalus or cerebral edema), loss of doll's eye movements, nystagmus (unilateral and horizontal suggestive of seizure activity), internuclear ophthalmoplegia (failure of adduction in one eye, nystagmus in the abducting eye from dysfunction of the medial longitudinal fasciculus), and loss of the caloric response. The caloric response should not be assessed if there is bleeding from the ear because of the risk of introduc-

ing infection into the cranial cavity. Loss of response to ice water calorics is an ominous sign, suggesting severe compromise of lower brainstem function.

6. **Leakage** of blood or cerebrospinal fluid from the nostrils is seen in base of skull fractures involving the anterior cranial fossa. Serous nasal discharge should not be confused with spinal fluid; the latter has a detectable concentration of glucose and a low protein content. Leakage of blood or cerebrospinal fluid from the middle ears suggests a base of skull fracture in the region of the middle cranial fossa. Ecchymosis behind the pinna is indicative of a fracture of the mastoid portion of the temporal bone (Battle's sign).

7. **Lateralizing deficits** (decreased spontaneous movements of one half of the body, tendon reflex asymmetry, a unilaterally dilated pupil or extensor plantar response) are seen with unilateral mass lesions (contusion/epidural hematoma/subdural hematoma).

8. All patients with head trauma should be considered as having **fracture/dislocation of the cervical spine**, until proven otherwise.

Management

1. The management of life-threatening systemic complications such as shock from chest or abdominal wounds takes precedence over the management of head injury.

2. If the patient is apneic or has shallow, inefficient respiration, the upper airway should be suctioned initially and the patient bagged with 50-100% oxygen. The neck should be kept immobile between sand bags.

3. A lateral x-ray of the cervical spine should immediately be obtained in the "swimmer's position" (arms fully extended overhead) in order to visualize the cervical spine for fractures/ dislocation.

4. Assuming there is no fracture/dislocation of the cervical spine, it is safe to flex the neck for endotracheal intubation. If a cervical spine lesion is present and intubation is not possible without flexing the neck, an emergency tracheostomy should be carried out. The pCO_2 should be kept between 22-25 torr to effect optimum cerebral vasoconstriction and to counteract cerebral edema.

5. Determine if the patient is herniating on the basis of progressive rostrocaudal deterioration of function. If herniation is suspected, administer mannitol 0.5-1.0 gm/kg IV push along with dexamethasone 0.2 mg/kg IV bolus, then 0.1 mg/kg/day in four divided doses.

6. Skull x-rays should be obtained in the anteroposterior, lateral, and tangential planes to rule out fractures. An open mouth view helps to visualize the odontoid process. Broad spectrum antibiotics are necessary in case of compound or base of skull fractures.

7. Non-contrast CT examination of the head is done to exclude disorders which require immediate neurosurgical intervention, e.g., epidural or subdural hemorrhage, intracerebral hematoma with midline shift, or acute hydrocephalus.

8. Once the blood pressure has been stabilized, fluids should be restricted to two thirds of the daily maintenance volume in order to counteract the tendency to develop post-traumatic inappropriate secretion of antidiuretic hormone.

9. Dilantin is the anticonvulsant of choice for seizures (10 mg/kg IV bolus at a rate not exceeding 30-50 mg/minute; may be repeated in a 10 mg/kg bolus if necessary).

10. If cerebral edema appears resistant to therapy on the basis of progressive rostrocaudal deterioration in brain function, or recurrent episodes of opisthotonus, consideration should be given towards insertion of an intracranial pressure monitoring device. Insertion of a cannula to monitor central venous pressure is also necessary in all patients if coma persists beyond 10-12 hours.

11. Lumbar punctures are contraindicated in head injured patients owing to the risk of precipitating herniation. Administration of morphine should also be avoided owing to its induction of miosis (which interferes with clinical assessment), respiratory depression, and lowering of seizure threshold.

12. After the initial 72-96 hours, mainly supportive care (with attention to nutrition, the skin, chest, bladder, and extremities) is called for.

CLOSED HEAD INJURY

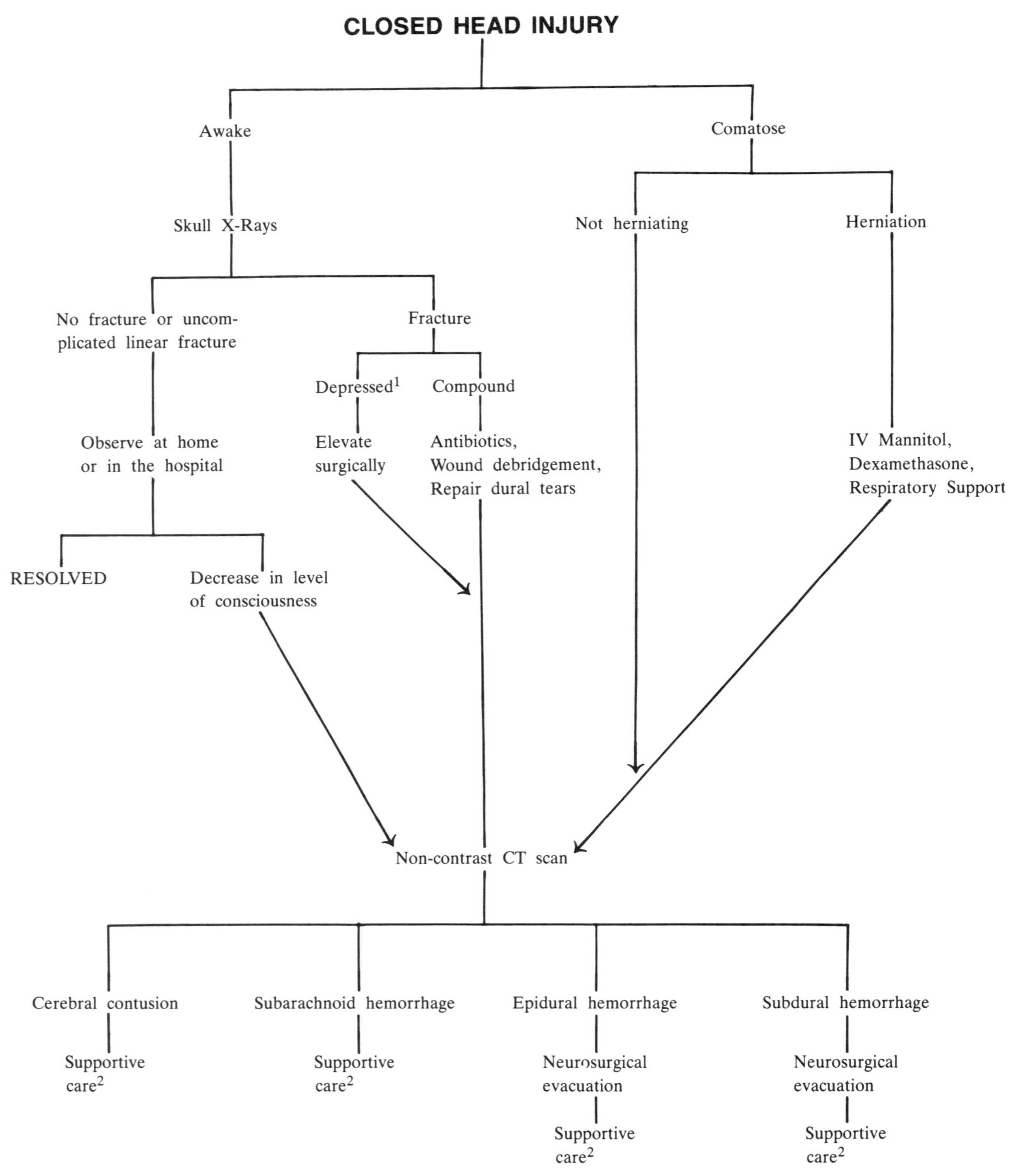

[1]Depressed by 5mm or more

[2]Fluid restriction to 2/3 of daily maintenance; respiratory support, pCO_2 kept between 22-25 torr; parenteral alimentation if comatose beyond 5-7 days; mannitol for cerebral edema; avoiding decubitus skin lesions; Dilantin for seizures.

Outcome

Between 53-85% of survivors have neurological sequelae. These vary from subtle cognitive and behavioral problems to hemiparesis, quadriparesis, language disorders, gait ataxia, cranial neuropathies and communicating hydrocephalus. Children under the age of five years are more liable to have severe sequelae. The incidence of severe neurologic impairment varies between 9 and 18%. The presence of coma of long duration (beyond 3-4 weeks) and episodes of increased intracranial pressure are associated with adverse outcome.

Gradual resolution of the neurologic deficit over a 2-3 year period is not uncommon in children.

Skull x-rays should be repeated 4-6 months after trauma in patients with parietal skull fractures to monitor for formation of a **leptomeningeal cyst**. This is an important late complication of linear skull fractures. The lesion evolves around a dural tear underneath the fracture site, with herniation of a sleeve of the arachnoid mater through torn edges of the dura. The encysted arachnoid sac then progressively enlarges over months, causing separation of the edges of the fracture and focal neurologic manifestations ("growing skull fracture").

BATTERED CHILD SYNDROME

This form of child abuse occurs in all socioeconomic strata. It is more prevalent in homes with high levels of stress from parental discord, unemployment, psychiatric illness, drug abuse, and in children with pre-existing neurologic disease. Parents who were themselves victims of abuse as children are more liable to inflict similar trauma on their offspring.

Clinical Manifestations

Suspicion of the battered child syndrome should be aroused when the historical account of trauma is far-fetched or out of proportion to the severity of the injury, e.g., skull fractures occurring following a fall from a couch onto a carpeted floor. The general physical examination may reveal other signs of injury inflicted by adults such as cigarette burns.

Direct trauma to the skull (being struck with a blunt object) can result in skull fractures and cerebral contusion.

Indirect trauma ("shaken infant syndrome") is the more common form of child abuse and occurs from vigorous shaking of the infant. This leads to tears in veins bridging the meninges and dural venous sinuses, with resulting subarachnoid or subdural hemorrhage. The subdural hemorrhage becomes loculated, enlarges gradually over time, and leads to signs of increased intracranial pressure (macrocephaly, full anterior fontanelle, impaired upward gaze, and vomiting). Retinal hemorrhages present along with the chronic subdural hematoma are diagnostic of recurrent trauma.

Skeletal radiological survey may disclose fractures in various stages of healing.

Management

The management of chronic subdural hematoma and cerebral contusion is discussed in Chapter X. The family should be reported to the appropriate legal authorities and the child not sent home until a safe environment can be guaranteed.

SUGGESTED READING

1. Brink JD and Woo-Sam J. Physical recovery after severe closed head trauma in children and adolescents. Pediatrics 97:721-727, 1980.

2. Feuer H. Early management of pediatric head injury. Physiological aspects. Pediatr Clin North AM 22(2):425-431, 1975.

3. Filley CM, Cranberg LD, Alexander MP, and Hart EJ. Neurobehavioral outcome after closed head injury in childhood and adolescence. Arch Neurol 44:194-198, 1987.

4. Mahoney WJ, D'Souza BJ, Haller JA, Rogers MC, Epstein MH and Freeman JM. Longterm outcome of children with severe head trauma and prolonged coma. Pediatrics 71:756-762, 1983.

5. Milhorat TH. Pediatric Neurosurgery. FA Davis Company, Philadelphia, 1978; 41-89.

CHAPTER XIX

NEUROLOGICAL EMERGENCIES

Status Epilepticus

Acute Elevation in Intracranial Pressure

    Brain Herniation Syndromes

Metabolic Coma

Toxic Coma

Acute-onset Paraplegia

STATUS EPILEPTICUS

Introduction

A series of seizures without recovery of consciousness in between or one continuous seizure of more than thirty minutes is termed status epilepticus. It is a neurological emergency. The mortality in one report[1] was 11% and 88 of 212 survivors (42%) had neurologic sequelae. When the overall mortality from epilepsy is considered, convulsive status epilepticus accounts for a third of all deaths. The exact prevalence is hard to estimate. However, it is responsible for up to 5% of all hospital admissions in patients with epilepsy in the United States.

Classification

Table 19-1 shows the classification of the various types of status epilepticus.

Table 19-1.

Convulsive status epilepticus
    Focal tonic, clonic or tonic-clonic
    Generalized tonic, clonic or tonic-clonic
    Status myoclonicus

Non-convulsive status epilepticus
    Absence status
    Complex partial seizure status

Epilepsia partialis continua

Pathophysiology

Seizure activity is associated with increased energy demands in the central nervous system. Reduction in cortical partial pressures of oxygen and cytochrome aa3 appear by twenty minutes after onset of seizure activity in experimental status epilepticus. Lactic and arachidonic acid, prostaglandins, and leucotrienes accumulate to toxic amounts within neurons, causing brain edema and cell death in selected regions. Permanent brain damage after sixty minutes of convulsive status has been noted in particular in the hippocampus, amygdala, cerebellum, thalamus, and middle neocortical layers. Repeated seizures in the newborn may lead to the development of a permanent seizure focus and overall reduction in both cell number and cell size.

Hypoxia and hypercarbia may develop in convulsive status epilepticus secondary to pooling of secretions in the oropharynx, prolapse of the tongue, laryngospasm, aspiration of gastric contents, or from the chest wall being held in tonic inspiration during the seizure. The ensuing hypoxia and hypercarbia further adversely impact central nervous system function.

Systolic hypertension, tachycardia, and cardiac arrhythmia may occur as a consequence of increased sympathetic activity during the seizure. Sudden death from cardiac arrythmia during the course of the seizure has been observed in experimentally induced status epilepticus.

Lactic acidosis may develop as a consequence of the convulsive activity and combination of systemic hypoxia. Rhabdomyolysis, myoglobinemia, myoglobinuria, and consequent acute renal failure may also occur in prolonged convulsive status. The longer status epilepticus continues, the more difficult it becomes to terminate, owning to depletion of inhibitory neurotransmitters. It is also more difficult to control in patients with pre-existing brain disease (symptomatic status) as compared to those who were neurologically normal prior to the event. In one study, the mean duration of convulsive status epilepticus in patients who did not have sequelae was 1.5 hours, 10 hours in those with sequelae, and 13 hours or over in those who did not survive.[3] The highest incidence of neurologic sequelae following convulsive status epilepticus is in infants. Hemiplegia, mental retardation, and long standing epilepsy are the most common deficits after convulsive status.

Clinical Features

Approximately a third of all children who develop status epilepticus do so by the age of one year. In one particular study, 85% of all episodes of status epilepticus had occurred by the age of five years.[1] The most common precipitants in childhood are high fever and a subtherapeutic serum anticonvulsant level in a child with pre-existing epilepsy (commonly from noncompliance, gastroenteritis, or a systemic febrile illness). Metabolic derangements (hypoglycemia, hyponatremia, hypernatremia), bacterial meningitis, and head trauma are other precipitating factors. More often than not, status epilepticus in infants and young children is characterized by one prolonged seizure rather than a series of small, frequent seizures.

Patients with non-convulsive seizure status are frequently mute, disoriented, and have associated eye blinking, lip smacking, facial twitching, and nonpurposive hand movements.

Investigations

1. **Serum electrolytes, glucose, blood urea nitrogen** in all patients, with the addition of **serum calcium** and **magnesium** in neonates and infants.

2. **Serum anticonvulsant levels** in any epileptic patient known to be on anticonvulsants; these studies should be obtained prior to administration of any anticonvulsant.

3. **Lumbar puncture** is performed in febrile patients (assuming a non-focal neurological examination and normal ocular fundi) to exclude bacterial meningitis, viral meningoencephalitis, or subarachnoid hemorrhage.

4. **CT head scan** in patients with focal findings or signs of increased intracranial pressure/ stupor/coma prolonged beyond a few hours in order to exclude cerebral contusion, infarction, intracranial hemorrhage, or abscess.

5. **Arterial blood gas studies** to monitor for hypoxia, hypercarbia, and metabolic and respiratory acidosis in all patients with convulsive status.

6. **Urine for myoglobin** in patients with prolonged convulsive status.

7. **EEG** to help diagnose non-convulsive status epilepticus and also to differentiate absence from complex partial seizure status (generalized spike-wave abnormalities are usually noted in the former, focal spike or sharp wave discharges in the latter).

Management

General Measures. Almost all patients with convulsive status epilepticus are hypoxic during the course of the seizure. Provision of oxygen for inhalation by mask or nasal cannula is essential. A good intravenous line and judicious suctioning of the upper airway area are also necessary. Auditory, visual, and tactile stimuli may lower seizure threshold and should therefore be kept at a minimum. Insertion of a nasogastric tube and emptying of the stomach is necessary in all older children to prevent aspiration pneumonitis.

Anticonvulsants. The anticonvulsant should be administered slowly via the intravenous route in a dose large enough to produce an immediate serum level in the "therapeutic" range. For both phenobarbital and phenytoin, the unbound (free) fraction is only approximately a tenth of the total serum level. It is only this free, circulating anticonvulsant that diffuses across the blood-brain barrier. Of the commonly used agents, intravenous **diazepam** has the most rapid onset of anticonvulsant action (within 1-2 minutes), followed by **phenytoin** (within 5-10 minutes), and then **phenobarbital** (within 15-20 minutes). However, the anticonvulsant action of intravenous diazepam is short-lived, lasting only 15-20 minutes. Diazepam, therefore, needs to be combined with a longer-duration anticonvulsant like phenytoin. **Lorazepam** (ATIVAN) is a longer-acting benzodiazepine (1-2 hours) and is believed to have less respiratory depressant and hypotensive action than diazepam. The author recommends the following anticonvulsant regimen:

I. Neonates

a. Phenobarbital 20 mg/kg slow I.V. bolus; if necessary, repeat 10 mg/kg I.V. after 10-15 minutes.

b. If seizures are uncontrolled: Phenytoin* 20 mg/kg slow I.V. at a rate not exceeding 20-30 mg/minute.

   ***Bradycardia and hypotension are common side effects of intravenous phenytoin, but can be avoided by slowing down the infusion rate.**

c. If seizures are still uncontrolled: Diazepam 0.1-0.2 mg/kg/dose. Two to three doses can be administered at 10 minute** intervals, if needed OR lorazepam 0.05-0.15 mg/kg/dose I.V.

   ****A combination of phenobarbital and diazepam may induce respiratory depression.**

II. Infants and young children (< 5 years)

a. Phenobarbital 10 mg/kg. I.V. may be repeated in a 10 mg/kg I.V. dose in 20-30 minutes if needed.

b. If seizures are uncontrolled: Phenytoin 10 mg/kg I.V. at a rate not exceeding 30-40 mg/minute; may repeat 10 mg/kg bolus in 10-15 minutes.

c. If seizures are still uncontrolled: Diazepam 0.1-0.2 mg/kg/dose times 2-3 doses at 10 minute intervals OR lorazepam 0.05-0.15 mg/kg/dose IV; may be repeated every 2-3 hours.

III. Children over 5 years and adolescents

a. Phenytoin bolus of 15-18 mg/kg slow I.V. at a rate not exceeding 30-40 mg/minute.

b. If seizures are uncontrolled: Diazepam 0.1-0.2 mg/kg/dose to a maximum of 10 mg/dose times 2-3 at 10 minute intervals OR lorazepam 0.05-0.15 mg/kg/dose

c. If seizures are still uncontrolled: Phenobarbital I.V. in a dose of 5-10 mg/kg slow I.V. push is recommended. Paraldehyde, 15 ml/metre^2 to a maximum of 15 ml/dose, mixed with an equal amount of mineral oil and administered as a retention enema is another alternative.

IV. Non-convulsive status epilepticus

Diazepam 0.1-0.2 mg/kg administered slowly I.V. usually terminates the disorder. Monitoring of the EEG at the time of I.V. diazepam administration is helpful in confirming seizure control. Ethosuximide for absence status and carbamazepine for complex partial seizure status should be commenced orally at the same time.

Skeletal muscle paralysis. This is indicated whenever convulsive activity has gone on for more than 2-3 hours and remains uncontrolled despite administration of anticonvulsants in adequate doses. **Pancuronium bromide** (PAVULON) or **curare** can be used. The patient is also intubated and placed on a respirator. Obviously, muscle paralysis does not abolish seizure activity in the brain, but it does help counteract some life threatening systemic complications of convulsive status epilepticus, i.e., hypoxia, hypercarbia, metabolic acidosis, and rhabdomyolysis. Frequent monitoring of central nervous system function with electroencephalograms is necessary for the duration of the skeletal muscle paralysis.

ACUTE ELEVATION IN INTRACRANIAL PRESSURE

Introduction

Prompt recognition and treatment of acutely raised intracranial pressure is essential for limiting mortality and morbidity in a variety of underlying acute neurological disorders. In contrast to disorders associated with subacute or long standing increased intracranial pressure, compensatory mechanisms for accommodating an acute rise in intracranial volume are limited and quickly exhausted. The intracranial contents can be divided into the brain, vascular system, and cerebrospinal fluid compartments—all are enclosed within the relatively rigid calvarium. Pathologic expansion of any one of these three compartments usually compromises function in the other two.

Table 19-2 lists the causes of acute increased intracranial pressure and groups them by categories.

Table 19-2. Causes of Acute Increased Intracranial Pressure

Trauma
  Extradural hemorrhage
  Sudural hemorrhage
  Intracerebral hemorrhage
  Cerebral contusion and laceration

Infection
  Bacterial meningitis
  Viral meningoencephalitis (especially
    herpes simplex)
  Fungal meningitis
  Brain abscess

Neoplasm
  Posterior fossa or paraventricular, particularly
    when associated with a recent increase in size
  Leukemic meningeal infiltration

Metabolic & Toxic
  Reye syndrome
  Lead encephalopathy
  Hypoxic ischaemic encephalopathy
  Diabetic ketoacidosis

Vascular
  Cerebral infarction
  Subarachnoid hemorrhage

Pathophysiology

The normal intracranial pressure is below 15 mm of mercury. Physiologic elevations exceeding 15mm are generally transient. Sustained or pathological increase in intracranial pressure beyond 15mm occurs generally in accordance with the pressure volume curve, i.e., the intracranial pressure remains normal during the initial phase of increasing intracranial volume. The horizontal portion of the pressure-volume curve represents this relationship. With further expansion in volume, however, there is a disproportionately greater increase in intracranial pressure. This exponential pressure-volume relationship is called compliance, and its inverse, elastance. Poor compliance may be more closely associated with outcome in children rather than the resting intracranial pressure.

Increased intracranial pressure impairs cerebral blood flow. The normal cerebral blood flow rate is between 50-55 ml/100 gms of brain tissue/minute. This relation is best expressed by the equation:

Cerebral perfusion pressure (CPP) = systemic arterial pressure (SAP) − intracranial pressure (ICP)

$$CPP = \frac{Systolic\ BP\ +\ 2(diastolic\ BP)\ -\ ICP}{3}$$

The normal cerebral perfusion pressure is above 55 mm of mercury. A drop below 50 mm is associated with ischemic cerebral injury. The above equation underscores the necessity of avoiding hypotension in a patient with increased intracranial pressure. The following vicious cycle must be avoided:

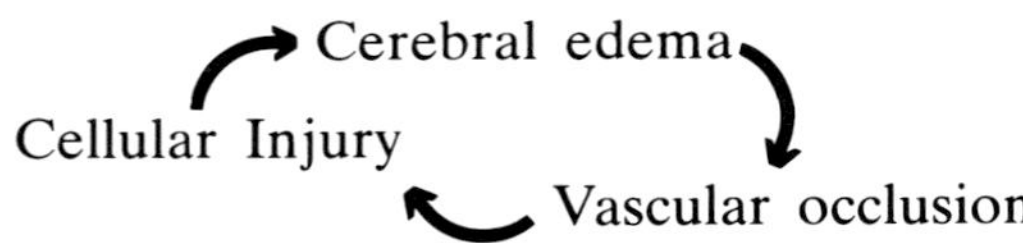

Sustained peaks in intracranial pressure to 25-40mm lasting between 2 and 10 minutes, are termed **plateau waves**. They are particularly liable to be triggered by fever, hypoxia, overzealous attempts at suctioning, and excessive handling of the patient. An increasing frequency of plateau waves leads to further ischemic cerebral injury, brain edema, and, ultimately, brain death.

Cerebral edema may be of the vasogenic or cytotoxic variety. Vasogenic edema is associated with opening up of capillary tight junctions in the blood-brain barrier and transudation of fluid into the brain. It is generally seen with inflammatory, traumatic, and neoplastic disorders as well as lead encephalopathy. It may be responsive to parenteral glucocorticoids. Cytoxic cerebral edema is characterized by failure of cell membranes to regulate the internal mileu, leading to hydropic cell swelling. It is commonly seen after hypoxic encephalopathy and generally is not steroid-responsive. Patients may have a combination of both forms of cerebral edema.

BRAIN HERNIATION SYNDROMES

Introduction

Protrusion of cerebral tissue through an intracranial opening as a result of increased pressure is termed herniation. The commonly observed syndromes are:

Cingulate or subfalcial herniation

Transtentorial herniation

Central herniation

Upward cerebellar herniation

Cerebellar tonsillar herniation

Cingulate, uncal, and central herniation are usually seen with supratentorial mass lesions.

Pathophysiology

Knowledge of anatomy of the dural structures helps to understand clinical features associated with the hernation syndromes. A relatively rigid fibrous structure, the tentorium cerebelli divides the cranial vault into the supratentorial and infratentorial compartments. On the anterior aspect, the tentorium is attached to the petrous temporal ridges and the anterior clinoid process. On the posterior aspect, this dural sheath is attached to the internal occipital protuberance. In the center of the tentorium is a semioval opening measuring 50-70 mms in the fronto-occipital axis, called the tentorial notch. The contents of the tentorial notch include the brainstem (midbrain portion), posterior cerebral and superior cerebellar arteries, the cerebral peduncles, and the occulomotor nerves.

The cerebellum is closely applied to the dorsum of the midbrain and occupies the posterior portion of the tentorial notch. Resting immediately above the free edge of the tentorium, in the middle cranial fossa, is the temporal lobe.

A combination of vascular and mechanical factors leads to the ultimate development of brain herniation. Mass lesions are commonly associated with edema in the adjacent cerebral tissue. **Autoregulation** (ability of regions of the brain to maintain fairly stable blood flow despite fluctuations in systemic blood pressure by regional vasoconstriction or vasodilatation, despite fluctuations in systemic blood pressure) **is frequently lost in the affected edematous area**, which becomes vulnerable to systemic fluctuations in blood pressure. Stretching and distortion of blood vessels because of the mass lesion leads to further brain injury and swelling, which in turn initiates a cycle of additional ischemia and edema. Eventually, the swollen, enlarged brain tissue is forced into potential spaces that exist beneath the falx, within the tentorial notch, or the foramen magnum. This ultimately results in compression of vital diencephalic and brainstem structures and death. Progressive rostro-caudal deterioration of neurological function is the hallmark of most brain herniation syndromes.

The Cushing response (elevated blood pressure and bradycardia) is not consistently present at the time brain herniation is evolving.

Cingulate Herniation

This is noted when an expanding hemispheric mass induces a shift across the midline. The cingulate gyrus (located on the medial aspect of the hemisphere) slips underneath the free edge of the falx cerebri, resulting in pressure on the internal cerebral vein and cerebral ischemia. The condition should be suspected in any comatose patient with decorticate posturing and progressive rostrocaudal deterioration of function.

Central Herniation

Symmetric downward displacement of the cerebral hemispheres with pressure initially on the diencephalon and midbrain, and ultimately on the pons and medulla, results in the clinical picture of central herniation. The clinical manifestations can be summarized as follows:

Early

Progressive deterioration in consciousness; Cheyne Stokes respiration

Intermediate

Small, reactive pupils; paratonia; decorticate posturing; extensor plantar response; brisk dolls eye movements; intact caloric eye movements

Late

Dilated, fixed pupils; loss of doll's eye movements; decerebrate posturing leading to flaccidity; central neurogenic hyperventilation evolving ultimately into irregular respiration and irreversible apnea; caloric responses initially preserved but ultimately lost

Uncal (Tentorial) Herniation

There is medial and downward displacement of a swollen temporal lobe, starting with the uncal portion, through a gap in the tentorium cerebelli. This results in pressure on the brainstem and its downward displacement. The occulomotor (III) nerve and posterior cerebral artery are compressed between the swollen uncus and the free edge of the tentorium, leading to a unilateral fixed pupil (from compromise of function of the pupilloconstrictor fibers carried in the occulomotor nerve). If the patient survives, blindness (from ischemic injury to the visual cortex owing to compression of the posterior cerebral artery) may result. The manifestations of uncal herniation can be summarized as:

Early

Unilaterally fixed, dilated pupil; deterioration in level of consciousness

Intermediate

Coma; loss of doll's eye movements; decerebrate posturing (ipsi or contralateral to the mass); intact caloric responses; central neurogenic hyperventilation

Late

Irregular respiration leading to respiratory arrest and irreversible apnea; pupils midposition and nonreactive; loss of caloric reflexes; flaccidity

Upward Cerebellar Herniation

Posterior fossa mass lesions may sometimes lead to upward displacement of the cerebellum through the tentorium cerebelli. The anterior lobe of the cerebellum is compressed against the dorsal brainstem. The hallmark of upward cerebellar herniation is absence of caloric response at a time when pupillary and oculocephalic responses are still present. Ultimately, pupillary responses and oculocephalic reflexes are also lost. This "caudorostral" change occurs as a consequence initially of pressure upon the lower brainstem and compromise of its function.

Cerebellar Tonsillar Herniation

Sudden descent and impaction of cerebellar tonsils in the foramen magnum may occur along with other herniation syndromes, or whenever there is sudden decompression of the infratentorial compartment in the presence of increased intracranial pressure, e.g., following lumbar puncture. It is usually heralded by opisthotonic posturing and relatively sudden respiratory arrest, followed by loss of caloric, pupillary, and oculocephalic responses.

Management of Brain Herniation Syndromes

The following steps should be taken immediately:

Supportive care. The patient should be intubated, placed on a respirator, and have close monitoring of blood gases to prevent hypoxemia and hypercarbia. **Hyperventilation**, with the pCO_2 being maintained between 22 and 25 torr, is a valuable adjunct in decreasing cerebral edema; it lowers cerebral volume by inducing vasoconstriction. Hypotension should be avoided at all costs.

Administration of hyperosmolar agents. When given as a bolus, such agents induce an acute increase in serum osmolality and decrease cerebral edema by creating an osmotic gradient across the blood-brain barrier which causes a fluid shift from the brain into the intravascular space. The most commonly used agents are:

1. Mannitol: 0.25-1.0 gms/kg/dose as an I.V. bolus over 15-20 minutes; doses at the lower end of the range are recommended for infants and young children.

2. Glycerol: 0.5-1.0 gm/kg/dose through nasogastric tube; hyperglycemia and diarrhea are side effects.

Glucocorticoids. Dexamethasone 2-8 mg/kg bolus followed by 2-4 mg/kg/day in four divided doses is useful in controlling vasogenic cerebral edema, as in head trauma or CNS inflammation. The onset of action may not be apparent for 2-3 hours, however.

Investigation into the cause of herniation. This should proceed simultaneously with other management steps. An emergency contrast CT scan will help determine the nature of the mass lesion.

Neurosurgical consultation. This should be obtained immediately for intervention in acute obstructive hydrocephalus, tumor, intracerebral hemorrhage, and brain abscess. Placement of an intracranial pressure monitor (extradural, subarachnoid, intraparenchymal, or intraventricular device) by the neurosurgeon should be requested.

METABOLIC COMA

Salient Features

1. Neurologic manifestations migrate from one anatomic locus to another.

2. Myoclonus; a common form of myoclonus is asterixis or flapping tremor at the level of the wrist.

3. Pupillary responses are preserved unless the disorder becomes complicated by brain herniation.

4. Presence of biochemical abnormalities indicative of fluid and electrolyte imbalance and/or altered osmolality.

5. Non-specific, generalized slowing of the electro-encephalogram.

Common Causes of Metabolic Coma

The most common causes of metabolic coma are:

    Hypoxia-ischemic encephalopathy
    Prolonged hypoglycemia
    Diabetic ketoacidosis
    Hypercalcemia, hypermagnesemia
    Water intoxication, hyponatremia
    Hepatic failure
    Renal failure
    Inborn errors of amino-acid or carbohydrate metabolism
    Reye syndrome

Reye syndrome is characterized by an acute encephalopathy associated with hepatic dysfunction. The disorder usually develops a few days after a systemic viral infection, especially varicella and influenza. There is acute onset of vomiting and decreased sensorium which may progress to coma, seizures, and hepatic dysfunction. Accompanying biochemical changes include hypoglycemia, hyperammonemia, a prolonged prothrombin time, and elevated serum transaminases. Certain inborn errors of metabolism (systemic carnitine deficiency, ornithine transcarbamylase deficiency, carbamyl phosphate synthetase deficiency, acyl coA dehydrogenase deficiency) may lead to identical clinical syndromes. The cerebrospinal fluid is invariably normal. The pathology consists of fatty infiltration of the liver and kidneys, and severe cerebral edema. The etiology is unclear, but it appears that the viral infection triggers a cascade of systemic biochemical derangements in genetically predisposed individuals. The incidence of Reye syndrome in North America has dropped significantly over the past four years with the decline in the prescription of aspirin for children with febrile illnesses of viral etiology.

The management of Reye syndrome is entirely supportive and consists of maintaining an appropriate fluid and electrolyte balance, supporting respiration artificially when necessary, using mannitol in case of severe brain edema, and anticonvulsants for seizures. The mortality rate in patients who have received intensive care is approximately 25-30%. There are no major neurological sequelae, unless the patient has suffered prolonged hypoglycemia or status epilepticus during the acute encephalopathy.

COMA OF TOXIC ETIOLOGY

Alcohol, barbiturate, and benzodiazepine intoxication generally lead to coma and depressed respiration. Patients who have ingested amitryptiline may develop coma, mydriasis, seizures, and cardiac arrythmia. **Physostigmine**, a centrally acting cholinergic agent, may be used to counteract amitryptiline related seizures if conventional anticonvulsants are unsuccessful (1.5 mg per meter,[2] this being repeated two to three times over a 4-6 hour period if necessary). Phencyclidine usually induces a state of agitation and psychotic behavior alternating with stupor. Nystagmus is frequently present. Theophylline levels above 15-20 ugm/ml may lead to jitteriness, irritability, recurrent vomiting, and status epilepticus. Besides aggressive use of anticonvulsants, theophylline intoxication also requires institution of gastric lavage and charcoal hemoperfusion. Coma due to lead encephalopathy is generally associated with signs of increased intracranial pressure and blood lead levels above 80 ugm/dl.

ACUTE-ONSET PARAPLEGIA

Prompt diagnosis and treatment of acute paraplegia are necessary if irreversible damage is to be avoided from progressive spinal cord dysfunction.

Causes

1. Trauma (with compression, contusion or transection of the cord due to fracture and dislocation)

2. Extradural hemorrhage or abscess

3. Tumor (generally extramedullary neuroblastoma, neurofibroma, metastatic medulloblastoma, ependymoma, or Ewing's sarcoma)

4. Spinal cord infarction (e.g., intraoperative anterior spinal artery occlusion during aortic surgery)

5. Acute transverse myelitis

Clinical Features

Weakness. The extent of the weakness will vary with the level of the lesion.

Sensory deficits and paresthesia, with a sensory level generally extending onto the trunk. The sensory change may not always be present, however.

Bowel and bladder dysfunction, such as constipation, acute retention of urine.

Pain. This is generally associated with extradural and extramedullary-intradural lesions. Point tenderness over the vertebrae may suggest an underlying epidural abscess, hematoma, or fracture.

Reflexes. Altitudinal changes in tendon reflexes, loss of abdominal reflexes or presence of extensor plantar responses.

All patients with head trauma should be treated as having an associated injury to the cervical spine until the neurological examination and radiographs have excluded this possibility.

Management

There should be a minimum of handling till fracture/dislocation of the spine have been ruled out in patients with trauma with antero-posterior and lateral radiographs of the appropriate region.

Emergency contrast CT or NMR study of the spine will help to determine the presence of extradural compressive lesions, such as neuroblastoma.

In non-traumatic disorders, if the CT or NMR studies are inconclusive and the patient's neurological status continues to deteriorate, myelography with the water soluble contrast agent metrizamide should be carried out for definitive exclusion of spinal cord compressive pathology.

Cerebrospinal fluid examination should be done. Acute transverse myelitis is characterized by pleocytosis (WBC count 50-100/c.mm) and moderate protein elevation in the 100-200 mg/dl range. The fluid should also be examined for tumor cells.

Treatment

1. Decompressive laminectomy for lesions causing pressure on the cord and application of direct skeletal traction to reduce any vertebral displacement.

2. Antibiotics for extradural abscess along with surgical drainage.

3. Periodic evacuation of the distended, atonic bladder by intermittent catheterization.

4. Frequent log-turning to prevent decubitus skin and pulmonary changes.

5. Dexamethasone 2 mg/kg bolus I.V. may help to decrease spinal cord edema.

6. Correction of bleeding diatheses in some patients with epidural hematoma, e.g., Factor VIII or IX administration in Hemophilia.

Differential Diagnosis

Guillain Barré Syndrome. This ascending, acute polyneuropathy is characterized by weakness, hypoactive or absent tendon reflexes, and the presence of an occasional distal sensory deficit. Bowel and bladder dysfunction is rare. The weakness also frequently involves the facial musculature. The cerebrospinal fluid rarely shows more than 10-12 WBC/mm, but there is a disproportionate increase in CSF protein (usually between 50-100 mg/dl).

Painful or inflammatory conditions affecting the lower extremities. In toddlers, acute septic arthritis of the hips or knees, or osteomyelitis may result in sudden inability to walk. Point tenderness can, however, be detected upon patient, gentle palpation. The bone scan may demonstrate a focal area of increased radioisotope uptake in osteomyelitis.

Tick paralysis. A tick bite can usually be found upon careful inspection of the skin. The cerebrospinal fluid is invariably normal.

SUGGESTED READING

1. Aicardi J and Chevrie JJ. Convulsive status epilepticus in infants and children: a study of 239 cases. Epilepsia 11:187-197, 1970.

2. Aicardi J. Status epilepticus in infants and children: consequences and prognosis. Int Pediatr 2:189-195, 1987.

3. Delgado-Escueta AV, Wasterlain C, Treiman DM and Porter RJ. Management of status epilepticus. N Engl J Med 306:1337-1339, 1982.

4. Treiman DM, Delgado-Escueta AV. Complex partial status epilepticus. Adv Neurol 34:69-81, 1983.

5. Soffer D, Melamed E, Assaf Y, Cotev S. Hemispheric brain damage in unilateral status epilepticus. Ann Neurol 20:737-740, 1986.

Introduction

Between 10-30% of school children are unable to meet the expected standards of academic achievement. A decline in school grades, failure, and the consequent development of emotional problems may occur if the cause is not recognized early enough and if timely intervention is not initiated.

CAUSES OF SCHOOL FAILURE

Learning disabilities

An inability to learn despite the presence of normal intelligence, normal motivation, and adequate exposure to teaching is termed learning disability. It encompasses a heterogeneous category of perceptual and motor disorders. The selective disability is most often in auditory comprehension, reading, arithmetic, or handwriting. More than one modality of intellectual function may be impaired in the same patient. Reading problems may be related to difficulties in spatial recognition or impaired visual and auditory memory, sequential analysis of speech sounds and rhyming judgements. Learning disabilities have a multifactorial etiology, being based partly upon a genetic predisposition and partly upon subtle central nervous system insults in infancy and early childhood. The result is a **maturational lag** in one or more specific areas of academic function, despite the overall presence of normal intelligence. Psychometric tests such as the Wechsler Intelligence Scale for Children-Revised demonstrate a disparity between scores on the verbal and performance sections, and often a scatter in the results of the subtests.

Dyslexia, or selective reading disability, can be the consequence of immaturity in development of a variety of interrelated mechanisms: visual inattention, left-right confusion, defective matching of written words with speech sounds, poor auditory or visual memory, and defective auditory/verbal synthesis. **Writing difficulty, attentional deficit disorder, and impaired calculation ability may be superimposed.** Contrary to general belief, there is no increased incidence of reading handicaps amongst ambidextrous and left-handed individuals in the absence of gross brain damage. Reading scores two grade levels below the expected level on standardized psychometric tests are diagnostic.

Attentional Deficit Disorder (Minimal Brain Dysfunction, Hyperkinetic syndrome) is characterized by poor concentration and impulsivity. Motor restlessness (hyperactivity) may or may not be consistently present. In those who are hyperactive, this overactive behavior can sometimes be traced back to infancy and early childhood. The child may be disruptive in the classroom, have difficulty in completing his schoolwork due to lack of concentration, and manifest poor social interaction. While the attention span breaks down in the normal classroom setting, the child may be able to concentrate better in individualized, one-on-one situations with the school teacher and when disruptions in the daily schedule are kept to a minimum. The favorable response of such patients to treatment with methylphenidate (Ritalin), pemoline sodium (Cylert), or dextroamphetamine (Dexidrine) suggests altered catecholamine function as a neurochemical basis for the disorder.

Developmental language disorders

Developmental language disorders (developmental dysphasia) is defined as delayed language development in a child despite lack of a hearing deficit, gross brain damage, or emotional disorder. Another definition states that verbal skills are two years or more, or 50% below norms. The deficit may be predominantly in the interpretation of language, formulation of an appropriate motor program, or speech expression. Faulty synaptogenesis probably underlies most such disorders. While developmental language disorders generally become apparent prior to school entry in a child labelled as being "shy" or non-verbal, they may sometimes be diagnosed only at the first or second grade level due to impaired language skills. **Auditory verbal agnosia** (word deafness) is a form of developmental dysphasia characterized by inability to decode speech. Comprehension of gestures and facial expression remains normal. Seizures are a frequent accompaniment. Such children benefit from combined use of speech therapy and sign language (total communication). Other patients with developmental language disorders have trouble understanding discourse and their speech has a loose, tangential quality (**semantic-pragmatic syndrome**). Residual elements of autism may also retard verbal and non-verbal communication skills. Refer also to Chapter XV.

The severity of the language disturbance in most patients calls for placement in a special school program with a small teacher-to-pupil ratio in order to enhance both the verbal and non-verbal communication skills of the child.

Psychiatric Disorders

Patients with **depression** or **anxiety** states are often poorly motivated and unable to concentrate on academic activities. In those with an underlying anxiety state, the attention span remains unaltered (or sometimes is even worsened) by stimulant medicines like methylphenidate. School failure may lead to further lowering of self image, thereby worsening depression and making the individual even less inclined to improve performance in the classroom. The basis for the emotional and affective disturbance is often temporary and self-limiting, e.g., anxiety from moving to a new school environment or depressed affect from loss of loved one. Unsocialized aggressive, delinquent, and runaway children (personality disorders) are also invariably scholastic underachievers. The delinquent youth may have a superimposed element of learning disability which responds favorably to methylphenidate. Runaways and delinquents both have a tendency to act out rather than verbalize their fears and frustrations. Intensive individual and group counselling is necessary for patients with personality disorders.

Borderline Intelligence, Mild Mental Retardation

These patients are generally identified at the kindergarten or pre-kindergarten level, at which time most are placed in appropriate classrooms. They may sometimes, however, go undetected until academic failure becomes apparent at the elementary school level. Global impairment of mental, adaptive, and social faculties is present. They have a very limited capacity to think in abstract terms. Psychometric evaluation discloses an IQ generally between 60 and 90.

While mainstreaming such an individual along with with normal children during kindergarten or first grade is appropriate, subsequent placement in an appropriate special school program with a small teacher-to-pupil ratio and modified curriculum is recommended.

Seizure Disorders

Certain children with poorly controlled seizures (particularly those with complex partial and absence episodes) are at risk of developing academic difficulties. The neurological insult predisposing to seizure (e.g., contusion) may also lead to cognitive difficulties. Certain anticonvulsants such as phenobarbital and primidone impair cognitive function and memory even when serum anticonvulsant levels are in the "therapeutic" range. Unnecessary simultaneous use of more than one anticonvulsant may lead to cumulative sedative and hypnotic effects. Children with early onset of partial seizures (less than three years of age) perform significantly poorly on the Weschler Intelligence Scale for Children-Revised (WISC-R) as compared to those with late onset partial seizures (age 8-9 years). This relationship between age and academic function also holds true for generalized epilepsies. Patients with idiopathic epilepsy are less likely to demonstrate scholastic underachievement when compared to those with symptomatic epilepsy.

Excessive daytime sleepiness

Daytime drowsiness may impair concentration and academic performance. The most common causes of excessive daytime sleepiness in a school child are poor sleep hygiene (going to bed late) and iatrogenic disorders (such as the administration of stimulant mediation in the afternoon or evening hours; this interferes with sleep onset and leads to rebound daytime sleepiness). Narcolepsy also generally has onset in the early teens, and results in attacks of irresistible sleepiness, sleep paralysis, hyponogogic hallucinations, and cataplexy. Refer also to Chapter XIII.

Assessment

1. Determine by history, the age of onset and delay, if any, in acquisition of the various language parameters; hyperactivity in early childhood; and risk factors for intellectual dysfunction, e.g., seizures, central nervous system infections, trauma.

2. Ascertain the current level of school placement, the teacher-to-pupil ratio, school grades in various subjects, history of any concentration difficulty noted by the school teachers, the child's level of motivation, interaction with teachers and peers, whether any necessary additional assistance is being provided to the child at school and its frequency and impact on the child's academic performance.

3. Inquire about the child's interaction with parents and siblings, any recent traumatic changes in the family such as parental separation, divorce, or moving to a new neighborhood; also, whether the home environment is conducive to learning.

4. The examination should attempt to determine whether the poor school performance is secondary to attentional/motivational problems or a consequence of cognitive incompetence. If the latter, one should attempt to determine the modality/modalities most impaired (reading, writing, arithmetic) and the severity of this deficit. The Gray Oral Reading Test, visual-motor function assessment (copying of geometrical figures up to age 7 years, and the Bender Gestalt figures beyond that age), calculation ability using the serial seven addition and subtraction tests, and asking questions about the general fund of information (e.g., current affairs) are useful office guides in assessing the child's intellectual function.

5. Psychological evaluation (psychometrics and projectives) is useful in determining the nature and severity of emotional and organic factors that could adversely impact school performance. It helps in creating a plan for school teachers and parents to modify and manage the child's behavior.

6. The electroencephalogram is of limited value in assessing children with school learning problems and should be obtained only in the infrequent instance when an undiagnosed or poorly controlled seizure disorder is suspected.

Management

Provide individual and family counselling in patients suspected of having poor motivation as a consequence of depression/conduct disorders.

If the child has a learning disability, contact the school in order to arrange for additional remedial assistance in the areas of weakness through a resource room. If school performance does not improve despite this assistance, placement in a classroom for learning disabled children on a full-time basis is recommended whenever such a service is available.

All children with attentional and learning problems benefit from a regularly scheduled daily review of the day's school work at home and completing the assigned home work according to a set time schedule, at which time distracting stimuli are kept at a minimum.

When an attentional deficit disorder is present, a trial of stimulant medication may be helpful in enhancing concentration and academic performance and, thereby, self-image. Methylphenidate (Ritalin) in a dose of 5-20 mg/day is most commonly prescribed. The salutory effect upon concentration is generally short-lived (3-4 hours). This necessitates administration of the drug prior to leaving for school and once again at mid day. If the child is on a larger dose, the enteric-coated slow release 20 mg tablet may be prescribed. The most common side effects are nausea, abdominal discomfort, anorexia, and sleep disturbances. Pemoline sodium (Cylert) is a longer-acting agent which needs to be administered only once every morning. It is available in 18.75 and 37.5 mg tablets. The dose varies between 18.75 and 75 mg per day. Side effects are similar to those of Ritalin. The author does not recommend prescription of dextroamphetamine (Dexidrine), owing to its high abuse potential. One should be cautious in continuing stimulant medication beyond adolescence for the same reason.

Supportive efforts at home and school, and developing hobbies as an outlet to frustration also go a long way in helping the child.

SUGGESTED READING

1. Thompson RF. The neurobiology of learning and memory. Science 233:941-947, 1986.

2. Allen DA and Rapin I. Language disorders in preschool children: predictors of outcome — a preliminary report. Brain Dev 2:73-80, 1980.

3. Rapoport JL, Zemetkin A. Attentional deficit disorder. Psych Clin North Am 3:425-441, 1980.

4. Stores G, Hart J, Piron N. Inattentiveness in school children with epilepsy. Epilepsia 19:169, 1978.

5. Rapin I. Children with Brain Dysfunction. Neurology, Cognition, Language and Behavior. Raven Press, New York, 1982.

6. Ottenbacher K.J., Cooper M.M. Drug treatment of hyperactive children. Dev Med Child Neurol 25:358, 1983.

7. Damasio AR and Geschwind N. The neural basis of language. Ann Rev Neurosci 7:127-147, 1984.

8. Golden GS. Neurobiological correlates of language disorders. Ann Neurol 12:409-418, 1982.

9. Shaywitz SE, Shaywitz BA. Attention deficit disorder: current perspectives. Pediatr Neurol 3:129-135, 1987.

Index